8×8|14

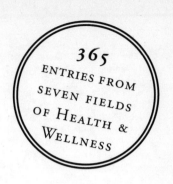

365 ENTRIES FROM SEVEN FIELDS OF HEALTH & WELLNESS

THE
INTELLECTUAL
DEVOTIONAL™

HEALTH

Revive Your Mind,

Complete Your Education,

and

Digest a Daily Dose

of Wellness Wisdom

DAVID S. KIDDER & NOAH D. OPPENHEIM
New York Times Best-Selling Authors of *The Intellectual Devotional*

AND BRUCE K. YOUNG, MD

RODALE

© 2009 by TID Volumes, LLC
All rights reserved. No part of this publication may be reproduced or transmitted in
any form or by any means, electronic or mechanical, including photocopying,
recording, or any other information storage and retrieval system, without the written
permission of the publisher.

Rodale books may be purchased for business or promotional use or for special sales.
For information, please write to:
Special Markets Department, Rodale Inc., 733 Third Avenue, New York, NY 10017

Printed in the United States of America
Rodale Inc. makes every effort to use acid-free ♾, recycled paper ♲.

Book design by Anthony Serge, principal designer;
initial interior creative by Nelson Kunkel, The Ingredient
For image credits, see page 375.

Library of Congress Cataloging-in-Publication Data
Kidder, David S.
    The intellectual devotional health : revive your mind, complete your education,
and digest a daily dose of wellness wisdom / David S. Kidder & Noah D. Oppenheim ;
with Bruce K. Young.
        p.   cm.
    Includes bibliographical references and index.
    ISBN-13 978-1-60529-949-5 hardcover
    ISBN-10 1-60529-949-9 hardcover
    1. Health—Miscellanea.   2. Intellectual life—Miscellanea.   3. Learning and
scholarship—Miscellanea.   4. Devotional calendars.   I. Oppenheim, Noah D.
II. Young, Bruce K., 1938–   III. Title.
    RA776.K4855 2009
    613--dc22   2009019525

Distributed to the trade by Macmillan
2   4   6   8   10   9   7   5   3   1   hardcover

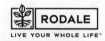

LIVE YOUR WHOLE LIFE™

We inspire and enable people to improve their lives and the world around them
For more of our products visit **rodalestore.com** or call 800-848-4735

To my dear family, let us share the best of health
—B. K. Young

To the eternal love and legacy of Robert and Luva Kidder
—D. S. Kidder

For Ascher
—N. D. Oppenheim

Contributing Editor

Alan Wirzbicki

Contributing Writers

Matt Blanchard

Caroline Einaugler

Sharon Liao

Introduction

Bedside devotionals have long been embraced as a means of maintaining spiritual health through the habit of daily reading. Therefore, it is especially appropriate that we have focused this volume on physical health. Like our previous devotionals, this book is divided into 365 passages that can each be completed in a short sitting. Each entry is an in-depth treatment of a topic vital to understanding the function of the human body.

There is no topic more important to more people than health. Without a basic understanding of biology and medicine, it is impossible to care properly for our families and ourselves. Too often, a trip to the doctor is like a trip to a foreign land. We leave baffled by the language, confused by the results. It is our hope that this book will empower readers to better understand their own bodies and better manage their health.

The following readings are divided into these fields of knowledge:

CHILDREN AND ADOLESCENTS
From the origins of life through the special circumstances of the developing body

DISEASES AND AILMENTS
The delicate human organism and all that can go wrong

DRUGS AND ALTERNATIVE TREATMENTS
Remedies both miraculous and mundane

THE MIND
The body's least understood and most powerful organ

SEXUALITY AND REPRODUCTION
The extraordinary process of perpetuating the species

LIFESTYLE AND PREVENTIVE MEDICINE
How to stave off disease and deterioration

MEDICAL MILESTONES
The march of progress in understanding and saving life

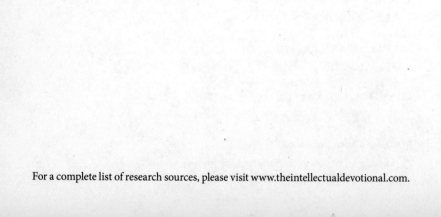

For a complete list of research sources, please visit www.theintellectualdevotional.com.

Apgar Score

Virginia Apgar (1909–1974) defied all odds to become a pioneering female physician. In spite of the financial hardships of the Great Depression, Apgar was one of the first women to graduate from Columbia University College of Physicians and Surgeons in New York City. She went on to become an anesthesiologist and the school's first female professor. In 1952, she developed the Apgar score, a quick evaluation of a newborn's condition during the first critical minutes after birth. This scale has saved countless lives and is still used today.

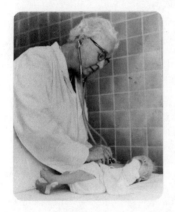

Doctors and nurses perform the screening at 1 and 5 minutes after an infant's birth. They evaluate five vital signs—skin color, heart rate, reflexes, muscle tone, and breathing—on a scale of 0 to 2, then add up the ratings for a total ranging from 0 to 10. (Medical students often remember these signs using the mnemonic APGAR: appearance, pulse, grimace, activity, and respiration.) If the score is 7 or above, the baby is deemed in stable condition. But if it's lower, physicians and nurses will reevaluate every 5 minutes until 20 minutes have passed or until two consecutive scores of 7 or higher are recorded.

If the infant has a score of 6 or lower, some resuscitation is needed, which may involve suctioning the airway and administering oxygen. Sometimes this is because of a heart or lung condition, or another medical issue. A newborn with a score of 0 to 3 requires immediate resuscitation, usually with assisted breathing. But an initial low score may be harmless: Some babies, especially those born after a high-risk pregnancy, Caesarean section, or complicated delivery, may just take a little longer to adjust to life outside the womb. Experts say that the Apgar test isn't a predictor of a child's long-term health, unless after 20 minutes the score remains 0 to 3.

ADDITIONAL FACTS

1. *At age 50, Virginia Apgar embarked on a second career. She earned a master's degree in public health and became an executive for the March of Dimes.*

2. *About 10 percent of newborns require medical intervention.*

◆◆◆

Immunity

Since the moment you rolled out of bed this morning, you've probably encountered thousands of viruses, bacteria, parasites, and fungi. But thanks to immunity, your body is able to fight off these foreign invaders and protect itself.

Like a high-tech security system in a bank or store, the body's immune system is multifaceted. The first line of defense is called nonspecific, or innate. This type of sweeping protection fends off all encroaching pathogens in the same way. It consists of a number of mechanisms, including the skin and the sticky mucous linings, such as those in the nose, lungs, and stomach, that trap small particles. If viruses or bacteria break through this initial barrier, white blood cells, natural killer cells, and other defending cells rush to destroy them. During this process, tissues react with an inflammatory response, bringing more blood into the affected area to attract defender cells that clear out the harmful particles and other types of cells that repair damaged areas. As another security measure, body temperature often rises, because most viruses and bacteria can't thrive in hot temperatures.

The other type of immunity is a finely tuned adaptive system that releases specialized cells whose main purpose is to destroy a particular pathogen. Once exposed to a certain offending virus or bacteria, such as the chicken pox virus or *Streptococcus* bacterium, the body produces white blood cells called T lymphocytes (T cells) and tailor-made antibodies to fight off microbes of that type. That's why people are typically safe from measles for the rest of their lives after one bout: These specialized cells are persistent in your body, and when you're reexposed to that same virus, they rush to fight it off before it can make you sick. Vaccines essentially capitalize on this process. By introducing tiny amounts or harmless pieces of certain pathogens, such as the agents that cause the flu, measles, or whooping cough, vaccines prompt the body to produce focused antibodies that safeguard the body without its undergoing an illness.

ADDITIONAL FACTS

1. *The phlegm that causes your runny nose and congestion is made up of mucus and dead white blood cells.*

2. *Stress, an unhealthy diet, and lack of exercise can weaken the immune system.*

3. *Although nearly all organisms have nonspecific immune systems, only higher-order vertebrates have an adaptive one as well.*

✦✦✦

Morphine

One of history's most important yet dangerous discoveries was morphine—a derivative of the opium poppy plant. German scientist Friedrich Wilhelm Adam Sertürner (1783–1841), who first produced the water-soluble, crystalline white powder in 1804, named it after Morpheus, the Greek god of dreams, because of its trancelike effect on patients. With the invention of the hypodermic needle in 1853, doctors put morphine into widespread use as a painkiller.

A narcotic, morphine relieves pain and anxiety, but also impairs mental and physical performance. It can decrease hunger and sex drive, inhibit the cough reflex, and interfere with a woman's menstrual cycle. Useful in treating pain caused by cancer and other conditions for which other analgesic medicines have failed, morphine also has a calming effect that protects the body against traumatic shock, internal bleeding, and congestive heart failure.

When it was first introduced, morphine was erroneously used as a cure for opium and alcohol addictions because doctors believed that addiction to morphine was less harmful than other chemical dependencies. Morphine quickly replaced opium as a medical cure-all and was readily available at drugstores as an over-the-counter and recreational drug throughout the late 19th century.

Like other narcotic drugs, however, morphine is very addictive. It produces feelings of euphoria, quickly causing cravings and tolerance—that is, the need for higher and higher doses in order to achieve the same results. Physical and psychological dependence is also common, and withdrawal from morphine can cause nausea, chills, sweating, and even stroke or heart attack. Self-detoxification can be dangerous. Experts agree that the best way to get off—and stay off—morphine is in an inpatient drug rehabilitation center. Treatment may result in addiction to other drugs (such as methadone) used to control withdrawal symptoms. However, medical maintenance is preferable to illegal addiction and can lead to complete withdrawal from drug dependency.

Today morphine is tightly regulated, and more than 1,000 tons of the drug are extracted from opium plants annually. Morphine can be converted into the illegal drug heroin and into other prescription painkillers, including methylmorphine (codeine).

ADDITIONAL FACTS

1. *During the American Civil War, in which morphine was frequently used to treat wounded soldiers, up to 400,000 veterans became addicted to the drug, a condition that became known as soldier's disease.*

2. *It's estimated that more than 1 million people worldwide are on methadone maintenance programs to treat a narcotics addiction.*

3. *Morphine's physical impact is so powerful that babies born to women who took the drug during pregnancy may suffer withdrawal symptoms after leaving the womb.*

◆◆◆

Circle of Willis

In 1664, the British scientist Thomas Willis (1621–1675) wrote about a circle of arteries at the base of the brain that act as a traffic circle for the blood flowing to the head. The two major arteries in the neck, the left and right carotids, meet at this circle and branch out into smaller blood vessels that nourish the face and brain. Because of Willis's thorough illustrations and explanation of this structure, it is known today as the circle of Willis.

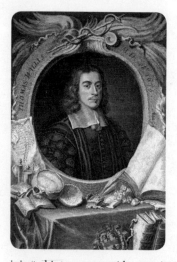

Located on the underside of the brain and encircling the pituitary gland, the circle of Willis joins the carotid and basilar arteries with smaller arteries such as the anterior cerebral artery, the middle cerebral artery, and the posterior cerebral artery, which travel to all parts of the brain. The circle is anastomotic, meaning that its stems branch out and then reconnect, so all the different blood vessels are connected like roads that merge into a traffic circle.

Scientists had observed this circle as early as the 16th century, but it was Willis who first noted its importance in directing the flow of blood. He showed that people could go on living even if one carotid artery was completely blocked or didn't work, and that when dye was injected into one carotid artery in animals, it stained all the vessels of the brain. This proved that the circle of vessels could redirect blood to both sides of the brain if one major artery became constricted by physical pressure, blocked by fat deposits known as plaque, or interrupted by disease or injury. This ensures that the brain will have the best possible blood supply.

ADDITIONAL FACTS

1. *Thomas Willis was an inaugural member of London's Royal Society, largely considered the oldest scientific society in existence. His definitive work,* Cerebri anatome *(the title is Latin for* "Anatomy of the Brain"*), coined the term* neurology.

2. *Willis attributed much of his knowledge and discovery to the English physician and writer Sir Thomas Millington (1628–1704) and to the scientist and architect Sir Christopher Wren (1632–1723).*

3. *The circle of Willis varies greatly from person to person; the structure described in anatomical textbooks appears in only about 35 percent of patients.*

◆◆◆

Ovum

An ovum, or egg, is merely the size of a pinhead, but it's the only cell in the entire human body that can be seen with the naked eye. At birth, a girl has about 2 million immature egg cells stored in two ovaries, but less than a quarter of the cells exist by the time she reaches puberty. Of those, only 300 to 400 are released during her reproductive years, from about ages 12 to 50.

Inside the ovary each immature egg lies dormant for years in its own fluid-filled cavity called a follicle. About once a month—in the ovulation phase of the menstrual cycle—a handful of these follicles arise from their slumber and begin maturing into fully formed eggs. During the process, a large cell is created. Its nucleus holds 23 chromosomes, or half of the number that comprises a human's DNA, which is the genetic blueprint for each individual. Surrounding the nucleus is cytoplasm, as well as the zona pellucida (clear zone), a membrane that encloses the cytoplasm and must be penetrated by a sperm to fertilize the egg. Usually only this one large cell is released per menstrual cycle.

That precious cell is coated with three protective layers when released in the process of ovulation. The inner one is a thin cellular membrane that is covered with the second, the microscopic zona pellucida. Finally, there's the corona radiata (radiating crown) of cells. After the egg is released from the ovary into one of the fallopian tubes, it lives for about 3 days before it begins deteriorating. The sperm usually have about 72 hours to fertilize the egg.

ADDITIONAL FACTS

1. *The word* ovum *(plural ova) is Latin for "egg."*

2. *Eggs are released from either ovary at random; the ovaries don't alternate months.*

3. *Human sperm can survive for up to 7 days in the female reproductive system.*

◆◆◆

Amino Acids

Amino acids are the basic units that combine to form proteins. When you eat foods that contain protein, the digestive juices in your stomach and intestines break down the protein into amino acids. Then your body uses the amino acids to build the specific proteins your body needs for your muscles, bones, blood, and organs.

Proteins are made up of many different amino acids, but 22 of them are necessary for your health. Your body can synthesize 13 of these amino acids, known as nonessential amino acids, through the regular breakdown of proteins.

You can obtain the other nine amino acids, called the essential amino acids, only by eating the right foods. The essential amino acids are found in the protein of meat, milk, cheese, eggs, vegetables, nuts, and grains. However, only protein from animal sources (meat, dairy, and eggs) contains all nine essential amino acids. Most vegetable protein is incomplete, because it lacks one or more essential amino acids.

It's important that you eat enough protein from a variety of sources to make sure you take in all the essential amino acids. Adults require about 60 grams of protein a day, and children need about 0.5 gram of protein daily for every pound they weigh. Your body cannot store extra amino acids for later use, so you must eat foods that contain all the amino acids every day for optimal health.

The nine essential amino acids are histidine, isoleucine, leucine, lysine, methionine, phenylalanine, threonine, tryptophan, and valine. Nonessential amino acids include aspartic acid, glutamic acid, and glycine, as well as 10 others.

ADDITIONAL FACTS

1. *In addition to eating animal proteins, you can get all the essential amino acids by combining certain vegetarian foods, such as peanut butter and whole grain bread, or red beans and rice.*

2. *Amino acids are molecules that contain both amino (NH_2) and carboxyl (COOH) chemical groups.*

3. *Because they're made up of long strings of amino acids joined together, proteins are described as necklaces of amino acid beads.*

◆◆◆

Celsus: Calor, Dolor, Rubor, and Tumor

The word *inflammation* comes from the Latin word *inflammare*, which means "to set on fire." In the 1st century, the Roman medical writer Aulus Cornelius Celsus is credited with first documenting the four cardinal signs of inflammation: *calor*, *dolor*, *rubor*, and *tumor*.

These four words mean, respectively, "heat," "pain," "redness," and "swelling." The symptoms make up what's considered the classic inflammatory response that may occur a few minutes or hours after an injury, such as a muscle tear, or during an infection. Today, we know that inflammation is the body's way of protecting us: White blood cells release chemicals to ward off foreign substances and increase the flow of blood to the area, causing redness and warmth. Some of the chemicals cause fluid to leak into the tissues, resulting in swelling, and nerves are stimulated in the process, causing pain. In the case of a muscle strain or sprain, the patient can lessen inflammation by applying ice or elevating the affected limb above the heart to keep blood from rushing to the area.

Celsus's description of inflammation emphasized the importance of clinical observation, rather than philosophy-based medicine. A century later, the Greek physician Galen (AD 129–216) elaborated on the theory of inflammation, suggesting that inflammation and pus were necessary parts of the healing process. In 1871, the German pathologist Rudolf Virchow (1821–1902) added a fifth sign of inflammation: *functio laesa*, or "loss of function" (although some sources attribute this addition to Galen as well). Virchow was also the first to make a connection between inflammation and cancer, writing that inflammation was a predisposing factor to the formation of tumors.

ADDITIONAL FACTS

1. *The five signs generally appear when acute inflammation occurs on the surface of the body, while internal inflammation usually does not cause all five symptoms. Pneumonia, or inflammation of the lungs, for example, typically does not cause pain.*

2. *Inflammation—especially in the case of an infection—may also be associated with flulike symptoms such as fever, chills, headache, and muscle stiffness.*

3. *In his writings, Celsus also described many 1st-century Roman surgical procedures, including the removal of a cataract, treatment for bladder stones, and the setting of fractures.*

✦✦✦

Prematurity

The average pregnancy lasts about 9 months, or 40 weeks. But for one in eight moms-to-be, the baby is born at least 3 weeks before the due date. That's called a premature, or preterm, birth.

Because the infant has less time to develop in the womb, premature babies are at greater risk for medical and developmental problems. In fact, premature birth is the leading cause of death among newborns; dangerous conditions, such as bleeding in the brain and breathing trouble, can occur. Some infants may require special care in a neonatal intensive care unit. Because of immature skin, poorly developed temperature control by the autonomic nervous system, and a lack of body fat, they are kept in an incubator—an enclosed plastic bassinet—to regulate their body temperature.

In about 40 percent of premature births, the cause is unknown. But scientists have identified some causes: Preterm births can be brought on by bacterial infection within the womb and inflammation in the mother, whether it's caused by a sexually transmitted disease or systemic infection. Physical or mental stress possibly is another factor, because stress hormones can stimulate the release of other hormones that trigger uterine contractions and premature delivery. An incompetent cervix; rupture of the amniotic sac; preeclampsia (serious complications occurring late in pregnancy); injuries or diseases that cause uterine bleeding; and the overstretching of the uterus due to anatomical abnormality, excessive amniotic fluid, or a multiple pregnancy can also lead to contractions.

If a mother begins preterm labor, physicians will try to keep the fetus in the womb so it has more time to develop and so that steroids can be administered to mature its lungs. For instance, women who aren't undergoing contractions but have a widening cervix may undergo a cervical cerclage. During this surgical procedure, the cervix is stitched closed with sutures. For those undergoing contractions, medications that stop or slow them may be administered. After birth, a baby is released from the hospital when he or she can breathe without support, maintain a stable body temperature, breast- or bottle-feed, and gain weight steadily.

ADDITIONAL FACTS

1. *One of the smallest babies to live, Rumaisa Rahman, was born 14 weeks early in 2004. She weighed 8.6 ounces, or a little more than half a pound.*

2. *The number of premature births in the United States has increased 36 percent over the past 3 years.*

❖❖❖

White Blood Cells

Without white blood cells (WBCs), or leukocytes, we would be defenseless against sickness and disease. These cells play a critical role in the immune system, fighting off the viruses, bacteria, toxins, and other foreign organisms that regularly invade our bodies.

Like guards on patrol, WBCs float through the bloodstream until they receive a chemical message from an area of tissue that requires protection. They then pass through the blood vessels to destroy the harmful organisms. Most WBCs live for only a few days.

Because of this short life cycle, people produce about 100 billion WBCs a day. Grown in the bone marrow, the soft tissue found inside the bone, they develop into one of five major types that vary by size, shape, and function. For example, basophils secrete markers to signal the area of infection, while eosinophils, lymphocytes, and neutrophils attack the invading parasite, bacterium, fungus, or virus. Monocytes act as the body's cleanup crew, devouring bacteria and dead or damaged cells.

In medicine, physicians count WBCs as a way to detect disease and monitor recovery from illness. The standard scientific measure is the number of cells per microliter of blood; a healthy adult has 4,500 to 10,000 WBCs per microliter. A low WBC count, or leukopenia, is usually caused by a bone marrow disorder and raises the risk of infection. A high WBC count, or leukocytosis, is often the result of the body fighting off an infection. But a consistently elevated number may signal an underlying problem of the immune system, such as allergies, arthritis, or leukemia, a cancer of the blood.

ADDITIONAL FACTS

1. *The word* leukocyte *is derived from the Greek* leukos *("white") and* cytes *("cell").*

2. *WBCs make up only about 1 percent of your blood; the majority consists of red blood cells and plasma.*

3. *A French professor of medicine, Gabriel Andral (1797–1876), and an English physician, William Addison (1802–1881), separately reported the first descriptions of WBCs in 1843, more than 200 years after the discovery of red blood cells.*

❖❖❖

Cephalosporins

Cephalosporins, which were discovered in the 1950s, are a type of antibiotic related to penicillin. Like penicillin, the medicines are derived from a fungus—in their case, *Cephalosporium acremonium*. Based on that original drug, scientists have created dozens of similar antibiotics to treat a wide range of diseases, from meningitis to gonorrhea.

Both cephalosporins and penicillin are beta-lactam antibiotics, meaning that their molecular structure includes a beta-lactam ring consisting of three carbon atoms and one nitrogen atom. They are bactericidal, which means that they kill bacteria. They work by breaking down peptidoglycan, a polymer that's needed for building cell walls. Because of the similarities between the two drugs, cephalosporins are often prescribed to people who have infections that are resistant to penicillin. Among their many capabilities, cephalosporins are used to treat ear, nose, throat, skin, or sinus infections; pneumonia; staph infections; and bronchitis. They are available in prescription-strength tablets, capsules, and liquids, as well as injectable forms.

First-generation (and newer, fourth-generation) cephalosporins are moderate- to broad-spectrum antibiotics generally effective against many different types of ailments. Gram-positive bacteria with high amounts of peptidoglycan in their cell walls—so named because they turn dark blue or violet when stained with dye in a process known as Gram staining—respond well to cephalosporins, as do many gram-negative bacteria that have just a thin peptidoglycan layer. For bacteria that are resistant to the first-generation cephalosporins, second- and third- generation drugs were developed. Allergic reactions to cephalosporins can include shortness of breath, a pounding heartbeat, a skin rash or hives, cramps or stomach pain, fever, diarrhea, and unusual bleeding or bruising.

ADDITIONAL FACTS

1. *The ability of many cephalosporin derivatives to penetrate the cerebro spinal fluid makes them effective in treating meningitis.*

2. *Cephalosporins named before 1975 are spelled with ph (cephalexin, for example), while those named later are spelled with f (such as cefadroxil).*

3. *A newly developed drug called ceftobiprole has been described as a fifth-generation cephalosporin.*

◆◆◆

Cerebral Ventricles

A clear fluid in the brain called cerebrospinal fluid (CSF) forms a crucial component of the central nervous system, distributing nutrients, removing waste, and providing a shock-absorbing layer for fragile brain tissue. This multipurpose substance is stored, and primarily produced, in four hollow chambers deep inside the skull called ventricles.

The four ventricles are connected to each other, and surround the central column of the spinal cord, through a system of ducts. Together, this network comprises what is known as the ventricular system.

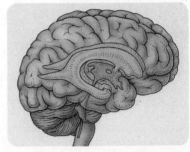

In addition to its other roles, CSF provides buoyancy to the brain—in essence, allowing it to "float" in the skull surrounded by fluid. This reduces the stress that the weight of the 3-pound brain would otherwise place on the spine and prevents compression of the brain against the bony skull and spine.

Each ventricle plays a somewhat different role. The left and right ventricles are located in the cerebrum, near the front of the brain, and produce 70 percent of the body's CSF. The third ventricle, in the middle section of the brain, also produces CSF and serves a different section of the organ. The fourth ventricle, at the back of the brain, provides openings allowing CSF to flow into the space surrounding the brain and into the spinal cord.

Just as our blood stream should not be too high or too low, neither should CSF pressure. To keep this pressure at a normal level (between 100 and 150 millimeters of water), CSF is absorbed back into the bloodstream through structures called arachnoid villi at roughly the same rate it is produced in the ventricles. If something prevents the circulation and absorption of CSF and it backs up in the brain, however, the ventricles will swell and push on the surrounding tissue—a condition called hydrocephalus, or water on the brain.

ADDITIONAL FACTS

1. *CSF typically contains high amounts of salt, sugar, and lipids, but low amounts of protein. Large amounts of protein in a sample of CSF (collected by a lumbar puncture, or spinal tap) may indicate that the body's blood-brain barrier is not working properly.*

2. *The third ventricle divides the thalamus into symmetrical halves.*

3. *The total volume of CSF in the body at one time is usually 125 to 150 milliliters.*

◆◆◆

Sperm

Since the advent of medicine, there has been a vast and wild array of theories about what, exactly, sperm is. The ancient Greeks believed that semen was a vital life force made partly of brain fluid, while 17th-century physicists thought that each individual sperm contained a "little man." Today, we know that the male reproductive cell is neither of these things. The smallest cell in the body, at 0.002-inch long, a sperm consists of a cell nucleus encased in a bulletlike or oval head and a whiplike tail, or flagellum.

Every day in a man's testes, about 300 million to 400 million sperm reach maturity. A steady stream of male sex hormones, including testosterone, triggers the sperm's production, which takes place over 72 days. During the process, male sex cells compact 23 chromosomes—half of a person's full number—into a single nucleus. (The woman's egg provides the other half of the chromosomes, but it's the sperm that carries the X or Y chromosome that determines whether a child will be male or female.) Surrounding the head of each sperm is a protective cap called an acrosome, which contains special chemicals that help the sperm penetrate the egg. After the sperm are fully formed, they're stored in the vasa deferentia (singular: vas deferens), the pair of sperm ducts that connect the testes to the penis, and in seminal vesicles that lie alongside the prostate gland.

During ejaculation, muscles in these structures power hundreds of millions of sperm—along with seminal fluid from the prostate—into and through the urethra, in the penis. Then the flagella power the sperm through the female reproductive tract in search of an egg to fertilize. Once released, a sperm can live for up to 7 days.

ADDITIONAL FACTS

1. *The sperm of crawfish, millipedes, mites, and worms do not have flagella, or tails.*

2. *Sperm that have been frozen for months or even years can be thawed and still effectively fertilize an egg.*

3. *One milliliter of average semen contains 50 million to 200 million sperm cells.*

✦✦✦

Protein

Protein is an essential nutrient for building and maintaining the bones, muscles, and skin. We get protein in our diets from meat, dairy products, nuts, grains, and beans.

The protein you obtain from meat and other animal products is complete, meaning that it contains all the amino acids your body cannot synthesize. Protein from plants is incomplete because it does not contain all the amino acids your body needs. Therefore, you must combine plant proteins to get all the amino acids you require.

The average adult needs 50 to 65 grams of protein daily. This is equivalent to eating 4 ounces of meat and a cup of cottage cheese. Most people who follow a reasonable diet will take in enough protein. You should eat a variety of foods to make sure you get all the amino acids you need.

When making protein choices, try to avoid saturated fats, found in fatty meats and whole-milk dairy products. Try to limit red meat to less than 18 ounces per week and skip processed meats altogether, as they have been linked to higher cancer risks. Beans, fish, and poultry are healthier choices that provide lots of protein. Soy and tofu should be eaten in moderation, about two to four times a week. Eating a balance of carbohydrates and proteins is ideal. Cutting back on processed carbohydrates and increasing protein intake improves blood levels of triglycerides and HDL cholesterol, potentially reducing your risks of heart attack, stroke, and other kinds of cardiovascular disease.

ADDITIONAL FACTS

1. *Six ounces of steak provides about 38 grams of protein and 44 grams of fat, 16 grams of which is saturated fat. That is nearly 75 percent of the recommended daily intake of saturated fat.*

2. *Six ounces of salmon provides 34 grams of protein and 18 grams of fat, 4 grams of which is saturated. That amounts to only 18 percent of the recommended daily total of saturated fat.*

3. *A cup of lentils has 18 grams of protein and less than 1 gram of fat.*

✦✦✦

Hippocrates

Anyone who knows medicine has probably heard of the Hippocratic oath—a pledge doctors make to always do what's best for their patients' health. What people may not be as familiar with is the person for whom this oath is named: the Greek physician Hippocrates, traditionally regarded as the father of modern medicine.

Hippocrates lived from approximately 460 to 377 BC on the island of Kos. He was known in his lifetime as a notable doctor and teacher. But it wasn't until about 100 years after his death that he became so well known. The Museum of Alexandria in Egypt at that time gathered a collection of medical writings that became known as the Hippocratic Corpus (the works of Hippocrates). Although it is accepted that the doctor did not actually write all these papers himself—they were probably compiled by several of his students and followers—that detail has proved insignificant in the grand scheme of history. Hippocrates' reputation as the model physician grew out of this collection.

The Hippocratic writings are known for their simplicity, directness, and emphasis on the practical problems of medicine. They discuss a range of basic tasks like setting broken bones, treating wounds, and making diagnoses. They also establish medicine as its own distinct profession and field of science, separate from philosophy or alchemy. The most famous document, the Hippocratic oath, deals largely with ethical issues in medicine. Others include a famous story about Greek history called "The Embassy." These articles mixed fact and fiction, and some may not even have been written by Hippocrates himself; still, they formed the basis of the mythology that evolved after his death.

Hippocrates is credited with being the first physician to reject superstitions that held that illness stemmed from supernatural or divine forces. Under the influence of Hippocrates' supposed works, surgery, pharmacy, and anatomy advanced in the Hellenistic period. While other physicians and schools of medicine gained and lost popularity in the centuries that followed, the simple theories presented in the works of Hippocrates continue to inspire physicians through the modern day.

ADDITIONAL FACTS

1. *Most medical schools today administer some form of Hippocratic oath, but most no longer use the original version, which forbade surgery, abortion, and euthanasia.*

2. *It has been suggested that scientists and engineers should pledge a code of ethics similar to doctors' Hippocratic oath.*

3. *Hippocrates is given credit for first describing of clubbed fingers (also called Hippocratic fingers), a telltale symptom of chronic lung disease, lung cancer, and cyanotic heart disease.*

◆◆◆

Respiratory Distress Syndrome

To delivery room physicians and nurses, the first wail of a newborn is a welcome sound. It means that the infant's lungs are strong and healthy—and chances are the child is safe from respiratory distress syndrome (RDS). Once the leading cause of death among premature infants, RDS is a breathing disorder in which the lungs' air sacs don't remain open. As a result, the baby is unable to breathe.

Premature babies, in particular, are at risk for RDS because a substance called surfactant isn't produced in the lungs until the final 3 months of fetal development. Surfactant is a type of protein that's secreted by cells in the respiratory membrane and lowers the surface tension of the fluid that coats the lungs. Without it, the water molecules cling together, causing the lungs to stiffen and the air sacs to collapse. Symptoms of RDS include a bluish color in the skin and membranes, rapid or shallow breathing, grunting, and rapid heartbeat.

Until the discovery of this surfactant in the 1950s, RDS claimed the lives of 10,000 babies in the United States every year. Fortunately, pregnant women going into premature labor today can receive injections of steroids, such as betamethasone and dexamethasone. These drugs cross the placenta into the fetus, accelerating its production of surfactant. Premature infants with RDS are also treated with supplemental oxygen delivered through an oxygen hood, tube, or other method. Natural or artificial surfactants may also be administered to aid breathing. Thanks to these medical advances, the number of RDS-related deaths has dwindled to roughly 1,000 infants each year.

ADDITIONAL FACTS

1. *Respiratory distress syndrome is also called hyaline membrane disease.*

2. *Besides premature birth, which is the leading cause, other risk factors for RDS include gestational diabetes, Caesarean delivery, and multiple pregnancy (carrying twins or more).*

◆◆◆

Germs

When most people think of germs, cold-causing microorganisms are usually the first things that spring to mind. While many of these bacteria, viruses, fungi, and protozoa *do* make you sick, the truth is that some of these microbes keep you healthy, too.

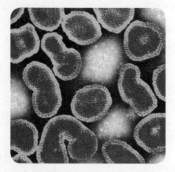

Bacteria are tiny, one-celled organisms shaped as rods, spheres, or spirals. Although they grow and reproduce on their own, they gather nutrients from the environment they're in. In some cases, that means the human body; bacterial infections include strep throat, dental cavities, and pneumonia. On the flip side, good bacteria live in the intestines and aid in food digestion.

Another germ form is the virus, which is essentially a capsule containing genetic material. Unlike bacteria, viruses require a host in order to reproduce. When a virus, such as those that cause the flu or the common cold, enters the body, it hijacks host cells in the body to reproduce itself.

Some fungi also are single-celled organisms, although they're slightly larger. Others, such as molds, yeasts, and mushrooms, live in the air, water, and soil and inside the body. Fungi are important for making some foods, such as bread, yogurt, and certain cheeses. But certain types can also lead to yeast infections and diaper rash.

The last major category of germs is protozoa, single-celled animals that thrive in moisture and can spread diseases through water. There are other germs that are sort of in between, such as mycoplasmas and rickettsias, and they cause illness, too.

Because there are so many different varieties of microbes, physicians examine blood and urine samples to determine what type of germ is causing illness in order to treat the problem accordingly. Because germs can live on surfaces for days, the most effective way of avoiding infection is to wash your hands frequently, and always after using the toilet.

ADDITIONAL FACTS

1. *One thousand bacteria placed next to each other would stretch across a pencil eraser.*

2. *The antibiotic penicillin is derived from a fungus.*

3. *In 1993, a type of protozoan infiltrated the water system in Milwaukee and eventually made some 400,000 people sick.*

❖❖❖

Aspirin

Around the 5th century BC, the Greek doctor Hippocrates (c. 460–c. 377 BC) described a miraculous powder that dulled muscle and joint pain, cured headaches, and reduced fever. Hundreds of years later, scientists discovered that this bitter substance, which in Hippocrates' time was extracted from willow tree bark, contained a compound now known as salicin, which the body converts into salicylic acid. This chemical, in turn, was the basis for modern-day aspirin, a medication that one of its manufacturers has called "the wonder drug that works wonders."

Salicylic acid in its purest form was indeed an effective pain reliever and fever reducer, but it also upset stomachs and led to bleeding in the digestive tract. In the late 1800s, the German scientist Felix Hoffman (1868–1946) set out to find a new compound that would help his father's arthritis without causing stomach distress. Working for the Bayer company, Hoffman created acetylsalicylic acid (ASA)—a modified version of salicylic acid that worked just as well but was much gentler on the stomach. In 1899, the company began marketing the new drug as aspirin.

Today, Americans take about 80 billion aspirin tablets a year. The drug is used to relieve pain from headaches, menstrual cramps, colds, toothaches, and muscle aches, as well as symptoms of lupus and other rheumatologic conditions in which the immune system attacks part of the body. Because aspirin can help prevent blood clots from forming, many people who have suffered heart attacks or strokes now take a low-dose aspirin a day to prevent recurrence. Aspirin can also reduce fever, possibly by affecting the brain's hypothalamus, which controls body temperature. The drug travels through the bloodstream to all parts of the body and is filtered out in the urine within 4 to 6 hours.

Aspirin works by binding to cyclooxygenase-2 (COX-2) enzymes, stopping them from producing chemicals called prostaglandins that play a role in pain, swelling, and blood clotting. COX-2 enzymes are often found in tissue that has been damaged by injury or sickness. But aspirin also inhibits a similar enzyme, COX-1, that helps protect the stomach lining; this is one reason why aspirin and its relatives can cause nausea and damage the digestive tract.

ADDITIONAL FACTS

1. *Aspirin comes in both prescription and nonprescription strengths and is available as plain tablets, enteric-coated tablets, delayed-release formulas, chewable tablets, gums, and rectal suppositories.*

2. *People who have asthma, frequently stuffed or runny noses, or nasal growths called polyps are at higher risk for an allergic reaction to aspirin.*

3. *In children, aspirin can cause a life-threatening condition called Reye's syndrome, in which fat builds up in the brain, liver, and other organs.*

✦✦✦

Carotid Arteries

Touch your finger to your neck along your trachea: That pulsing you feel comes from your common carotids, two large arteries that pump oxygen-rich blood to the face and brain.

Each side of the body has a carotid artery; the right common carotid originates in the neck from the brachiocephalic trunk, while the left arises directly from the heart's aortic arch. From there, the two sides follow nearly identical paths.

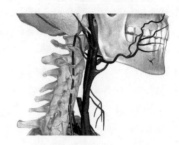

Both arteries split into two branches at the base of the skull. The internal branch carries blood to the brain, while the external branch spreads out around the face.

If a carotid artery becomes blocked by fat and cholesterol buildup (called atherosclerosis or plaque), brain function and vision can be affected and a stroke can occur. Plaque in a carotid artery may cut off the flow of blood, or it may cause blood to flow abnormally and form a clot. Blockage can be detected by an ultrasound, CT scan, or angiography, in which dye is injected into the artery and x-rays are taken.

Patients whose carotid arteries are between 75 and 99 percent blocked usually have surgery to clear them out and restore blood flow to the brain. (A complete blockage, however, is too dangerous to be operated on.) A doctor may insert a plastic tube called a shunt into the artery above and below the blockage to reroute bloodflow while the plaque is removed. Narrowed or blocked arteries can also be treated with changes in lifestyle—implementing a low-fat, low-cholesterol diet and getting regular physical activity—and medications such as blood thinners and cholesterol-lowering drugs.

ADDITIONAL FACTS

1. *Doctors may listen with a stethoscope against the throat for something called a carotid bruit—an abnormal sound that indicates the presense of a fatty buildup and a higher stroke risk.*

2. *A clot that stays in one place and blocks the flow of blood in an artery is called a thrombus. A clot that travels and wedges itself into a smaller vessel is called an embolism.*

3. *A significant cause of stroke among middle-aged adults is carotid artery dissection, in which a small tear forms in the arterial lining and blood seeps into the space between vessel layers. Dissection usually results from blunt trauma to the head or neck, although spontaneous tears occur as well.*

✦✦✦

Ovary

Although each ovary is roughly the size of a walnut, these two pearl-colored lumps of tissue serve as the center of the female reproductive system. Not only do they house the egg supply, but they also pump out the sex hormones estrogen and progesterone. These bodily chemicals influence almost every aspect of a woman's physiology: In addition to controlling ovulation and menstruation, they help keep the bones, heart, breasts, skin, and vagina healthy.

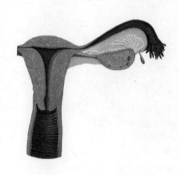

Attached to the top of the uterus by ligaments, the ovaries are located at the sides of the uterus and about an inch away from it. An ovary is composed of two main parts: the medulla (a core of fibrous connective tissue, nerves, and blood vessels) and the cortex (a thick outer layer). Making up the cortex are tens of thousands of fluid-filled egg sacs called follicles. Every month during a woman's reproductive years, the pituitary gland, at the front of the brain, releases follicle-stimulating hormone (FSH) into the bloodstream. This triggers up to 20 follicles to start maturing and secreting estrogen, priming the rest of the body for a potential pregnancy.

Once the follicles are fully developed, usually only one follicle from one of the two ovaries rises to the surface. Then there is a surge of FSH and luteinizing hormone (LH), the ovary bursts open, and the egg is expelled on a wave of fluid. As the ovary's exterior layer heals, progesterone-producing cells temporarily grow in its place. (Excess progesterone is to blame for the bloating, breast tenderness, and mood swings of premenstrual syndrome.) As a result, a woman's ovaries become more scarred and pitted with age; by menopause, they're mainly made of a white, fibrous tissue.

ADDITIONAL FACTS

1. *Each ovary is about 1.6 inches long; the set weighs less than 0.3 ounce.*

2. *The ovaries are the female gonads, or the glands that produce reproductive cells. The male gonads are the testes.*

3. *In childhood, the ovaries are only tiny structures with minimal function. They elongate and develop during puberty.*

✦✦✦

Carbohydrates

Carbohydrates are one of the three major kinds of foods, along with proteins and fats. Your saliva, stomach, and liver break down carbohydrates into glucose, which is the simplest type of sugar and the form in which sugar circulates in the bloodstream. This sugar gives your body's cells the energy they need to function properly.

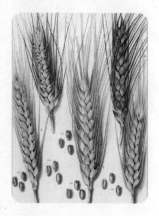

Carbohydrates are either simple or complex, depending on how quickly your body digests them. Fruits, milk products, and refined sugar provide simple carbohydrates that are digested quickly. Whole grain breads and cereals, starchy vegetables, and legumes are made up of complex carbohydrates, which are digested slowly.

Foods like soda, candy, and cake, which contain refined carbohydrates such as white flour and added sugar, have high calorie counts and cause rapid changes in blood sugar. These are simple carbohydrates and are sometimes referred to as bad carbs. It's a good idea to limit these food choices.

Generally, complex carbohydrates are healthier food options than simple carbohydrates. Complex carbohydrates, such as whole grains, and some simple carbohydrates, including fruit and milk products, are sometimes referred to as good carbs, because they contain vitamins, minerals, and fiber. You should emphasize these nutrient-rich carbohydrates in your diet for optimal health.

ADDITIONAL FACTS

1. *Your body either uses glucose immediately or stores it in your liver and muscles for later use.*

2. *The term* whole grains *refers to grains that contain all the parts of the grain seed or kernel, including the dietary fiber and other important nutrients. Refined grains are produced when manufacturers process whole grains in ways that remove some of the dietary fiber, folic acid, and iron. Enriched grains are refined grains, such as white rice and white bread, that have had the folic acid and iron added back. Fortified grains are enriched grains that have extra nutrients added.*

3. *Date sugar and dark brown sugars are good alternatives to white sugar, as they contain much higher levels of antioxidants.*

◆◆◆

Trepanation: Ancient Incan Brain Surgery

It may seem as though brain surgery is a product of the 20th century; after all, doctors need advanced surgical technology to perform such a delicate, dangerous procedure, right? According to a recent and surprising discovery, this may not be the case.

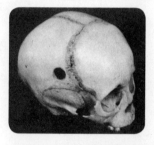

In 2008, researchers at Southern Connecticut State University in New Haven and Tulane University in New Orleans published a study of 411 ancient Incan skeletons recently unearthed in the Peruvian Andes. Human skulls dating back to AD 1000 showed evidence of undergoing a type of primitive yet effective surgery to treat head injuries. Specifically, small portions of the skulls had been removed by a procedure known as trepanation (also called trephination).

This procedure, archaeologists believe, was performed mostly on men who had been wounded in combat. By boring a hole in the skull, the surgeon aimed to drain excess fluid that built up in the skull after a head blow. Marks on the skeletons indicated that the Incan doctors created the hole by scraping away at the skull until they reached the brain. Evidence suggests that it took many years to perfect the method, and that few wounded soldiers survived the first wave of trepanations.

By the time European explorers arrived in South America, however, Incan surgeons had largely perfected the technique and boasted survival rates of nearly 90 percent. Incan surgeons used wild tobacco, maize beer, and medicinal plants to relieve pain and reduce the likelihood of infection. Though doctors today have anesthesia, x-rays, and better surgical tools, a similar procedure in which a piece of skull is removed to reduce bleeding and pressure on the brain caused by severe head trauma is still commonly performed.

ADDITIONAL FACTS

1. *Although trepanation was most common in men, remains of some women also show signs of the procedure. It is believed that the Incas may also have used the surgery for cases of epilepsy.*

2. *The coca plant, used as an anesthetic by Incan doctors, is still widely chewed across the Andean region and acts as a mild stimulant. It can also be processed into cocaine.*

3. *After trepanation surgery, Incan warriors who survived the procedure sometimes wore the removed section of their skulls as good-luck amulets.*

✦✦✦

Necrotizing Enterocolitis

When it comes to language, necrotizing enterocolitis (NEC) is fairly straight-forward. *Necrotizing* means causing the death of tissue, *entero* refers to the small intestine, *colo* denotes the large intestine, and *itis* signals inflammation. But in life, this medical condition is far more complicated—and dangerous. Striking 25,000 infants every year, the gastrointestinal infection and inflammation can destroy part—or all—of the intestinal tract.

More than 85 percent of NEC cases occur in babies born prematurely. Symptoms, which usually appear within the first 2 weeks of life, include bloody stools, greenish vomit, a bloated or red abdomen, and poor tolerance of feedings. Less common signs are diarrhea, lethargy, and fluctuating body temperature. If NEC is suspected, a physician will use an x-ray to look for gas bubbles in the intestines and abdominal cavity. Treatments for the condition include antibiotics, nasogastric drainage (inserting a tube through the nose into the stomach to remove air and fluid), and intravenous fluids for nutrition. In more severe cases, surgery to remove the damaged intestine is necessary.

Although NEC has been studied extensively, the exact cause is still unknown. Some experts believe that premature infants are simply born with weaker intestinal tissue. When they begin to feed, the stress of digestion may cause usually harmless bacteria to attack and damage the digestive organs. Meanwhile, other researchers believe that babies who have low oxygen levels due to respiratory distress syndrome are suscep-tible, because the available oxygen is routed to the vital organs instead of the gastro-intestinal tract. A more debatable theory is that NEC may be infectious and spread among newborns, as it often affects a number of infants in the same nursery.

ADDITIONAL FACTS

1. *Necrotizing enterocolitis is rare, affecting only 1 in 2,000 to 4,000 births. Those odds spike for prema-ture births; some 10 percent of newborns weighing less than 3 pounds, 5 ounces experience NEC.*

2. *Babies fed breast milk are at lower risk of NEC than those given infant formula.*

◆◆◆

Virus

Viruses are the freeloading vampires of the body. Not a plant, animal, or bacterium, these infectious agents are unable to live on their own. Instead, they hijack other cells to help them reproduce and carry out metabolic activities.

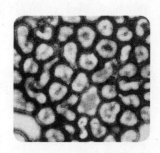

First identified in 1892 by the Russian scientist Dmitry I. Ivanovsky (1864–1920), viruses get their name from the Latin word meaning "poison" and "slimy liquid." Today, scientists have identified more than 5,000 different types of viruses. Some of them, such as those that cause the common cold and flu, multiply rapidly and kill the host cell, while others, such as the genital herpes virus, can lie dormant in the body for years. Still others, such as the one that leads to AIDS, are slow viruses, meaning that they remain in the cells and replicate slowly over years.

Essentially, viruses consist of nucleic acids—either DNA or RNA—surrounded by a protein shell, or capsid. Most viruses are shaped as either rods or spherical, 20-sided polygons. Because they lack enzymes for energy production and ribosomes for protein synthesis and reproduction, viruses latch onto a host cell. Like a needle, they inject their genetic material into the new cell. At that point, the viral nucleic acid takes over the cellular machinery, producing new virus particles. Often, this process destroys the host cell. This releases new viruses to infect other cells.

Because viruses are embedded in the cells, they're much more difficult to kill than bacteria. Some antiviral medications attack viruses, while vaccines are also effective in stimulating the immune system to produce white blood cells that target specific viruses.

ADDITIONAL FACTS

1. *Viruses range from 20 to 400 nanometers in size. Only the largest viruses can be seen under a powerful microscope on the highest resolution.*

2. *Some experts theorize that a virus is to blame for the extinction of dinosaurs.*

3. *The viruses that cause the common cold can live on surfaces outside the body for a few days.*

✦ ✦ ✦

Chiropractic

Chiropractic is an alternative form of medicine based on the theory that adjustments to the spine can treat health problems and improve general well-being. Studies have shown chiropractic to be effective in easing lower-back pain and some types of headaches. The benefits for nonspinal conditions—such as high blood pressure, attention deficit disorder, and ear infections, for example—have been suggested but not scientifically proven.

An Iowa doctor, Daniel David Palmer (1845–1913), is credited with founding modern chiropractic medicine in 1895. The word is derived from the Greek terms for *hand* (*cheir*) and *action* (*praxis*). Palmer believed that the body has a powerful self-healing ability, but that misalignments of the spine interfere with its natural flow of energy.

Chiropractic treatments involve manipulating the joints and bones in a person's spine beyond their passive range of motion by using sudden twisting, pulling, or pushing movements. The goal of such treatments is to reverse damage caused by accidents, bad posture, or other spinal problems.

Potential side effects resulting from spinal manipulation include temporary discomfort, headache, and fatigue. Serious complications are rare but include lower-back pain or weakness from damaged nerve roots and blockage of blood supply to the brain from damaged arteries.

Some chiropractors use heat or ice, electrical stimulation, acupuncture, or ultrasound to help relax a person's muscles before spinal adjustment. They may also incorporate healing strategies such as dietary supplements, rehabilitative exercise, and nutrition and weight-loss counseling.

About 20 percent of Americans have received chiropractic care at some point in their lives, a 2002 national study found. Compared with other forms of alternative medicine, chiropractic is frequently covered by insurance: Many health care plans, including Medicare and Medicaid in some states, cover chiropractic services.

ADDITIONAL FACTS

1. *Doctors of chiropractic (DCs) must complete 3 years of undergraduate study plus 4 years of accredited chiropractic school.*

2. *Half of all working Americans say they have back pain. It is the second most common reason for a visit to the doctor in the United States.*

3. *The "backbone" is made up of 33 doughnut-shaped bones called vertebrae.*

✦✦✦

Autonomic Nervous System

Many of our bodies' major organs and muscles are regulated by the autonomic nervous system (ANS). In most cases, the ANS functions involuntarily: Our blood vessels narrow or our heart rates increase, for example, to help us respond to our environment. The system works without our conscious effort or, in many cases, even our awareness.

The ANS regulates muscles in the skin, eyes, heart, lungs, and stomach. It also controls the intestines, salivary glands, secretion of insulin, urinary function, and sexual arousal. The autonomic nervous system's main goal is to maintain homeostasis, or proper balance, in the body through two main components: the sympathetic nervous system and the parasympathetic nervous system.

During periods of perceived danger or emergency, the sympathetic nervous system helps our bodies exhibit a fight-or-flight response. When faced with a threat—either physical or emotional—the brain responds to protect the body from danger: Blood vessels constrict to divert bloodflow away from the gastrointestinal (GI) tract and skin. Pupils dilate, letting more light enter the eyes. Lungs open up, allowing for greater oxygen exchange.

Conversely, the parasympathetic nervous system reverses many of these functions during calmer times. This allows us to rest comfortably, breathe easier, and digest food, absorbing more nutrients thanks to greater bloodflow to the GI tract. The parasympathetic nervous system is also involved in producing erections in males.

ANS problems include erectile dysfunction, excessive dizziness, incontinence, and inability to sweat. These disorders may arise with age or can be caused by an illness like diabetes. In such cases, treatment of the underlying medical issue may alleviate the disorder. If not, drugs are available to treat the symptoms of many autonomic disorders.

ADDITIONAL FACTS

1. *Some people can be trained to control functions of the ANS, such as heart rate or blood pressure, through practices such as meditation and biofeedback.*

2. *The ANS is made up of neurons in the lower brain stem, in the brain's medulla oblongata. If the central nervous system is damaged above that level, involuntary processes such as cardiovascular, digestive, and respiratory functions will continue, and life, although possibly in a vegetative state, can be sustained.*

3. *When parts of the ANS stop functioning involuntarily, disorders such as decreased sweating, urinary retention, constipation, and erectile dysfunction can occur.*

◆◆◆

Fallopian Tubes

Around 1544, an Italian priest named Gabriele Falloppio (1523–1562) decided to switch careers and become a surgeon, with somewhat disastrous—and a few fatal—results. That experience spurred him to step away from patients and concentrate his efforts on the study of medicine, which was a profession, as opposed to surgery, then considered a trade. It was a fortuitous choice: Falloppio went on to become one of the most renowned anatomists in history by shedding light on the female reproductive system. Most notably, he discovered the two ducts that transmit eggs from the ovaries to the uterus; these ducts were later named fallopian tubes in his honor.

These soft, flexible, 2- to 3-inch-long wands of pink tissue play a crucial role in the fertilization process. Extending from the upper edges of the uterus, they stretch toward the ovaries but aren't attached to them. Instead, each tube fans out in short, finger-like tentacles called fimbriae. When an egg is released, these fimbriae sweep over the ovary to capture the egg. Once the egg is inside, the fallopian tube's muscles and tiny hairlike projections, or cilia, guide it slowly downward toward the uterus; in total, the journey takes about 6 days. Fertilization by sperm, which travel to the fallopian tubes through the uterus, typically takes place within the first 2 days.

Because the fallopian tubes are essential for reproduction, one method of permanent birth control is to cut and seal them so that the eggs can't enter the uterus. This method, called tubal ligation (also known as having one's tubes tied), is virtually foolproof; each year, more than 750,000 women opt for the surgery. There is a procedure to reverse it, but success rates for reversal are low.

ADDITIONAL FACTS

1. *Fallopian tubes are also called oviducts.*

2. *To reduce the transmission of syphilis, Gabriele Falloppio invented a rudimentary condom. It was a medicated sheath that was placed over the foreskin of the penis and tied with a pink ribbon to make it more appealing to women.*

✦✦✦

Sugar

Sugar usually refers to the simple sugars or simple carbohydrates that are one of the two major kinds of carbohydrates (simple and complex carbohydrates). The sweet taste of sugar makes us crave foods that contain it, and sugar is often added to foods and drinks for this reason. However, consuming too many simple sugars can be unhealthy.

Your body processes carbohydrates, including sugars, by breaking them down into their simplest form, simple sugar. This sugar is then absorbed into your bloodstream. As the sugar level rises in your blood, your pancreas releases a hormone called insulin, which helps move sugar from your blood into all the cells in your body for use as energy. Simple sugars are a source of quick energy. Some foods, such as candy, soda, cookies, cake, frozen desserts, and some fruit drinks, already contain simple sugar. Other foods are made with refined grains, such as white flour and white rice. Because both simple sugars and refined grains are broken down by your body easily and quickly, they cause rapid spikes in your blood sugar levels. Eating too much of these foods may increase your risk of developing diabetes and heart disease.

Consuming simple sugars in excess can also lead to weight gain and contribute to dental cavities. Many of the foods that contain simple sugars, such as candy and soda, provide concentrated calories. The calories your body doesn't use are stored as fat, which is one reason added sugar should be limited in a healthy diet.

An easy way to immediately cut down on simple sugars in your diet is to eliminate soda and other sugar-sweetened beverages. A 12-ounce serving of sugar-sweetened soda contains the equivalent of 10 teaspoons of sugar, 150 calories, and no vitamins or fiber.

ADDITIONAL FACTS

1. *Examples of simple sugars are fructose, glucose, and lactose.*

2. *The largest source of added sugar in the diets of children in the United States is soda.*

3. *Consuming just one sweetened soft drink per day increases a child's risk of obesity. Juice intake should also be limited in children under 12.*

4. *Not all simple sugars or carbohydrates are bad. Some simple carbohydrates are found in nutritious foods, such as fruits, vegetables, and dairy products.*

◆◆◆

Aesculapius

Aesculapius is known today as the Greco-Roman god of medicine, although his legend may be based on the life of a real physician who lived around 1200 BC.

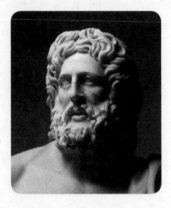

In Greek mythology, Apollo—the god of healing, truth, and prophecy—had a son with Coronis, a mortal princess. Coronis was unfaithful to Apollo and was killed and burned on a funeral pyre, but her baby was rescued from her womb and named Asklepios, meaning "to cut open." Asklepios learned the art of healing from a wise centaur named Chiron and became a healer so skilled that he could bring the dead back to life. This caused Hades, ruler of the underworld, to complain to Zeus (king of the gods) that Asklepios was depriving him of subjects. Zeus was also concerned that Asklepios was assuming godlike powers and that he might make all men immortal. So Zeus killed Asklepios with a thunderbolt and then, at Apollo's request, made Asklepios the god of medicine.

A cult developed around his following and became very popular around 300 BC, spreading throughout Greece and to Rome, where Asklepios was known as Aesculapius. Because people supposed that Aesculapius cured the sick while they slept—or visited them and offered treatment advice while they dreamed—his followers frequently slept overnight in temples built in his honor. These temples were staffed with physicians and functioned as health care facilities and medical schools. Snakes, which Aesculapius held to be sacred, were a common fixture in his temples; followers believed that the reptiles might carry healing powers or messages from the gods. Aesculapius is frequently pictured standing, dressed in a long cloak and holding a staff with a serpent coiled around it. This is similar to today's symbol of medicine, a winged staff with intertwined serpents that is called a caduceus.

ADDITIONAL FACTS

1. *Aesculapius was often worshipped along with Hygeia, the Greek goddess of health. The two are sometimes referred to as father and daughter or as husband and wife.*

2. *In* The Iliad, *Aesculapius is mentioned as a "blameless physician" and the father of two Greek doctors at Troy, Machaon and Podalirius.*

3. *The plant genus* Asclepias *(commonly known as milkweed) is named after Aesculapius and includes the medicinal plant called "pleurisy root."*

◆◆◆

Respirator Therapy

In 1929, the American physician Philip Drinker (1894–1972) unveiled the first mechanical respirator, a machine meant to provide artificial respiration for a person who was unable to breathe properly. The large metal tank was built so that a child or adult could fit inside the pressurized environment, on his or her back with a rubber collar around the neck. In the decades following the advent of the Drinker respirator, scientists refined and improved this process, but the application of respirator therapy—or the use of an outside device to aid in breathing—continues.

Today, doctors mainly use positive-pressure ventilators to aid breathing in newborns with respiratory distress syndrome and premature babies who are administered an anesthetic for surgery. (Ventilators are also used for adults suffering from respiratory arrest, coma, apnea, respiratory muscle fatigue, or abnormally slow or weak breathing.) These machines, which consist of a turbine, oxygen supply, and reservoir, deliver air to the patient. For infants, the most common ventilator methods involve a face mask attached to a continuous positive airway pressure, or CPAP, machine. If only a small amount of additional oxygen is needed, the patient wears a nasal cannula—a tube with plastic prongs that are inserted into the nose. A specific amount of oxygen is released through the tubes and into the nose each minute.

Mechanical ventilator machines also measure peak airway pressure, which is the amount of pressure needed to overcome the natural respiratory resistance caused by the lungs and chest wall. Trained professionals known as respiratory therapists keep tabs on the amount of pressure to apply. Too much pressure can damage the lungs or airways, while too little can deprive the lungs of the oxygen that's needed throughout the body.

ADDITIONAL FACTS

1. *The Drinker respirator was also known as an iron lung.*

2. *Modern-day ventilators became popular during the polio epidemics of the 20th century.*

◆◆◆

Antibodies

Antibodies are the foot soldiers of the immune system. These proteins latch onto foreign invaders called antigens that are present on the surface of or inside the illness-causing microorganisms and toxic substances. The antibodies then attach to the offending substance and help white blood cells remove it from the body.

When white blood cells called B lymphocytes, or B cells, come in contact with an antigen, they release millions of antibodies into the bloodstream. These antibodies bind to a microbe and destroy it by causing it to burst, a process called lysis, or they flag down another cell to consume it through phagocytosis. Antibodies often circulate for more than a week and can linger in the body for several months to several years.

Each antibody molecule is made up of two parts: The surface is specially formed to attach to a specific antigen. Like a key inserted in a lock, this section attaches to a section of the antigen's surface called the epitope. The stem of the antibody molecule is one of five structures that determines the type of antibody—immunoglobulin M, G, A, E, or D. The different types of antibodies reflect what the protein does and where in the body it resides: IgM (immunoglobulin M) is the first responder to an antigen and circulates only in the blood. But on second exposure to the antigen, IgG—the most prevalent class—is released; these antibodies are smaller and faster than IgM and can leave the bloodstream to enter the tissue. IgA antibodies, on the other hand, are produced by B cells in the mucous membranes and are most often found in bodily secretions such as tears and saliva. IgE antibodies trigger allergic reactions and fight certain parasites. The last group, IgD, is the least common antibody; scientists aren't sure about its function.

ADDITIONAL FACTS

1. *The study of antibodies began in 1890, when scientists transferred blood from animals with diphtheria to healthy animals. The researchers discovered that the second group became immune to the disease.*

2. *Antibodies are also called gamma globulins.*

♦♦♦

Quinolones

Quinolones are broad-spectrum antibiotics derived from nalidixic acid that are effective against urinary tract infections, bacterial prostatitis, bacterial diarrhea, bronchitis, and gonorrhea. They work by destroying bacterial DNA components called gyrase and topoisomerase IV, enzymes that are essential for cell replication.

The first generation of quinolones arose from the discovery of nalidixic acid in the 1960s and the development of norfloxacin, a fluoridated quinolone compound, in 1986. These early drugs had poor distribution throughout the body and were used primarily for urinary tract infections. Since then, more effective quinolones have been developed, and there are now nine varieties available in the United States.

Fluoroquinolones are often prescribed because their relatively long half-lives (the time it takes for the drug to leave the body) allow them to be administered only once or twice a day. They also have a relatively low incidence of serious side effects, although they are not completely without risks: Caffeine, nonsteroidal anti-inflammatory drugs, and corticosteroids enhance fluoroquinolones' toxicity, while antacids, warfarin, antiviral agents, and other medications can interact dangerously with them. As with other types of antibiotics, resistance to quinolones can evolve quickly, and the drugs have been rendered ineffective against several pathogens around the world. Distribution of the drugs through widespread veterinary and livestock use, especially in Europe, has been implicated.

ADDITIONAL FACTS

1. *In 2008, the Food and Drug Administration requested that manufacturers place a black box warning on fluoroquinolone medications describing their increased risk of tendinitis and tendon rupture.*

2. *Quercetin, an antioxidant vitamin occasionally used as a dietary supplement, competitively binds to DNA gyrase and may make quinolones less effective. But the effect on the drugs of foods that contain high levels of quercetin, such as apples and garlic, is not clear.*

3. *Quinolones are usually administered orally but can also be given intravenously or applied topically for certain types of infections.*

◆◆◆

The Limbic System

In a real sense, it is the limbic system that gives humans humanity—the ability to love, to laugh, to cry, to remember.

The system within the brain that controls our emotions and behavior, the limbic system, comprises three main parts, the hypothalamus, the hippocampus, and the amygdala. Several other parts of the brain are also associated with the limbic system, including areas that store associations for different smells and the part of the brain that appears to be responsible for orgasms.

These parts are interconnected by a network of neural pathways, forming a web that produces complex emotions and allows us to interact with the world around us.

The hippocampus, a seahorse-shaped structure (*hippocampus* comes from the Greek word for seahorse), turns experiences into memories. A damaged or malfunctioning hippocampus can make it impossible for a person to form long-term recollections andimmediately forget the name of a person he or she has just met, for instance.

Fear and sexual arousal are controlled by the amygdala, which comprises two clusters of nerves next to the hippocampus.

The hypothalamus is one of the busiest parts of the limbic system—indeed, of the entire brain. It controls feelings of hunger and thirst and processes our reactions to pain and pleasure. It is the hypothalamus that is thought to generate rolling, uncontrollable laughter. The hypothalamus also sends signals to the rest of the body via the pituitary gland, which pumps hormones into the bloodstream. Both are located at the front of the brain, above and between our eyes.

Because natural pleasures are an important part of (and reason for) survival, the limbic system creates an appetite for things that will provide sensory rewards. A part of the brain called the ventral tegmental area responds to positive experiences—being praised for a job well done, sexual intercourse, ice cream—by releasing a chemical called dopamine, which produces feelings of happiness and contentment.

ADDITIONAL FACTS

1. *The limbic system contributes to the production of uncontrollable laughter, the formation of friendships, and the expression of love and affection.*

2. *Some antidepressants work by lowering the "reuptake" of dopamine, thus allowing this pleasure-inducing chemical to stay in the brain longer,*

3. *Drugs such as nicotine, cocaine, and marijuana may cause intense feelings of pleasure—and spark an addiction—by flooding the brain with dopamine. Similarly, people whose limbic systems are damaged have trouble enjoying life and may turn to drugs, alcohol, food, or gambling to provide the thrills they're missing.*

◆◆◆

Uterus

When you think of powerful muscles, bulging biceps or rippling abdominals are probably the first things to come to mind. But some of the strongest muscles in a woman's body are found in her uterus, a 3-inch-long reproductive organ shaped like an upside-down pear. Consisting mainly of smooth muscle, the uterus primarily provides a place for a pregnancy to develop. These muscles stretch like taffy to accommodate a growing fetus and then contract forcefully to push the baby out during labor and delivery.

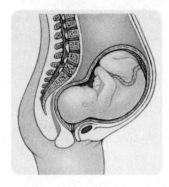

Also known as the womb, the uterus rests between the bladder and the rectum. The womb's top stretches toward the ovaries and their egg supply, accessed via the fallopian tubes; the bottom of the uterus curves into the narrow cervix, which leads to the vagina. (Science has debunked many theories regarding these organs over the centuries: In the 6th century BC, Egyptian, Greek, and Roman physicians believed that the uterus could detach and roam around the body.)

Lining the interior of this hollow organ is the endometrium, a layer of pink cells placed next to each other like tiles. After entering the uterus, a fertilized egg (now an embryo) attaches itself to the endometrium. Then the endometrial cells, which are in a tissue rich with blood vessels, gradually cover the precious embryo as it burrows into this layer of cells, seeking blood vessels to supply it with oxygen and nutrients. But if fertilization doesn't occur, the endometrium's top layers are expelled from the body during a 3- to 5-day menstrual period. The uterus contracts to shed the unused lining, sometimes causing the woman to have cramps and back pain. New endometrial cells then grow in the uterus, ready for the next cycle of ovulation.

ADDITIONAL FACTS

1. *In the late 19th century, experts believed that "the evils of masturbation" could lead to uterine diseases and abnormal periods.*

2. *The word* uterus *is Latin for "belly" or "womb." When describing more than one uterus, both* uteri *and* uteruses *are correct.*

◆◆◆

Folic Acid

Folic acid is a B vitamin that is essential for helping your body make new cells. It is found in its natural form (called folate) in many foods, including leafy green vegetables, fruits, dried beans, peas, and nuts. The synthetic form, folic acid, is added to enriched and fortified breads, cereals, and other grain products. You can also take it as a dietary supplement.

Folic acid is necessary to keep your blood healthy. When you have a folic acid deficiency, you can develop anemia, a condition in which the body may have too few red blood cells. This makes it hard for your blood to carry enough oxygen throughout your body. If you are diagnosed with anemia, you should have your folic acid level checked.

It is especially important for pregnant women to take in enough folic acid both before and during pregnancy to prevent birth defects of the infant's brain and spine, including anencephaly (the failure of most or all of the brain to develop) and spina bifida (a deformity of the spine). Most women need 400 micrograms of folic acid daily. When women are pregnant, they should take 400 to 800 micrograms daily. You should check with your doctor to determine how much you need, especially if you are taking medications that may affect how your body uses folic acid.

You cannot get too much folic acid from food, but it is possible to consume too much from supplements. Taking more than 1,000 micrograms of folic acid a day may cause nerve damage and mask pernicious anemia in people who do not have enough vitamin B_{12} in their bodies. People at risk of a B_{12} deficiency include vegans and people over 50.

ADDITIONAL FACTS

1. *Folic acid may also help prevent Alzheimer's disease, age-related hearing loss, and some cancers.*

2. *Since 1998, the United States government has required that folic acid be added to cereals and breads to help prevent birth defects.*

3. *Folic acid supplements have been reported in one study to increase the occurrence of colon cancer.*

◆◆◆

The Black Death

In the early 1300s, an epidemic known as the Black Death broke out in China or Egypt and soon spread to Europe via flea-infested rats. Within 5 years, it had killed 25 million people—one-third of Europe's population.

The plague arrived in Europe in 1347, when a trade ship returning from the Black Sea landed in Sicily. Most people on board were already dead from the disease, and the survivors soon infected the entire town. From Sicily, the sickness spread north through Italy and into other countries. The plague spread especially quickly in Britain because of its crowded cities and squalid living conditions. Homes were quarantined (*quarantina* in Italian means "40 days," the original required isolation period) if even one family member showed symptoms, and others living there were left to their fate. There was not enough room or enough healthy people to dispose of all the dead, and bodies piled up in the streets. Ironically, cats were suspected as a cause and driven out of town—though they were the one instrument that possibly could have controlled the infected rat population. It was believed that the Black Death was a punishment from God, and Jews, foreigners, lepers, and beggars were blamed and persecuted in the period of social upheaval triggered by the mass deaths.

Today, most doctors believe the Black Death was caused by the bubonic plague bacterium, *Yersinia pestis*. Both the Black Death and the bubonic plague are characterized by chills, fever, vomiting, diarrhea, and the formation of black boils (from which the Black Death gets its name) on the neck, groin, and armpit from bleeding into lymph nodes. Bubonic plague is almost always fatal within a week if not treated, especially when the bacteria spread to a victim's lungs. The plague still exists in some parts of the world today, although antibiotics are now available to treat it.

Some scientists, however, believe that the Black Death was not, in fact, the bubonic plague. They suggest that the Black Death spread from person to person rather than through infected rats and argue that it was caused by some other unidentified infectious agent.

ADDITIONAL FACTS

1. *Bubonic plague returned to Europe several times over the next few centuries. More than 300 years after the initial outbreak, an epidemic broke out in London in 1665. As many as 100,000 people died in 1 year, before winter and a massive fire killed the infected fleas and the plague tapered off.*

2. *The children's song "Ring around the Rosy" is rumored to have originated during the 14th century. "Ring around the rosy" is thought to refer to a reddish rash and "We all fall down" to symbolize death. Most experts, however, doubt that this is true.*

3. *The Italian writer Giovanni Boccaccio (1313–1375) lived through the plague as it ravaged the city of Florence in 1348. In his book* The Decameron—*a story of 10 people who escape the disease by fleeing to a villa outside of town—he gives a graphic description of the epidemic's effects on his city.*

◆◆◆

Sudden Infant Death Syndrome

The fact that sudden infant death syndrome (SIDS) can strike without warning or explanation is what makes the condition so frightening. Not a particular condition or disease, SIDS is a diagnosis that's given when a baby passes away without any discernible cause. In many cases, a sleeping baby simply never wakes up. SIDS is the leading cause of death for children under the age of year, striking 2,500 infants each year.

Despite years of research, scientists have yet to pinpoint the exact biological reason for SIDS. Experts believe that it's a combination of a physical problem, such as a heart or brain defect or an immature autonomic nervous system, and an environmental trigger, such as sleeping facedown. Recent studies have suggested that having long QT syndrome, a heart problem that can lead to an abnormal heartbeat, may play a role.

While there's no magic bullet that fends off SIDS, experts have found that certain habits can help protect infants. The most important move is to place a baby on its back, rather than its belly or side, during sleep if the infant can't roll over on its own. One theory is that a stomach-sleeping baby nestled into a thick mattress may wind up breathing in exhaled air, lowering oxygen to dangerous levels. That, coupled with a defect in the area of the brain that controls breathing during sleep, may result in SIDS.

Because infants born to mothers who smoke are more likely to die of SIDS, it's important to stamp out smoking in the household. Using a crib and lightweight bedding can also protect an infant, as thick comforters or adult beds may lead to suffocation. Lastly, giving a baby a pacifier to suck on at bedtime may also lower the chances of SIDS.

ADDITIONAL FACTS

1. *SIDS occurs more frequently in boys than in girls.*

2. *Babies who are born in fall or winter months, are born to mothers who smoke or do drugs, or are African American or Native American are all at higher risk of SIDS.*

3. *Breastfeeding may protect an infant from SIDS by reducing the risk of infections that may lead to the condition.*

◆◆◆

Red Blood Cells

Red blood cells (RBCs) give blood its crimson hue. Making up nearly half of blood's volume, some 4 million to 5 million are crammed into every cubic-millimeter-size drop. These tiny cells, which are also called erythrocytes, are responsible for ferrying oxygen throughout the body.

A mere 7.5 micrometers in diameter, RBCs are the only cells in the body that lack a nucleus; the organelle leaves the cell as it matures. As a result, they look like bagels without holes—round disks with flattened or sunken-in centers—and are highly flexible, often bending and folding to pass through small blood vessels. Inside the cell's membrane sheath are lipids, proteins, and hemoglobin, the iron-rich substance that binds to oxygen as the cells pass through the lungs. As these RBCs circulate throughout the body, they diffuse oxygen through the capillary walls. Tissues and organs use the oxygen for energy, converting it into carbon dioxide during the metabolic cycle. Then the RBCs pick up this waste by-product and transport it to the lungs for disposal.

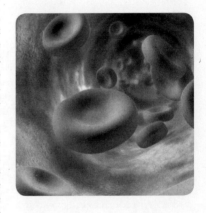

RBCs live for about 4 months before they die and are removed from the bloodstream by the spleen or liver. New cells, which are grown in the bone marrow, replace them. If tissues aren't receiving sufficient amounts of oxygen, the body will pump out an excessive number of RBCs. Called erythrocytosis, this condition usually indicates poor heart or lung function due to causes such as heart disease, chronic obstructive pulmonary disease, or smoking. Rarely, a high RBC count indicates a disease called polycythemia. A physician can administer a simple blood test to count RBCs.

ADDITIONAL FACTS

1. *RBCs die at a rate of 2 million per second.*

2. *Being at a high altitude, where there's less oxygen in the air, causes the body to produce more RBCs.*

3. *The hemoglobin molecule with its iron content turns red when binding to oxygen. This is what gives the blood cell its red color.*

◆◆◆

Digitalis

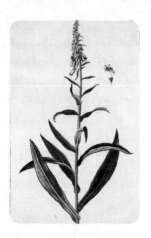

The Foxglove's leaves, with caution giv'n,
Another proof of favouring Heav'n
Will happily display;
The rapid pulse it can abate;
The hectic flush can moderate;
And blest by Him whose will is fate,
May give a lengthen'd day.

These words were written around 1820 by the poet Sarah Hoare (1777–1856) and published in the ninth edition of *An Introduction to Botany* (1823). The poem refers to foxglove, a plant that's been used for hundreds of years to slow down and strengthen contractions of the heart muscles. An extract obtained from foxglove's dried leaves, called digitalis, is commonly used today to restore circulation in patients with congestive heart failure.

Digitoxin and digoxin are the most commonly prescribed forms of digitalis—available as either oral or intravenous medications—and belong to a class of drugs called cardiac glycosides. The drugs work by slowing a rapid heartbeat, decreasing the size of a swollen heart, and increasing the strength of the heart muscle's contractions and thus the heart's output.

Too much digitalis, however, can lead to a dangerous condition known as digitalis toxicity. Symptoms include heart palpitations, vomiting and diarrhea, and visual disturbances: Some patients see lights or bright spots, see halos around objects, or experience changes in color perception. Toxicity can be caused by a single large dose of digitalis or by an accumulation of medication over time and is more frequent in patients with kidney disorders. Often, people with heart failure who take digitalis are also prescribed diuretic medications, which help reduce blood pressure by expelling sodium and excess fluid from the body. But diuretics can cause dehydration and potassium deficiency, both of which increase the risk of digitalis toxicity. To avoid this problem, potassium supplements or potassium-sparing medications are often prescribed as well.

ADDITIONAL FACTS

1. *Digitalis was first prescribed in the late 1700s by the English physician William Withering (1741–1799), who used it to treat of dropsy, a condition that "puffed [people's] bodies into grotesque shapes, squeezed their lungs, and finally brought slow but inexorable death." Dropsy is now known as edema, an overaccumulation of fluid in the body.*

2. *Digitalis toxicity can cause an abnormal heartbeat (arrhythmia) severe enough to be fatal.*

3. *In the 18th century, digitalis concoctions were often used—with little or no success—in attempts to treat asthma, epilepsy, hydrocephalus, insanity, and other conditions.*

✦✦✦

Cerebral Cortex

The largest part of the brain is the wrinkly outer layer, called the cerebral cortex. This region is responsible for conscious experience, including perception, reasoning, memory, and planning. The cerebral cortex also coordinates all sensory and motor activities by analyzing nerve signals and sending out responses to nerve cells all over the body.

If the cerebral cortex were removed from the brain and all of its folds spread out, it would be roughly the size of a large hand towel. It is ¼ inch thick and six layers deep and makes up about 40 percent of the brain by weight. This outer covering is mostly gray matter, made up of unmyelinated neurons (cells that are not covered with a protective layer of white insulation, or myelin). It is divided into two hemispheres, left and right, and each hemisphere is divided into several lobes.

The frontal lobe is the largest cerebral lobe and contains the precentral gyrus; specific areas in this region control most of the movements of the opposite side of the body. Parts of the frontal lobe are also involved in speech, emotions, and problem solving. The parietal lobe receives and translates sensory information related to touch, pressure, temperature, and pain. The temporal lobe regulates sensations of hearing and smell and contains the hippocampus, which helps form new memories. And the occipital lobe is responsible for vision. Two internal lobes, the insular and limbic lobes, not visible from the surface of the cerebral cortex, are thought to be involved in taste perception and autonomic (involuntary) behaviors.

Besides having sensory and motor areas, the cerebral cortex also has regions called association areas. These regions work to organize the jumble of perceptions gathered by the senses into a coherent understanding of our surroundings. Language and mathematical abilities are concentrated in these areas, mainly in the left hemisphere. That's why it's said that if people are good at language (and math or science, as opposed to art), they are "left-brained," and if they are creative, it means they are "right-brained."

ADDITIONAL FACTS

1. Cortex *is Latin for "bark" or "rind."*

2. *Thicker cerebral cortexes are often found in people who suffer migraine headaches, but it is unclear whether thicker cortexes cause the headaches—or vice versa.*

3. *The crest of a single convolution on the cerebral cortex is called a gyrus, and the fissure between two gyri is called a sulcus.*

✦✦✦

Cervix

In Latin, the word *cervix* means "neck." While that description may seem inappropriate for an organ in the female reproductive system, it makes sense when you consider its appearance: This continuation of the lower uterus narrows into a 1.5- to 2-inch tube before it connects to the vagina. Sperm must swim up this channel to fertilize the egg, and menstrual blood must pass through it to leave the body.

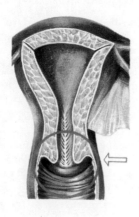

Made primarily of connective tissue, the cervix comprises three parts: the external os, the endocervix, and the internal os. The outer opening is the external os, which opens to the vagina and looks like a small, pink doughnut. (After childbirth, it widens and changes shape.) It is the entrance to the endocervix, pierced by the endocervical canal, which runs the length of the cervix. This ends at the internal os, which is the area that opens into the main part of the uterus, the corpus.

The inside of the cervical canal is lined with a moist mucous membrane that has nooks and crannies like an English muffin. Cells within this layer secrete mucus and project cilia, or tiny hairlike extensions, that help move sperm to the uterus. The cervical fluid also contains enzymes that help destroy infection-causing bacteria before they reach the uterus. This mucus becomes extremely thick during pregnancy and acts as a plug that helps seal off the uterus from infection. During labor, the mucus plug is expelled and the cervix widens to about 4 inches in diameter to allow the baby to pass.

ADDITIONAL FACTS

1. *While the cervix is technically part of the uterus, it has an entirely different function and its own array of possible diseases.*

2. *Most cases of cervical cancer are caused by human papillomavirus, a sexually transmitted disease that affects more than half of sexually active men and women.*

3. *During the female orgasm, the cervix and uterus contract.*

◆◆◆

Enriched Foods

Enriched foods have had nutrients added that were lost during processing. Examples of enriched foods are foods made from enriched white flour, such as bread, pasta, and tortillas. They are enriched with iron, B vitamins such as folic acid and niacin, and other nutrients that the flour lost when it was processed.

Enriched foods usually have lower vitamin and mineral levels than unprocessed foods do, because many more nutrients are lost during processing than are replaced. For example, the fiber that's stripped from grains when they're processed into white flour is not usually replaced in enriched white flour. So even enriched white flour contains less fiber and other nutrients than unprocessed brown flour does.

Eating only foods that have been enriched is not likely to ensure that you take in all the nutrients you need on a daily basis. For example, for most females ages 13 to 45 to obtain enough folic acid on a daily basis by consuming only enriched foods, they would need to eat a whole loaf of bread, 4 servings of cereal, 3½ servings of pasta, or 10 servings of rice. Most people will need to take a supplement to augment their nutrient intake with enriched foods. But eating enriched foods is still a better dietary choice than eating foods that have been processed and not enriched at all.

Some foods are enriched because the law requires them to be to ensure better health among the population. Manufacturers voluntarily enrich many other foods. In the United States, the federal government requires that each pound of enriched bread, rolls, or buns contains 1.8 milligrams of thiamin, 1.1 milligrams of riboflavin, 15 milligrams of niacin, 0.43 milligram of folic acid, 12.5 milligrams of iron, and 600 milligrams of calcium. Additionally, some salt must be enriched with iodine.

ADDITIONAL FACTS

1. *There is a difference between enriched foods and fortified foods. Fortified foods have had nutrients added to them in addition to what was lost during processing. Low-fat and fat-free milks are usually fortified with vitamin A, which is not found in unprocessed milk.*

2. *Pregnant women should take 400 milligrams of folic acid daily to reduce the risk of birth defects. In addition to using supplements, women who are pregnant should increase their intake of enriched grain products to meet their folic acid needs.*

◆◆◆

Paracelsus

The 16th-century physician and chemist known as Paracelsus (1493–1541) revolutionized medicine by proving that remedies containing copper sulfate, iron, mercury, sulfur, and other chemical compounds could play a role in treating diseases. Scornful of both many of his colleagues and ancient medical authorities, he also helped disprove many of the erroneous medical beliefs of his time.

Paracelsus—originally Theophrastus von Hohenheim—was trained as a young boy by his father, a German doctor and chemist. He also attended school for mining in Switzerland, where he learned about metals and minerals that came from the earth.

As a teenager, Theophrastus attended several universities across Europe, but he more highly valued advice from old wives, gypsies (the Roma), sorcerers, and outlaws. The University of Ferrara in Italy was one of the few places in Europe where it was acceptable to criticize the writings of the prominent 2nd-century Greek physician Galen (AD 129–216) and to question the widely held belief that the stars and planets controlled human health. Around this time, he adopted the name Para-Celsus, meaning "above or beyond Celsus," because he regarded himself as greater than the renowned 1st-century Roman medical writer Aulus Cornelius Celsus.

After graduating from Ferrara, Paracelsus held a variety of jobs across Europe, serving as an army surgeon in the Netherlands and Italy and learning about alchemy in Egypt and Constantinople. Eventually he returned to Switzerland to teach at the University of Basel. In one of his widely attended lectures, Paracelsus shocked the authorities by burning the books of ancient physicians.

In 1530, Paracelsus wrote the best clinical description of syphilis to date and suggested that the ailment could be treated with mercury compounds. He also provided an early explanation for miners' disease (silicosis), a lung disease triggered by exposure to toxic dust that many Europeans then believed was caused by vengeful mountain goblins. He was the first to suggest the fundamental idea of homeopathy, declaring that "what makes a man ill also cures him." And in 1536, Paracelsus published one of the first treatises on treating combat wounds caused by gunpowder—a growing problem in Europe as use of the explosive spread in the 16th century.

ADDITIONAL FACTS

1. *Goiters, painful growths on the front of the neck, perplexed medieval doctors until Paracelsus linked them to iodine deficiency. Iodine deficiency remains a problem in much of the developing world, even though the best means of prevention—iodized salt—costs pennies.*

2. *Dissatisfied with many of the universities throughout Europe, Paracelsus once wrote that he wondered how "the high colleges managed to produce so many asses."*

3. *After his lectures at Basel, Paracelsus spent many years in disfavor. When one of his patients died, Paracelsus was plagued by a disastrous lawsuit, and he fled the city in the middle of the night.*

❖❖❖

Febrile Seizure

Any parent who's soothed a feverish child knows that sickness can be worrisome.

But it can take an even more frightening turn when a child suffers a febrile seizure, full-body convulsions brought on by a spike in temperature. About 1 in 25 children experience them; of that group, more than a third have them more than once. The incidents occur most frequently in children between the ages of 6 months and 5 years, but particularly in toddlers.

While experts aren't certain what causes febrile seizures and why some children are more susceptible, they know that most who experience them have temperatures of 102°F or higher. Certain viruses may raise the risk: Most often, they're common childhood illnesses, such as a middle ear infection or roseola. Some cases may be the result of a more serious infection, such as meningitis, or may occur during the fever brought on by a childhood immunization.

Although scary, febrile seizures are generally harmless and don't increase the risk of epilepsy or brain damage. During the seizure, a child can lose consciousness, cry or moan, roll his eyes back in his head, vomit, and shake or twitch. Most seizures end within 15 minutes, but some can last longer or recur multiple times within a 24-hour span. Parents should consult a doctor if a child experiences seizures.

This is hard for a parent to see without panicking, so all parents should learn what to do in case a febrile seizure does occur.

ADDITIONAL FACTS

1. *The word* febrile *means "feverish."*

2. *The best way to protect against febrile seizures is to give a sick child plenty of fluids and children's medication to keep a fever in check.*

◆◆◆

Blood Clotting

When a blood vessel becomes damaged, the body sets off a chain of events to quickly repair it. The vessel immediately constricts so that the bloodflow slows and clotting can begin. The resulting clot, much like caulk on a pipe, seals the tissue until the vessel is healed.

Clot formation begins when injured collagen fibers in the vessel wall signal blood platelets to adhere to the wound. Before long, a group of platelets forms a temporary bandage and begins to release chemical SOS signals into the bloodstream. As a result, an enzyme called thrombin converts a dissolvable protein, fibrinogen, into long, sticky strands of fibrin. These threads weave together to form a net that holds in blood cells and platelets, sealing off the injured area. At this point, the platelets release other chemicals that aid in tissue repair. Once the injured tissue is undergoing repair, the clot dissolves as part of the healing process.

Although blood clots help heal the body, they can also cause serious harm if the system is interfered with and clotting becomes uncontrolled. Certain diseases can trigger clotting throughout the body, blocking bloodflow. More commonly, arteriosclerosis or inflammation can create a rough spot in a blood vessel where a large clot can develop; if it blocks an artery leading to the heart, a heart attack can occur. If the clot breaks off and clogs a blood vessel in a lung, that's called a pulmonary embolism, a life-threatening condition, while a clot that affects the brain triggers a stroke. Certain drugs that prevent clotting, called anticoagulants, are often prescribed to keep these large blood clots from forming.

ADDITIONAL FACTS

1. *Some people lack a clotting factor in their blood. As a result, they can bleed profusely from even a minor injury. This condition, called hemophilia, is hereditary and most often affects males.*

2. *The female hormone estrogen, often found in birth control pills, can increase the risk of clot formation.*

3. *Some people have a genetic defect that increases clotting, giving them a higher risk of phlebitis (an inflamed vein plugged by a clot), heart disease, pulmonary embolism, and stroke. This defect primarily affects females and, during pregnancy, may increase the risk of premature separation of the placenta and obstetrical hemorrhage.*

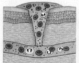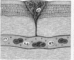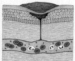

❖❖❖

Diuretics

Diuretics, or water pills, as the oral form of this medication is often called, are drugs that increase the flow of urine and help remove sodium and metabolic wastes from the body. They are often prescribed to patients with high blood pressure and congestive heart failure who have excess fluid (a condition called edema) in their tissues.

Simply put, diuretics cause the kidneys to allow less fluid to return to the bloodstream and to instead excrete it as urine. By lessening the amount of fluid entering blood vessels, the drugs decrease the pressure on artery walls.

The most convenient and commonly prescribed type of diuretic, hydrochlorothiazide, is available in pill form. Thiazide diuretics, as they are sometimes called, lower blood pressure in two specific ways: They moderately increase sodium excretion from the kidneys and also widen the blood vessels. For more serious cases, loop diuretics are prescribed to increase sodium and water excretion, especially for congestive heart failure patients who have severe fluid retention and edema (see Digitalis, page 38). Both of these drugs can have the dangerous side effect of lowering the potassium level in the body, so they are sometimes prescribed along with a third type of diuretic, called a potassium-sparing medication. Loss of potassium—which can cause heart rhythm disturbances and muscle cramps—can also be treated by taking a potassium supplement or eating a high-potassium food such as a banana or orange juice.

Urine flow usually increases within hours of taking a diuretic, and frequent urination can last for up to 6 hours per dose; it can still take several weeks, however, for a diuretic to successfully treat conditions such as high blood pressure. Dehydration, dry mouth, constipation, dizziness, and weakness are common side effects, especially in older people. In up to one-third of patients with heart failure (and in those taking painkillers or other drugs that can interfere with absorption by the kidneys), a diuretic will not remove enough sodium and fluid from the body—a condition called diuretic resistance.

ADDITIONAL FACTS

1. *A diet high in salt tends to counteract the effects of diuretics, forcing the kidneys to absorb more sodium than they should.*

2. *People with eating disorders sometimes use diuretics to compensate for food binges, so that they lose weight through loss of water. However, the weight returns rapidly as the person drinks to replace the lost fluid.*

3. *Diuretics are sometimes prescribed to treat severe menstrual cramps and bloating, which are caused by retention of sodium and water.*

◆◆◆

Cerebellum

The traffic cop of the central nervous system, the cerebellum is the part of the brain that coordinates and regulates motor movements. In the course of a single action—say, swatting a fly—the cerebellum computes a huge amount of information to execute the task, marshaling the muscles and movements needed to complete the motion with speed and precision.

This peach-size structure, known as the little brain because of its convoluted folds that resemble those of the cerebral cortex, is located at the lower back of the skull. The cerebellum can be compared to a powerful computer: It contains more nerve cells than the rest of the brain combined and can process information more quickly than any other region. It's connected to the highest level of the brain—the cerebral cortex—by about 40 million fibers that send down information from the sensory, motor, cognitive, language, and emotional areas all at once. (In contrast, the optic nerve, responsible for our entire field of vision, has only about 1 million fibers.)

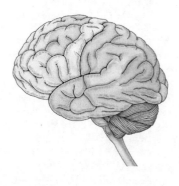

Traditionally, it was thought that the cerebellum was involved solely in motor functions such as walking and standing and that another part of the brain—the cerebrum—was in charge of mental development and intelligence. Indeed, the cerebellum does control coordination and balance; when it's damaged by a stroke or tumor, a person's motions may become jerky and unsteady, and he or she may unintentionally stop short of or continue past an object being aimed for. But modern studies suggest that the cerebellum is in fact closely intertwined with the cerebrum and that both regions play a role in cognitive functions such as planning, verbal fluency, abstract reasoning, and use of correct grammar.

ADDITIONAL FACTS

1. *The layer of white matter inside the cerebellum is known as the* arbor vitae *("tree of life") because of its branched, treelike appearance.*

2. *The reason people become dizzy, nauseated, and clumsy when they've had too much to drink is because alcohol penetrates the cerebellum and disrupts coordination.*

3. *Neurons that send motor signals away from the cerebellum, called Purkinje cells, are some of the largest, most elaborate cells in the human brain.*

◆◆◆

Testis

If you've ever watched a television courtroom drama, you know that defendants on the stand swear on the Bible before testifying. But in ancient Rome, men placed their right hands somewhere else—over their testes, according to some classical scholars. This may explain why the male gonads are named for the Latin word *testis,* or "witness." Truth-telling abilities aside, this set of plum-shaped organs' role in the body is to produce sperm and male hormones, called androgens.

Because sperm need a temperature of 97°F (2° lower than the normal body temperature) in order to grow, the testes reside in a scrotal sac that hangs from the body. Located behind the penis and in front of the anus, the scrotum has a built-in thermostat. If the body becomes too cold—from jumping in a chilly pool, for example—the cremasteric muscles in the scrotum pull the testes closer to the body for more warmth.

Also known as a testicle, each testis weighs less than an ounce and measures about an inch in diameter. Inside the scrotum, a thin, blue white membrane called the tunica albuginea surrounds each testis. Within this membrane, fibrous tissue partitions the interior into 200 to 400 wedge-shaped sections, or lobes. Each individual lobe contains up to 10 tubules, where the sperm develop; these tubules make up about 90 percent of a testicle's mass. Growing between the tubules are cells that secrete the all-important androgens, including testosterone. These hormones are responsible for driving the male reproductive system.

ADDITIONAL FACTS

1. *In animals that mate only during certain times of the year, such as sheep and goats, the testes descend from the body during breeding season; this process is called recrudescence.*

2. *Men who frequently perch laptop computers on their laps may have reduced fertility, because the heat from the computer can raise the scrotum's temperature.*

3. *Each year in Throckmorton, Texas, there is a World Championship Rocky Mountain Oyster Festival, at which people cook—and eat—bull testicles. One of the contests is a "tastes like chicken" event.*

◆◆◆

Artificial Sweeteners

Artificial sweeteners, or sugar substitutes, are generally considered safe alternatives to sugar. Sugar is high in calories, so it can cause weight gain. Artificial sweeteners are chemicals or natural compounds that are sweet like sugar without the added calories, making them an excellent part of a weight-loss or weight-control plan.

Generally, sugar substitutes are sweeter than the same quantity of sugar. Therefore, it takes a smaller amount to achieve the same level of sweetness. Foods made with artificial sweeteners are usually much lower in calories than their counterparts made with sugar.

Another benefit of artificial sweeteners is that they do not raise blood sugar levels, which makes them ideal for people with diabetes who want sweet-tasting foods that won't raise their blood sugar (although the food the artificial sweeteners are added to may still affect blood sugar). However, artificial sweeteners should be used sensibly, since they are empty calories. A diet made up of sugar-free drinks and desserts would be severely lacking in healthy nutrients.

There are five artificial sweeteners approved for use in the United States and considered safe for both children and adults. They are acesulfame potassium (Sunett, Sweet One), aspartame (Equal, NutraSweet), neotame, saccharin (SugarTwin, Sweet'N Low), and sucralose (Splenda). There are recommended limits on how much of any of these should be consumed on a daily basis. However, the average person takes in less than 2 percent of the limit per day, so it is extremely unlikely that someone would ingest too much through normal eating and drinking. Even the acceptable daily intake is intended to be 100 times smaller than the minimum amount that might cause health concerns. There is no scientific evidence that any of the sugar substitutes approved for use in the United States cause cancer.

ADDITIONAL FACTS

1. *Some foods are considered sugar free but actually contain one or more of the sugar alcohols mannitol, sorbitol, and xylitol. These are not artificial sweeteners and, in addition to raising your blood sugar, they may cause diarrhea.*

2. *Aspartame is not safe for people who have a rare hereditary disease called phenylketonuria (PKU). Foods that contain aspartame must carry the warning label "PKU."*

◆◆◆

Vesalius and Anatomy

In the early 1500s, medical schools in Europe taught anatomy using the methods of the 2nd-century Greek physician Galen (AD 129–216). Students and professors rarely performed dissections themselves, instead simply reading from and trusting Galen's ancient texts. That is, until a Belgian-born anatomist in Padua, Italy, dramatically rejected Galen and insisted that doctors must perform their own dissections to learn how the body truly worked.

Andreas Vesalius (1514–1564) began his career as a believer of Galen's teachings. But unlike most professors of the time, he developed a habit of dissecting corpses himself to show students anatomical details. (Most lessons of the time involved a professor reading from Galen's texts while a surgeon stood by with the body of an executed criminal on which to show the relevant body parts.) But Vesalius was mystified when he found that several basic anatomical facts, like the number and relative size of bones, where often wrong in Galen's writing. Eventually, Vesalius came to the realization that Galen, the source of authority in Western medicine for more than a thousand years, had never actually dissected a human body. Because religious law had not allowed such a practice, Galen had based his writings on the anatomy of cattle, primates, and other animals.

For the next 4 years, Vesalius worked on his masterpiece: a collection of works completed in 1543 and titled *De Humani Corporis Fabrica Libri Septem,* or *The Seven Books on the Structure of the Human Body,* commonly known as the *Fabrica*. This was the first profusely illustrated record of human anatomy and included detailed drawings of bodies with their skin stripped away—muscles, tissues, and bones exposed—in lifelike poses, such as walking, leaning against a table, and hanging from a noose.

The exquisite art and bold medical theories in *Fabrica* made Vesalius famous across Europe—he was later made a count by Holy Roman Emperor Charles V (1500–1558)—and contributed to a profound medical and intellectual shift across Europe. Vesalius had proved that the ancient texts were fallible and that doctors should trust their own observations and experiments. Vesalius himself died on a Greek island during his return from a pilgrimage to Jerusalem.

ADDITIONAL FACTS

1. *Early in his career, Vesalius made a name for himself by drawing detailed anatomical charts of the circulatory and nervous systems for his students to study. The criminal court judge of Padua took interest and made sure Vesalius had a steady supply of cadavers from the gallows.*

2. *Though it's known today that Galen himself emphasized the importance of personal observation (as opposed to the blind following of ancient texts), this detail seems to have been lost in the many translations of his work by the time it reached 16th-century Europe.*

3. *Controversial modern-day exhibits such as Bodies: The Exhibition and Body Worlds, which display plasticized human cadavers in lifelike poses, have been called continuations of Vesalius's work.*

◆◆◆

Autism

Autism is the most common condition in a group of developmental problems known as autism spectrum disorders (ASDs). Although the symptoms of these disorders vary, what they all have in common is that they cause poor communication skills, trouble with social relationships, and, sometimes, obsessions or repetitive body movements. Currently, there are 1.5 million Americans living with ASDs, and experts say that number is on the rise. Unfortunately, there are no clear diagnostic criteria, and many conditions, such as fragile X syndrome, may be lumped under this diagnosis.

The signs of autism begin as early as infancy; most cases are diagnosed before the age of 3. Signs of the disorder include constant movement, a tendency to make little eye contact, a resistance to cuddling or holding, and failure to respond when called by name. As autism sufferers progress through childhood, they seem unaware of other people's feelings, speak in singsong or robotic tones, and are unable to start conversations. Some people with mild cases of autism can lead normal lives, while others with more severe cases require constant care and possibly antidepressants or antipsychotic medications to help control symptoms.

Despite years of study, scientists aren't sure of the exact cause of autism. But they suspect that both genetics and environment play a role. Families who have one autistic child, for instance, have a 5 percent chance of having a second child with the disorder. Researchers are also examining whether viral infections and pollution may lead to autism. Other risk factors include the age of the father (children born to men age 40 or older are six times more likely to have an ASD) and the child's sex (boys are three times likelier to be autistic than girls are).

Perhaps one of the most publicized—and controversial—possible causes is a preservative called thimerosal, which contains trace amounts of the heavy metal mercury and is found in certain childhood vaccines. Although these vaccines have not contained thimerosal since 2001, a debate over the safety of vaccinations still goes on, despite numerous studies and government reports disproving any relationship between vaccines and ASDs.

ADDITIONAL FACTS

1. *The lifetime cost of raising a child with autism is estimated to range from $3.5 million to $5 million.*

2. *Research shows that children who are diagnosed with autism early on have better outcomes than those diagnosed later.*

3. *Pediatricians recommend seeing an expert if an infant doesn't babble, coo, point, or wave by age 1.*

◆◆◆

Anemia

In Greek, the word *anemia* means "without blood." The description is apt enough, because although people with anemia aren't completely "without blood," the condition develops when there aren't enough healthy red blood cells in the body. Symptoms of anemia, such as fatigue, dizziness, headaches, and pale skin, occur because tissues aren't receiving sufficient amounts of oxygen. The most common blood condition in the United States, anemia affects some 3.5 million people. Women and those with chronic diseases are at a higher risk for having the condition.

Although more than 400 different types of anemia exist, there are really three main culprits—a loss of blood, a decrease or defect in red blood cell production, and the destruction of red blood cells. The most common form is the result of an insufficient amount of iron in the body. Without iron, the bone marrow can't produce enough hemoglobin for red blood cells. Along with this mineral, the body also requires vitamin B_{12} and folate to manufacture red blood cells. In some cases, people may have an intestinal disorder or other problem that interferes with B_{12} absorption; this condition is called pernicious anemia.

Less common are chronic diseases that interfere with the growth of red blood cells, such as cancer, kidney failure, and bone marrow diseases. One genetic cause, which affects mainly those of African descent, is called sickle-cell anemia: Instead of a round, disklike shape, the red blood cells adopt a crescent form and die prematurely.

To diagnose anemia, physicians usually run a series of tests, including a complete blood count to assess the number and type of red blood cells. Treatments depend on the cause and can vary from something as simple as taking a vitamin B_{12} or iron supplement to receiving a blood transfusion.

ADDITIONAL FACTS

1. *Some 25 percent of women, nearly half of pregnant women, and 3 percent of men suffer from iron-deficiency anemia.*

2. *In the case of iron-deficiency anemia, red blood cells appear paler and smaller than normal.*

3. *Because meat is a major source of iron and vitamin B_{12}, vegetarians and vegans are more likely to be anemic.*

❖ ❖ ❖

Sulfa Drugs

The first antimicrobial drugs that were used to treat bacterial infections in humans were known as sulfa drugs—synthetic medications created from a crystalline compound called sulfanilamide. Sulfa drugs saved countless lives in the 20th century and paved the way for modern antibiotics.

In the early 1930s, German scientists realized that a red dye called prontosil prevented the growth of *Streptococcus* bacteria in mice. In fact, the dye seemed to protect against all types of infections, including blood diseases, childbed fever (infection of the uterus), and the skin condition erysipelas (also known as St. Anthony's fire). The researchers discovered that the active ingredient in this reaction was sulfanilamide. Over the next decade, medicines derived from the sulfanilamide molecule, commonly known as sulfa drugs, became the only widely available antibiotics. They were standard in first-aid kits during World War II and are credited with saving the lives of tens of thousands of patients, including Franklin Delano Roosevelt's son, Franklin Delano Roosevelt Jr. (1914–1988), and Winston Churchill (1874–1965).

Unlike antibiotics, sulfa drugs do not kill bacteria—they merely limit their growth. This is called bacteriostatic activity, and it allows the body's immune system to fight them more readily (see Immunity, page 2). The drugs disrupt the synthesis of folic acid, a B vitamin present in all living cells. This can stop the growth of invading bacteria (which need to make their own folic acid to survive) without harming healthy host cells (because humans and other mammals obtain folic acid through their diets instead of making it internally)—a principle known as selective toxicity.

Sulfur, by itself, is not toxic to the body. However, about 3 percent of people are highly allergic to relatives of sulfur, such as sulfites and sulfa drugs. For these people, sulfa drugs can cause skin rashes, high fever, headache, fatigue, and gastric problems. With the introduction of less-toxic derivatives and the mass production of penicillin in the 1940s, the widespread use of sulfa drugs declined. Today, they are used to treat pneumonia in AIDS patients, acne, urinary and vaginal infections, skin burns, and malaria and are receiving renewed interest in light of newer, drug-resistant strains of bacteria.

ADDITIONAL FACTS

1. *The German company IG Farben (which then owned what's now Bayer) hoped to exclusively market sulfanilamide, but the compound had actually been used in the dye industry since 1906. Its patent had expired, making the drug available to anyone.*

2. *Hundreds of manufacturers tried to strike it rich in the 1930s by producing tens of thousands of tons of sulfa drugs, sometimes with little care for safety or quality. As a result, at least 100 people were poisoned with diethylene glycol in the Elixir Sulfanilamide disaster of 1937, leading to the passage of the Federal Food, Drug, and Cosmetic Act in 1938.*

3. *The first recorded use of a sulfa drug in the United States was for a 10-year-old girl with meningitis in July 1935. After an apparent cure, the patient suffered a relapse a few months later and died.*

◆◆◆

Medulla Oblongata

The medulla oblongata is a bulbous structure in the brain that controls a variety of basic body functions, including digestion, sleep, breathing, and heartbeat. It is one of the parts of the brain responsible for the autonomic nervous system, which regulates such essential activities without our active awareness. Located at the base of the skull, the medulla oblongata is also the connection between the brain and the spinal cord.

Composed of both white matter and gray matter, the medulla oblongata is roughly triangular in shape, tapering from a wider section at the midbrain to a relatively narrow band where it joins the spine. Seven cranial nerves emerge from the medulla oblongata and help control sensory and motor functions, along with arousal and sleep.

The medulla also contains two clumps of motor nerves called pyramids, which control skeletal muscles. The neurons connecting the pyramids to the muscles cross each other in an X-shaped formation, meaning that the right side of the medulla controls the left side of the body. Therefore, injury or disease affecting one side of the medulla may produce paralysis or loss of senses on the other side of the body.

Another part of the medulla, two oval structures called olives, contain cells that are involved in balance, coordination, and the modulation of sound impulses from the inner ear.

Since the medulla oblongata is essential to basic body functions, damage to this part of the brain often causes instant death. In some cases, people with damaged medulla oblongatas can remain alive, but will need to be put on life-support machines to maintain breathing, heartbeat, and other functions.

ADDITIONAL FACTS

1. *Injury to or disease of the medulla may cause vertigo, vomiting, loss of the gag reflex, difficulty in swallowing, loss of the ability to sense pain and temperature, or loss of concentration.*

2. *General anesthesia works in part by suppressing wakefulness and arousal in the medulla oblongata—but if too much is administered, autonomic functions, such as heartbeat and breathing, are in danger of stopping.*

3. *Studies have shown that autistic children tend to have smaller brain stems and medulla oblongatas.*

◆◆◆

Seminal Vesicle

Even though a single drop of semen contains hundreds of millions of sperm, the majority of it consists of a fluid made by the seminal vesicles. This pair of small, fingerlike glands behind the bladder secretes a thick, yellowish liquid that mixes with the sperm and prostate fluid before ejaculation. The fluid contains sugars to fuel the sperm's journey, enzymes to increase their speed, and chemicals called prostaglandins that thin the mucus that guards the entrance to the woman's cervix.

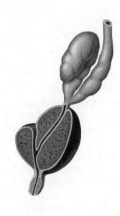

Although each seminal vesicle measures only 2 inches in length, it houses a 6-inch-long coiled tubule surrounded by a layer of connective tissue. The tubule comprises an inner lining, a mucous membrane, and a thin layer of muscle. The mucous membrane secretes the seminal fluid. Like an expanding suitcase, the membrane remains folded up when there's little liquid, but grows to accommodate the fluid during sexual activity. At ejaculation, the muscular tissue contracts to empty the vesicle into the ejaculatory ducts. There, the fluid mixes with the sperm that have recently been released from the vas deferens. This liquid then travels up to the man's urethra, where it joins with fluids from the prostate before being expelled from the body.

ADDITIONAL FACTS

1. *In rare cases, infections and disorders of the seminal vesicles can cause infertility.*

2. *Seminal vesicles produce about 60 percent of the semen.*

✦✦✦

Fats

Along with carbohydrates and proteins, fats are one of the three primary types of foods. An important source of energy, fats also help your body absorb vitamins and are essential for growth, development, and good health. Fats are especially important for infants and children.

There are three major types of fats: saturated fats, trans fat, and polyunsaturated and monounsaturated fats. Saturated fats are sometimes referred to as the solid fats in your diet. This is because this kind of fat sometimes forms a solid layer of fat at the top of food. Saturated fats are found in cheeses, meats, whole milk and cream, butter, ice cream, and palm and coconut oils.

Diets that are high in saturated fats have been linked to coronary heart disease. Saturated fats also affect your cholesterol levels. No more than 10 percent of your daily calories should be from saturated fats.

Trans fat is found in vegetable shortenings, some margarines, crackers, cookies, snack foods, and foods made with partially hydrogenated oils. Partially hydrogenated oils are created through the process of hydrogenation, in which liquid oils are converted to solid fats. The trans fat in partially hydrogenated oils raise your LDL ("bad") cholesterol and decrease your HDL ("good") cholesterol, both of which increase your risk of heart disease.

Fortunately, some companies have altered how they manufacture foods to decrease the amounts of trans fat in their products. Check the labels of the processed foods you buy to see whether they contain trans fat. It's recommended that you reduce the amount of trans fat in your diet as much as possible.

Most of the fat you eat should be polyunsaturated fats and monounsaturated fats. These are the good fats. Unsaturated fats are found in avocados, flaxseeds, nuts, herring, salmon, trout, and the following oils: canola, corn, olive, safflower and high-oleic safflower, soybean, sunflower, and vegetable.

ADDITIONAL FACTS

1. *Fats make food tasty and help you feel full.*

2. *Eating too much fat of any kind will cause you to gain weight.*

❖ ❖ ❖

Ambroise Paré and Surgical Ligature

When the French surgeon Ambroise Paré (1510–1590) entered the army in the mid-1500s, gunshot wounds were typically treated with amputation of the affected limb and cautery of the amputation site with boiling oil. Realizing that this method was ineffective and even dangerous, Paré later introduced the technique of surgical ligature—the predecessor of today's modern surgical technique.

Paré was a surgeon in Paris and served four French monarchs in his lifetime. On one occasion when treating soldiers' gunshot wounds, he ran out of hot oil and instead dressed some of their wounds with a cloth soaked in egg yolk, rose oil, and turpentine. To his surprise, he noticed that these soldiers recovered more quickly and did not suffer from the infection or fever that affected many of the cauterized soldiers. He determined that the gunshot wounds were not inherently poisonous, as previously believed, but that infection was carried into the body from the outside. He began recommending debridement, the opening and cleansing of the wound, to assist the healing process. To perform amputations without cautery, he revived the use of the tourniquet—tying off extremities with a cord above the amputation site to reduce blood loss and sensation. Even with the use of a tourniquet, however, no fewer than 53 ligatures were required for a proper thigh amputation, and the practice required trained assistance. Each artery had to be separately tied, prolonging the surgery in an unanesthetized patient. Only after the invention of anesthesia could this approach be widely used.

In 1545, Paré described these practices in the book *La méthod de traicter les playes faites par les arquebuses et aultres bastons à feu*, or *The Method of Treating Wounds Made by Harquebuses and Other Guns*. In addition to improving the way wounds were treated, Paré helped to popularize the use of crude prosthetic devices like gold eyes, wooden teeth, and artificial limbs. He also made many contributions to the field of obstetrics, first describing the technique of podalic version in childbirth, in which the baby is rotated so that it comes out feet first. Today, he is often referred to as the father of modern surgery.

ADDITIONAL FACTS

1. *After amputating the limbs of wounded French soldiers, Paré noticed that many of them would complain about pain and other sensations in the arms and legs that they had lost. He was the first to describe this puzzling neurological oddity, now called phantom limb syndrome.*

2. *Paré's* Method of Treating Wounds *became an important text and has been translated into many languages. But it was ridiculed when it was first published because Paré wrote in conversational French rather than Latin, the language of scholars and doctors.*

3. *Paré was originally trained as a barber and offered haircuts in addition to surgery. This was a common combination in Europe, where such practitioners were called barber-surgeons. The red-and-white-striped poles still found at many barbershops have their origins in the bloody rags that barber-surgeons once draped across their doorsteps.*

◆◆◆

Birthmarks

Many newborns have bumps or splotches that appear at birth or shortly after. These birthmarks come in a variety of sizes and shapes: They can be flat or raised; have regular or irregular borders; and come in shades of red, pink, purple, gray, tan, or brown. They're mainly harmless and may shrink or even disappear over time.

A completely random occurrence, birthmarks aren't influenced by anything done or eaten during pregnancy. There are two main types: Pigmented birthmarks are caused by an overgrowth of the cells that produce pigment in the skin. The most common kind is a café au lait, or tan-colored, spot. Others include Mongolian spots, which are bluish gray patches that often appear on the lower back or buttocks; and moles, which should be closely monitored, as changes in their shape or appearance may indicate the skin cancer called melanoma.

The other kind of birthmark is vascular, and they appear when there is a tangle or overgrowth of blood vessels. About 10 percent of all infants have a vascular mark. One of the most common is a macular stain, which is also known as a stork bite, angel kiss, or salmon patch. Red or pale pink in color, these often fade during the first 2 years of life. Hemangiomas, or strawberry marks, are slightly raised and bright red or even blue. They appear on the head or neck and usually disappear when a child is between 5 and 9 years old. Finally, there are port-wine stains, named after the dark red color they eventually turn. These patches of malformed blood vessels grow and darken with time. Because they're permanent, many people opt to undergo laser therapy to remove them.

ADDITIONAL FACTS

1. *Famous birthmarks include the port-wine stain on former Soviet president Mikhail Gorbachev's (1931–) forehead and the mole near supermodel Cindy Crawford's (1966–) mouth.*

2. *Large moles that children are born with are more likely than smaller ones to develop into melanoma later in life.*

◆◆◆

Common Cold

There are few things that people have in common like the cold virus: Each year, Americans come down with 1 *billion* colds. Adults average 2 to 4 colds each year, and children suffer through 6 to 10. The majority of these occur during the late fall and winter months, because people tend to spend more time indoors—and in close contact with each other, spreading germs.

Colds aren't caused by just one virus; more than 200 types cause symptoms of the common cold. Rhinoviruses account for about 35 percent of them; coronaviruses and viruses that cause other, more severe illnesses are also culprits. These viruses are typically spread by inhaling drops of mucus that contain the virus (by breathing in someone else's sneeze, for example) or by touching an infected surface, then an eye or nose. (Cold viruses aren't spread through oral contact.) Because cold viruses can live outside the body for a day or more, experts recommend washing your hands with soap and water frequently to protect yourself.

A handkerchief in time

saves nine

and helps to keep the nation fighting fit

COUGHS and SNEEZES SPREAD DISEASES

Symptoms take about 2 to 3 days to develop after infection and include a sore throat, runny nose, fatigue, and a mild cough. Although they clear up within 4 to 7 days, the stuffiness can last for weeks. For the first 3 days, colds are contagious. Although colds themselves aren't dangerous in children and adults, they can wear down the immune system, making the body more vulnerable to bacterial infections, such as strep throat.

When it comes to recovery, nothing works better than getting plenty of fluids and rest. Taking over-the-counter pain relievers and decongestants, as well as gargling with salt water, can help relieve symptoms. The jury's still out on other popular remedies, such as vitamin C, zinc, and echinacea; results of scientific studies on their effectiveness have been mixed.

ADDITIONAL FACTS

1. *Each year, the average child loses 22 school days because of colds.*

2. *The term* rhinovirus *is derived from the Greek word for "nose,"* rhin.

3. *Chicken soup can soothe colds. Research has found that both homemade and canned versions have anti-inflammatory effects and may help relieve congestion.*

◆ ◆ ◆

Penicillin

The drug penicillin ranks among the most important discoveries—medical or otherwise—of the 20th century. Introduced just before World War II, this "miracle drug" saved countless lives during the war by allowing doctors to prevent infections in combat wounds and to effectively control for the first time diseases like gonorrhea and syphilis. The drug was the second after sulfa, of a powerful class of medicines called antibiotics, which are now used to treat countless illnesses. Penicillin was the first bactericidal antibiotic, capable of actually killing bacteria, unlike sulfa, a bacteriostatic antibiotic that stopped their growth, allowing the body's immune system (see Immunity, page 2) to kill them more easily.

Penicillin was discovered in 1928 by Alexander Fleming (1881–1955), a British doctor who would go on to win a Nobel Prize for the discovery in 1945. It is derived from a fungus called *Penicillium*, which Fleming noticed was able to kill bacteria in a petri dish. Tests showed that penicillin worked against many other disease-causing bacteria, and it was soon developed into an injectable form and later into tablet form for treating bacterial infections in humans.

In the years since penicillin's discovery, many other fungi and microorganisms have also been found to yield antibiotics, and medications derived from those microorganisms have replaced penicillin for many uses. However, penicillins remain widely prescribed for diseases like pneumonia and meningitis.

Penicillin is not effective against viral infections such as the common cold, however, and it does not work against certain types of bacteria. Like all antibiotics, penicillin can also cause a severe and occasionally fatal allergic reaction in some people. Other side effects include skin rashes, hives, and swelling.

In addition, the overuse of antibiotics such as penicillin in today's society has paved the way for more antibiotic-resistant pathogens, rendering the drugs ineffective at fighting a growing number of infections. Failure to finish an entire prescription of penicillin, even after symptoms have gone away, can contribute to drug resistance. A current example of such bacteria is methicillin-resistant *Staphylococcus aureus* (MRSA), which has developed such strong resistance that it is largely unaffected by traditional antibiotics. Ironically, it was in a dish full of this very same bacterium— long before it had developed resistance—that Fleming made the fateful discovery of penicillin's powers in the first place.

ADDITIONAL FACTS

1. *Roughly 300 to 500 people die each year from a severe allergic reaction to penicillin, called penicillin-induced anaphylaxis.*

2. *Penicillin V can make birth control pills less effective.*

◆ ◆ ◆

Reflexes

To perform some of the body's most primitive actions, there just isn't time for a signal to make it all the way to your brain and back. If you put your finger in boiling water, for instance, your hand jerks away even before pain consciously registers in your mind. For these responses, called reflexes, signals travel to and from the spinal cord instead—shortening the time needed for your body to react.

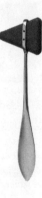

Reflex pathways typically involve information flowing from a sensory neuron (in your fingertip, for example) that connects to a motor neuron in the spinal cord. Reflexes are involuntary, meaning that we don't typically control them or decide to do them consciously. They include blinking or jumping in response to a sudden noise and sneezing or coughing when irritants enter the nose or mouth. Reflexes are also the reason you gag when something threatens to block your throat and airway and why your pupils get smaller when a bright light comes on.

One commonly known reflex is the knee-jerk response, also known as the patellar or deep tendon reflex. When a doctor taps an area under the knee with a rubber hammer, the patellar tendon—and a connected muscle in the thigh—stretches slightly. A message is sent to the spinal cord, which instructs the muscle to contract, causing the lower leg to kick outward. The entire process takes about 50 milliseconds and is important for maintaining balance and standing upright. Deep tendon reflexes can also be checked along the outsides of the elbows, in the crooks of the arms, and at the wrists and ankles.

In this process, the brain acts as an interested observer of reflex responses, collecting information about what is happening in the body. That way, you can learn from these involuntary reactions and better protect yourself from threats (like that boiling water) in the future.

ADDITIONAL FACTS

1. *People typically blink about 15 times per minute—or 14,400 times a day if they spend 16 hours awake.*

2. *Doctors aren't sure why, but some people sneeze when they look at a bright light or walk outside into the sunlight.*

3. *Babies are born knowing how to suck milk from a breast (the rooting reflex), how to tightly grab onto objects placed in their hands (the grasping reflex), and how to move their extremities and cry out when startled by a loud noise (the Moro reflex).*

◆◆◆

Prostate Gland

In many ways, the prostate gland is Grand Central Station for the male reproductive and urinary systems: Both urine and semen must pass through this walnut-size gland, located directly beneath the bladder, before leaving the body. The prostate surrounds the urethra, the passageway for both of these bodily fluids.

Inside the prostate itself are 30 to 50 saclike glands that secrete fluids that make up about 20 percent of semen. The two ejaculatory ducts, which transport the semen and seminal vesicle liquids, converge in the prostate and join with the urethra; there, the prostate fluid is added to the mix. Containing zinc, citric acid, calcium, and more, it gives semen its milky color and helps the sperm survive in the female vagina, primarily by neutralizing the vaginal acids.

The prostate becomes fully developed during puberty, at around age 12 or 13, and remains the same size for the next 30 to 40 years. At that point, more than one in two men experience a midlife growth spurt in their prostate size. This condition, called benign prostatic hypertrophy (BPH), is a nonmalignant enlargement of the prostate. The gland can grow to the size of a plum; in very severe cases, it can become the size of a grapefruit. In most instances, BPH does not have to be treated, but the enlarged prostate may press against the urethra and cause urinary incontinence or difficulty in urination. Prescription medications or a minimally invasive procedure can help alleviate the symptoms.

ADDITIONAL FACTS

1. *Prostate cancer is the most common type of cancer in males.*

2. *An Australian study found that men who masturbated more than five times a week during their twenties were one-third less likely to develop aggressive prostate cancer later in life. That's because frequent ejaculation may prevent carcinogens from building up, say the researchers.*

◆◆◆

Cholesterol

Cholesterol is a waxy, fatlike substance that occurs naturally in your body and is made by your liver. Your body uses cholesterol for various functions, including protecting nerves, making tissues, and producing hormones. You take in extra cholesterol from the food you eat.

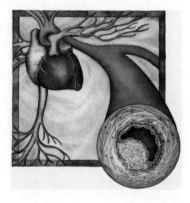

High levels of cholesterol in your blood can raise your risk of heart disease, including heart attack and stroke. This is because the higher the level of cholesterol in your blood, the more likely you are to develop plaque in your bloodstream. Plaque occurs when the cholesterol in your blood sticks to the walls of your arteries, blood vessels that carry blood from your heart throughout your body.

As plaque builds up, it can narrow your arteries and eventually block bloodflow. If an artery that supplies blood to your heart itself is blocked, you can have a heart attack. If an artery that supplies blood to your brain is blocked, you can have a stroke.

Men ages 35 and over and women ages 45 and over should have their cholesterol checked annually. You may need to have it tested more often if you have other risk factors. You are more likely to have high cholesterol if it runs in your family, if you are overweight, or if you have a high-fat diet.

If you do have high cholesterol, you may be able to lower it by exercising, eating more fruits and vegetables, and possibly taking medication. Smokers should stop smoking. If you are overweight, losing as little as 5 to 10 pounds can help. You should avoid eating saturated and trans fats and limit your overall cholesterol intake to less than 300 milligrams daily. Also steer clear of high-cholesterol foods such as eggs, fatty meats, and high-fat dairy products.

ADDITIONAL FACTS

1. *LDL and HDL are specific types of cholesterol that are important to measure. LDL delivers cholesterol to your body, while HDL removes cholesterol from your bloodstream. Too much LDL is bad for your body, whereas a high level of HDL is good.*

2. *A total cholesterol level of less than 200 is best, 200 to 239 is considered borderline high, and 240 or higher indicates an increased risk of heart disease.*

◆ ◆ ◆

Van Leeuwenhoek and the Microscope

The earliest microscopes were essentially high-powered magnifying glasses developed by eyeglass manufacturers around 1600 and consisting of a tiny bead of glass held in a tube or between two metal plates. While many scientists used these tools to get a closer look at the world around them, the work of one particular Dutch researcher contributed much to the field of microbiology.

A draper from the city of Delft, the Netherlands, Antoni van Leeuwenhoek (1632–1723) initially made microscopes as a hobby. It is rumored that he was inspired by the English scientist Robert Hooke's (1635–1703) book *Micrographia,* an illustrated description of fleas, flies, plant cells, and Hooke's own microscopes. In 1674, Van Leeuwenhoek began to do investigations of his own. Peering through his homemade lenses at specimens magnified more than 200 times, he observed what he called "very little animalcules," objects that would later be identified as bacteria and protozoa. The population density of these animalcules, he estimated, was more than 1 million in each drop of liquid.

Wood, plants, insects, and crustaceans all found their way under Van Leeuwenhoek's microscopes over the next several decades. He studied the bones, hair, teeth, eyes, muscles, and blood vessels of different animals and was the first person to give an accurate description of red blood cells. He was also the first to observe spermatozoa in human semen, fueling debate about the origins of conception. Van Leeuwenhoek's studies showed that insects, vermin, and shellfish did indeed hatch from tiny eggs, an observation that helped refute the widely held doctrine of spontaneous generation.

Most of Van Leeuwenhoek's discoveries were made public in the Royal Society of London's publication *Philosophical Transactions*—including one of his illustrations, the first recorded visual representation of bacteria. But he carefully guarded the secret designs of his microscopes themselves, which would not be rivaled in quality until the 1800s.

ADDITIONAL FACTS

1. *Grinding glass to produce microscopes was a dangerous occupation. Although Van Leeuwenhoek lived to age 90, the toxic dust produced by glass grinding may have contributed to the death of another well-known Dutch lens maker, the philosopher Baruch Spinoza (1632–1677).*

2. *Simple, single-lens microscopes were preferred during Van Leeuwenhoek's time because the compound microscope—made with two lenses—increased chromatic aberration, in which colored fringes appear around the edges of the image because different wavelengths of light bend at different angles.*

3. *Robert Hooke coined the term* cell *after noticing similarities between the cells of dried cork under a microscope and monks' living quarters, called cells, in monasteries.*

✦✦✦

Barker Hypothesis

In the late 1980s, a British physician and epidemiologist named David Barker (1938–) happened across an interesting correlation in his data: He noticed that a group of men who were born small had a higher incidence of heart disease. What if, Barker speculated, poor nutrition in the womb led to developmental disturbances that put an infant at risk for heart disease, diabetes, and obesity throughout life? This theory later became known as the Barker hypothesis.

According to the premise, a mother's weight, diet, and exercise habits can influence a baby's metabolism in the womb. In turn, this controls how organs form, genes become activated, and brain chemistry develops, and all these factors contribute to an individual's health.

Although the topic is still hotly debated, evidence in favor of Barker's hypothesis is mounting. Research reveals that being obese during pregnancy is associated with an increased risk of birth defects, including those of the spinal cord, heart, and limbs. Meanwhile, another study found that babies born to mothers with high blood sugar levels were twice as likely to become obese as those whose moms had normal levels. Fetuses may adapt to the constant exposure to sugar by increasing their production of insulin, say experts. As a result, these babies may be wired for insulin insensitivity as children and adults, raising their risk of becoming obese and developing diabetes.

To ensure a child's long-term health, experts recommend that expectant mothers gain the right amount of weight and eat a healthy diet full of fruits, vegetables, lean protein, and whole grains.

ADDITIONAL FACTS

1. *Research suggests that moms-to-be who follow a high-carbohydrate or a high-protein diet may give birth to children who are equally likely to be of normal birth weight. It's the calories that count.*

2. *Barker's idea was officially dubbed the Barker hypothesis in a 1995* British Medical Journal *article.*

♦♦♦

Sinusitis

The sinuses are cavities in the skull that are lined with mucous membranes. Thought to help with warming and moistening inhaled air, they are often over-looked—until they become infected. Yearly, some 37 million Americans endure this painful condition, called sinusitis.

Conditions that block the sinuses, such as allergies, colds, nasal polyps (small growths in the nose's lining), and a deviated septum (crooked carti-lage or bone in the nose), can all lead to sinusitis. This interferes with the drainage of mucus, which can result in facial pain, headache, greenish mucus, and congestion that lasts for more than a week.

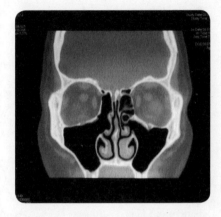

In acute sinusitis, these symptoms are a brief problem that comes on after a cold and responds well to antibiotics and decongestants. With chronic sinusitis, however, the sinus infection comes back and can last for 3 months or longer. An underlying problem, such as nasal polyps or allergies, is frequently the culprit and must be treated in order to relieve symptoms. A doctor can prescribe allergy medication or, if polyps or a devi-ated septum is to blame, a surgical procedure. Nasal steroids that shrink swollen membranes may also be prescribed.

To help relieve symptoms, experts recommend elevating the head during sleep to allow the sinuses to drain. Rinsing out the sinuses with a bulb syringe, inhaling steam, and drinking plenty of fluids to dilute mucus can also help.

ADDITIONAL FACTS

1. *Americans spend nearly $6 million in health care costs due to sinusitis every year.*

2. *Sinusitis caused by a bacterial infection tends to be more painful than that caused by a viral infection.*

3. *Sinusitis is one of the most common causes of headaches.*

◆◆◆

Tetracycline

One of the most widely prescribed antibiotic classes in the world, tetracyclines are used to treat a wide variety of bacterial infections ranging from acne to gonorrhea. Tetracyclines work by blocking the transfer of RNA needed to synthesize new protein, essentially preventing cell growth and multiplication.

The first tetracycline used in modern medicine was aureomycin, a yellowish substance that was discovered in 1948 by Benjamin Duggar (1872–1956), an American botanist studying bacteria in soil.

Tetracyclines do not actively destroy existing cells, but instead only work to prevent cultures from multiplying. The drug stops growth in both host and invading cells, although bacteria are naturally more susceptible to its harmful effects than human cells are. They are commonly used to treat skin problems like rosacea, sexually transmitted infections like chlamydia, and other infectious diseases. Along with several other types of antibiotics, they have also been added to livestock feed. Recently, however, researchers have begun to raise concerns about overuse of tetracyclines in animals and humans. The widespread use of these drugs, even in cases where they are not medically necessary, may be contributing to the development of antibiotic-resistant organisms and more-resilient infections.

Some people may experience hypersensitivity reactions to tetracyclines, including nausea, vomiting, and an unpleasant taste. The drugs can make skin more sensitive to sunlight and susceptible to sunburn, and can make birth control pills less effective. Tetracycline absorption in the gastrointestinal tract can be impaired by milk and other dairy products, multivitamins or iron supplements, and sodium bicarbonate or calcium antacids.

ADDITIONAL FACTS

1. *Although it wasn't used as a drug until the 1950s, archaeological researchers have discovered significant levels of tetracycline in mummies from Nubia (northern Sudan) and other African cultures from as far back as the 4th century. It's believed that the beer brewed at the time may have been the source.*

2. *Tetracycline is absorbed into bone and glows under fluorescent light, and thus can be used as a marker of bone growth for biopsies in humans.*

3. *Tetracycline can inhibit bone growth, damage tooth enamel, and cause permanent yellowing or graying of the teeth. It should not be prescribed to pregnant women or to children under age 8.*

✦✦✦

Taste

Our sense of taste is important not only for appetite and enjoyment of food, but also for survival: Taste provides an early warning system that can detect when something is spoiled or potentially poisonous.

The tasting process begins when molecules in food or drink stimulate gustatory (taste) cells in the mouth, tongue, or throat. The average person has about 10,000 goblet-shaped taste buds, each containing between 50 and 150 tall, skinny receptor cells. These cells transmit signals through nerve fibers and into the brain's medulla oblongata, where they meet other signals of temperature, flavor, and texture. The information ascends to the thalamus and then to taste-receiving areas in the cerebral cortex and the limbic system, where it is translated into the sensations we use to recognize and evaluate food.

The brain recognizes these basic tastes: sweet (organic compounds such as alcohols, sugars, and artificial sweeteners), sour (acids), bitter (alkaloids, such as quinine and caffeine), and salty. A more recently identified taste, umami, occurs when we eat foods that contain glutamate—such as potatoes, mushrooms, some cheeses, and meals made with monosodium glutamate, or MSG. Each receptor cell is especially sensitive to one taste, as are the different areas of the tongue where these cells are clustered. Most cells can, however, recognize at least two different tastes.

Taste is only one part of overall flavor, which includes extra details such as the sting of ammonia, the irritation of chile peppers, and the coolness of menthol. Flavor is largely drawn from the sense of smell: If you hold your nose, you may not be able to detect the difference in flavor between apples and pears, for example, but you can still taste that they're both sweet.

A rare condition, ageusia, causes the loss of taste. Congestion or allergies can cause temporary loss, as can certain medications, exposure to dangerous chemicals, or radiation treatment for cancer. Sensitivity to taste declines with age, because taste and smell cells (which are replaced every 1 to 2 weeks) regenerate at a slower pace as we age.

ADDITIONAL FACTS

1. *Some taste fibers in the tongue travel along the lingual nerve to the chorda tympani, a slender nerve that traverses the eardrum on the way to the brain. When an eardrum is injured and the chorda tympani is damaged, taste buds may begin to die, and sensitivity may be lost at the back of the tongue on the same side.*

2. *People generally seem to detect flavors best when food or drink is at or slightly below body temperature.*

3. *Taste partially controls even an infant's sucking response: Babies accept sweet solutions more readily than plain water, and bitter, salty, or sour stimuli tend to stop the sucking reflex.*

◆◆◆

Menstrual Cycle

During puberty, a girl's complex hormonal system begins to stir to life. These changes cause the development of breasts, feminine curves, and more. It's around this time that she experiences her first menstrual period, which concludes an approximately 28-day cycle of hormonal interaction readying the body for pregnancy and producing an egg for fertilization. Over the next few decades of her life, she'll experience this cycle about 450 more times.

The menstrual cycle begins when the brain produces hormones that stimulate the pituitary gland to release gonadotropins, including follicle-stimulating and luteinizing hormones. These bodily chemicals trigger a handful of follicles to begin maturing into eggs. Simultaneously, the hormones also cause the ovaries to begin pumping out estrogen, which stimulates the uterine lining (the endometrium) to thicken in preparation for a fertilized egg. After about 2 weeks, a full-grown egg is released from one of the ovaries into the neighboring fallopian tube, where the egg may join with a sperm. The empty follicle releases progesterone in addition to estrogen, a hormone important to the early stages of pregnancy. If the egg isn't fertilized, however, the inner lining of the uterus breaks down and is shed from the body during the 3- to 5-day span of menstruation, which occurs about 2 weeks after ovulation. Then the process starts over again.

ADDITIONAL FACTS

1. *The Museum of Menstruation and Women's Health was located for more than a decade in New Carrollton, Maryland, before it was shuttered. Today, its archive of menstruation history and advertisements lives on its Web site, www.mum.org.*

2. *Girls are beginning to menstruate at earlier ages than ever before. Although experts aren't sure exactly why, one reason may be the increased number of chubby girls; fat makes more estrogen, and girls are reaching the necessary minimum weight for menstruation at earlier ages.*

3. *After a girl's first menstrual period, it takes about 3 years for the menstrual cycle to become regular.*

◆◆◆

DHA and EPA

Docosahexaenoic acid (DHA) and eicosapentaenoic acid (EPA) are omega-3 fatty acids derived from fish and fish oils. Studies show that DHA and EPA in the form of fish or fish oil supplements reduce triglyceride levels, slow the buildup of atherosclerotic plaques (hardening of the arteries), and lower blood pressure. DHA and EPA also decrease the risk of death, heart attack, abnormal heart rhythms, and stroke in people with heart disease.

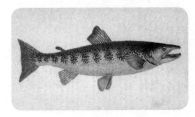

It's recommended that adults consume 0.3 to 0.5 gram of DHA and EPA each daily. However, the average American adult takes in only about 0.1 to 0.2 gram of DHA and EPA each per day. One way to increase your intake is to eat fatty fish at least twice a week. Examples of recommended fatty fish are anchovies, bluefish, carp, catfish, halibut, herring, lake trout, mackerel, pompano, salmon, striped sea bass, tuna (albacore), and whitefish. However, because fish may contain methylmercury, the amount of fish young children and pregnant or breastfeeding women consume should be discussed with a physician.

Another good way to increase your consumption of DHA and EPA is to take fish oil supplements. However, they should be used with caution. Dosages of DHA and EPA that are too high can be harmful, leading to an increased risk of bleeding. And supplements contain different ingredients and different amounts of ingredients, even within the same brand. You should discuss how much you should take with a qualified health care professional before using fish oil supplements. Fish oil capsules should not be given to children except under the direction of a physician.

ADDITIONAL FACTS

1. *DHA is thought to have greater benefits than EPA.*

2. *DHA and EPA have been found to be important for healthy pregnancies for both the mother and the fetus. Additionally, it is thought that infants whose mothers consume DHA in foods or supplements during pregnancy have better problem-solving skills and better-developed visual systems.*

3. *Alpha-linolenic acid (ALA) may provide benefits similar to those of DHA and EPA, although studies are less convincing. ALA is derived from some nuts and vegetable oils.*

❖❖❖

William Harvey and Blood Circulation

When the English physician William Harvey claimed in 1628 that the heart was responsible for pumping blood throughout the body, the medical community largely criticized him. Today, we know that his research laid the groundwork for our modern understanding of circulation and physiology.

Harvey (1578–1657) was a highly respected doctor in London and the personal physician of King James I (1566–1625) and his son Charles I (1600–1649). In 1615, Harvey became a lecturer for the College of Physicians, where he often discussed his controversial theory. His notions about the role of the heart were quite a departure from the commonly accepted belief that blood's movement through the body was caused by an innate pulsing in the arteries themselves. This traditional philosophy also held that there were two types of blood, venous and arterial, and that venous blood was produced in the liver and converted from food. It was assumed that, instead of circulating continuously, blood was simply absorbed by the body and new blood was constantly produced.

The culmination of Harvey's research came with the publication of *An Anatomical Essay Concerning the Movement of the Heart and the Blood in Animals,* a report that explained how blood was propelled through the arteries by heartbeats. It argued that in animal experiments, the amount of blood forced out of the heart in an hour far exceeded the blood's volume in the whole creature—thus suggesting that the blood must be circulating, otherwise the arteries would burst under pressure. Although he could not see the capillaries that branch out to nourish the body's tissues and connect the arteries to the veins, Harvey proposed the existence of such tiny blood vessels, as well.

Harvey's ideas were not trusted at the time, and his radical theories lost him many patients. But within his lifetime his ideas were eventually accepted, although they did not change common medical practices, such as bloodletting, for many years.

ADDITIONAL FACTS

1. *A second groundbreaking work published by Harvey in 1651,* Essays on the Generation of Animals, *is considered the basis for modern embryology.*

2. *Harvey was able to witness the way a human heart pumps blood firsthand when he met a young man who had a gaping hole in his chest as a result of a childhood injury. The man wore a metal plate over the wound, but he could remove it to expose to Harvey and other observers his heart beating through the scar tissue.*

3. *In one famous experiment, Harvey showed the existence and function of valves in the veins. He cut off circulation in a patient's arm with a tourniquet, then tried to push the blood in the swollen veins away from or toward the heart. He was able to empty the veins in only one direction (toward the heart), showing that the valves allowed blood to flow only one way.*

✦✦✦

Developmental Delay

The first babble, wobbly step, and "mama" make every parent swell with pride. For a pediatrician, however, these actions are all important milestones in a child's mental and physical development. If a child is significantly behind his or her peers in a certain area—such as motor, language, social, or thinking skills—that's called a developmental delay.

The developmental landmarks start as early as 1 month of age. For instance, by that time, an infant should move its head from side to side, clench its hands into tight fists, focus on objects at least a foot away, recognize sounds, and prefer sweet tastes. If the infant doesn't blink near a bright light, rarely moves its arms and legs, feeds slowly, or doesn't respond to loud sounds, that may be a sign of a developmental delay. Parents and pediatricians alike follow a baby's progression closely during the first 3 years of life.

There's no single cause of these delays. A wide variety of conditions, illnesses, and diseases may lead to slower-than-usual development. Some genetic causes, such as Down syndrome, or pregnancy or birth complications, such as infection or premature delivery, may be to blame. Other culprits, including hearing loss due to chronic ear infections or lead poisoning, may be curable. Experts encourage parents to consult their pediatricians if they suspect that their children may have a developmental delay; research shows that the earlier a delay is diagnosed and appropriate treatment is prescribed, the better the outcome later in life.

ADDITIONAL FACTS

1. *Experts believe that 3 percent of children do not meet developmental milestones; of those children, about 15 to 20 percent actually have abnormal development.*

2. *There is a wide range of "normal" development.*

3. *Premature babies usually catch up with full-term infants developmentally by 2 years of age.*

◆◆◆

Allergy

About 50 million Americans suffer from allergies, or an overzealous immune system. Instead of ignoring harmless particles, such as pollen and animal dander, the body of an allergic person flags them as intruders and releases inflammatory chemicals to combat them.

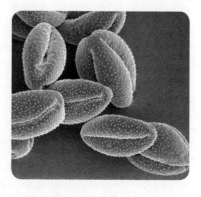

There are four categories of allergies. Type I, or anaphylactic, reactions are the most common and include hay fever, food allergies, and reactions to insect bites. Almost immediately after exposure to the allergen, the body releases a cascade of histamines and leukotrienes. Consequently, airways and nasal linings swell, resulting in congestion, wheezing, and foggy thinking. Treatments include antihistamines and desensitizing shots, in which increasing amounts of the antigen are injected over time until they no longer set off an allergic response. A severe form of type I allergy, called anaphylaxis, is life threatening, because air passageways close and blood vessels rapidly dilate. It's treated with the hormone epinephrine, which causes the airways to open and the arteries to constrict.

Type II, or cytotoxic, allergic reactions occur on a cellular level; the body is fighting off antigens attached to the surface of cells, such as when rejecting a blood transfusion. A type III, or immune-complex-related, reaction occurs when an antibody-antigen pair becomes deposited in the walls of small blood vessels and results in inflammation and cellular and vascular damage. The most common example of this is rheumatoid arthritis. Last but not least is type IV, or a cell-mediated response, which takes up to 2 days to manifest. This reaction is brought on by an excess of T cells and includes skin allergies and the rejection of transplanted organs.

ADDITIONAL FACTS

1. *The Austrian physician Clemens, Baron von Pirquet (1874–1929), coined the term allergy in the early 1900s from the Greek word* allos, *which means "other."*

2. *Although many people suspect that they suffer from food allergies, only 2 percent of Americans actually do.*

3. *Experts believe that one result of global warming will be an increase in ragweed growth, which will lead to an upsurge in seasonal allergies.*

✦✦✦

Blood Pressure Drugs

Nearly one in three US adults has hypertension, or high blood pressure—defined as 140/90 millimeters of mercury (mmHg) or higher. Because hypertension increases the risk of stroke, heart attack, heart failure, and kidney failure, it's important that people with this condition be treated. Some people can lower their blood pressure with diet and exercise, but most will need one (or more) of the following drugs.

Diuretics, or water pills, help the kidneys flush extra water and salt from your body, thereby decreasing blood volume. With less fluid pushing against vessel walls, the blood pressure may drop to a safer level. Diuretics cause frequent urination and can also lead to dehydration and dry mouth, among other side effects.

Angiotensin converting enzyme (ACE) inhibitors keep the blood vessels relaxed and blood pressure low by stopping the body from forming angiotensin II, a hormone that causes blood vessels to narrow.

Angiotensin II receptor blockers (ARBs), in contrast, work by protecting blood vessels from the effects of angiotensin II, rather than blocking the creation of the hormone itself. However, a 2008 study found that a newer ARB called telmisartan did not lower the rate of stroke, cardiovascular events, or diabetes any better than a placebo in patients who had had a stroke.

Beta-blockers are used to treat a wide variety of ailments, including high blood pressure. The drugs reduce the heart rate and force of cardiac contractions, causing blood pressure to drop. A 2008 study, however, found that beta-blockers don't prevent the development of heart failure in people with high blood pressure and should not be used as a first-line treatment.

Other drugs, such as calcium channel blockers (CCBs), alpha-blockers, vasodilators, and nervous system inhibitors, work by reducing certain effects of nerve impulses to the blood vessels, allowing the vessels to relax and blood to pass through more freely. These drugs are often prescribed with other types of blood pressure medications, or two different medications are combined in a single pill.

ADDITIONAL FACTS

1. *Chicken soup may help reduce blood pressure: Researchers have found that chicken contains a collagen protein that appears to act like an ACE inhibitor. However, the salt added to most chicken meals or soups may offset or even reverse this potential benefit.*

2. *Blood pressure drugs shouldn't be allowed to make a person's pressure too low: In a 2008 study on patients with coronary artery disease, bringing diastolic pressure (the bottom number in a blood pressure measurement) below 70 with medication doubled the risk of dying of a heart attack, stroke, or other cause.*

3. *Patients with high blood pressure are often encouraged to buy a home blood pressure monitor to check their levels more frequently than just during visits to the doctor's office.*

❖❖❖

Memory

One of the most important functions of the brain is to control memory, the ability to recall facts, people, events, and other information that was learned at an earlier time and stored for later use. The gray matter that makes up the brain's wrinkly outer cerebral cortex is filled with memories, much as a computer disk is full of files, waiting to be activated and pulled back into the conscious thought process.

The are two basic types of memory. To remember snippets of information you need soon, the brain relies on **short-term memory,** or working memory. You may need to make a deliberate effort to keep these thoughts fresh in your mind, such as when someone gives you a phone number but you can't write it down right away.

Long-term memory is forged when temporary memories are transferred to a more permanent vault in the brain. Not every piece of information becomes a long-term memory; in order for something to make the transition, the nerve pathways on which it travels must be strengthened and reinforced over time; that's why study guides often advise students to read things or recite information at least three times. Having a strong emotional association with a memory also helps you retain information. A good night's sleep seems to be important for transferring short-term memories into permanent ones, as well.

Long-term memory can be further divided into three subtypes: explicit memories, implicit memories, and semantic memories. An explicit memory is something that you trained yourself to know, such as the periodic table of the elements in a chemistry class, but which you must "ask" your brain to retrieve for you. Implicit memory includes tasks like typing or driving a car, which your brain has trained itself through experience to do automatically. A semantic memory might be something like the memory of your own name—an item of information that you (hopefully) can recall instantly and without effort.

As adults reach middle age and beyond, it's normal for them to experience a small amount of memory loss—these experiences are sometimes called senior moments. But too frequent forgetting, especially of important details such as where one lives or how to use a telephone, can be a sign of a stroke, Alzheimer's disease, or another form of dementia. Memory problems can also result from alcohol and certain medications. Regular exercise and consumption of healthy fats (such as omega-3 fatty acids) seem to keep the brain nourished and help prevent age-related memory loss.

ADDITIONAL FACTS

1. *Memory tricks called mnemonic devices may help you remember facts better. For example, "Every good boy deserves fudge" is a popular way to remember the letters (E, G, B, D, and F) corresponding with the lines on the treble clef in music.*

2. *After a traumatic brain injury, a person may suffer amnesia, or loss of memory. Memory usually returns over time.*

3. *Sleep apnea, a condition in which a person's airway is blocked and he or she stops breathing during sleep, damages the brain's ability to transition memories from short-term to long-term. People with untreated sleep apnea may have trouble remembering things for longer than a few hours.*

◆◆◆

Fertilization

The miracle of life begins with fertilization, or the moment when sperm meets egg. Like a chain of dominoes, this phenomenon is a well-choreographed sequence of events. If there's any interruption in the chain, fertilization will not occur.

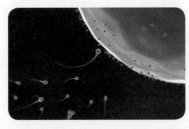

The first factor is timing: Once a month, a woman ovulates and her egg is viable for 24 to 72 hours as it travels down one of the fallopian tubes. During this window, sperm must enter the body. Millions of ejaculated sperm then swim through acidic vaginal fluids, push through cervical mucus, and pass through the uterus into a fallopian tube to reach and fertilize the ovum. Along the journey, each sperm begins to shed its outer layer of proteins until the tip of its head, called the acrosome, is revealed. When the sperm finally reach the egg, many of them release a barrage of powerful acrosomal enzymes to break down the egg's tough zona pellucida layer. Once one sperm plunges through and reaches the egg's inner membrane, the egg destroys its receptors and blocks any other sperm from entering.

When the sperm arrives at the center of the egg, the sperm's chromosomes begin to swell and line up with those already present in the egg. Both the egg and sperm nuclei have merged their genetic messages by aligning the male and female chromosomes; it's at this point that the egg graduates to a zygote, or preembryo. The zygote must still travel for another week down the fallopian tube to the uterus. During that time, it divides and grows into a fluid-filled ball of cells called a blastocyst, which will grow into an embryo. At that point, it will implant in the uterus.

ADDITIONAL FACTS

1. *The blastocyst attaches to a sticky protein surface inside the uterus. About a week later, the endometrial cells lining the uterine cavity completely cover the embryo.*

2. *It takes 36 hours for the newly fertilized zygote to cleave into two new cells.*

✦✦✦

Trans Fat

Trans fat, or trans fatty acid, also called partially hydrogenated oil, is most commonly produced by a manufacturing process that adds hydrogen to liquid vegetable oils to make them more solid. Companies and restaurants use trans fat because it is inexpensive to produce, lasts a long time, and makes food tasty.

Trans fat is in many foods, including fried foods, such as french fries and doughnuts, and baked goods, such as pastries, pie crusts, biscuits, pizza dough, cookies, crackers, stick margarines, and shortenings. You can find out how much trans fat is in commercially packaged foods by reading their nutrition facts labels. In ingredient lists, trans fat is often called partially hydrogenated oil. Small quantities of trans fat occur naturally in some meat and dairy products, such as beef, lamb, and butterfat.

Trans fat is unhealthy because it raises your LDL ("bad") cholesterol level, lowers your HDL ("good") cholesterol level, and increases your risk of coronary heart disease, stroke, and type 2 diabetes. The amount of trans fats you eat should be limited to less than 1 percent of your total daily calories. So if you need 2,000 calories a day, no more than 20 calories a day should come from trans fat. This means that you probably should not eat commercially manufactured goods with trans fat in them at all. It's best to replace trans fat with monounsaturated or polyunsaturated fat.

ADDITIONAL FACTS

1. The health effects of trans fat were not known before 1990. Now the United States government requires food manufacturers to list trans fat on nutrition facts labels.

2. Coronary heart disease is one of the leading causes of death in the United States, with 12.5 million Americans suffering from the disease.

3. Some dietary supplements, energy bars, and nutrition bars contain trans fat from hydrogenated vegetable oil. It's wise to read the nutrition information and ingredient lists on these products.

✦✦✦

Blood Transfusion

Although blood transfusion has been practiced successfully for less than a century, the idea that fresh blood gives new life has been around for much longer.

The first authentic attempt at transfusion may have been the case of Pope Innocent VIII (1432–1492) around 1492. An unknown illness left the pope semicomatose, and he was transfused with the blood of three young boys. All three donors died, as did the pope shortly afterward.

In the 17th century, the English physician William Harvey (1578–1657) discovered that blood flowed through arteries in one direction and veins in another, paving the way for new theories about transfusion. The English physician Richard Lower (1631–1691) performed one of the first successful animal-to-human transfusions in 1667, by putting blood from a sheep into the vein of a man's arm. The French physician Jean-Baptiste Denys (1640–1704) wrote that he preferred animal donors to humans because their blood was less likely to be "rendered impure by passion or vice." However, in 1668, Denys performed a calf-to-human transfusion and his patient became sick to his stomach and urinated black liquid—then died after a second transfusion a few months later. A lawsuit followed, and the practice of blood transfusion was banned by the Catholic Church and abandoned by scientists. (It is understood today that animal and human blood are incompatible, and that anything more than a very small transfusion can cause a deadly "hemolytic transfusion response.")

It wasn't until the 19th century that interest in blood transfusion was renewed, most notably by the physician James Blundell (1790–1877), the "father of modern blood transfusion." Blundell determined that blood from one animal could not be substituted with blood from another, and he introduced the idea of using a syringe for human-to-human transfusions. In 1829 he performed what is considered the first successful transfusion, on a woman with severe postpartum bleeding.

The discovery of the different blood types and the development of anticoagulants greatly reduced the mortality and complications associated with blood transfusions. Human blood was first classified by Karl Landsteiner (1868–1943) as type A, B, AB, or O. Further typing by Alexander Wiener (1907–1976) in the 1950s showed that some people, about 85 percent, share a factor with rhesus monkeys, the Rh factor. The immune systems of women who lack it can react with their Rh-positive babies' blood during pregnancy, causing "Rh disease" in the newborn. Today, Rh immuno globulin injections for pregnant women prevent this from happening.

ADDITIONAL FACTS

1. *The development of electrical refrigeration allowed the first blood bank to open in Barcelona in 1936. Methods of freezing and storing blood helped increase availability in the following years.*

2. *In 1985, after dozens of Americans developed AIDS after receiving tainted blood transfusions, the first blood-screening test to detect the presence of HIV antibodies was licensed and adopted by blood banks and plasma centers.*

◆◆◆

Oppositional Defiant Disorder

At some point, every single child shows a flash of rebellion by arguing with or deliberately disobeying a parent, teacher, or other authority figure. But when this behavior seems excessive and lasts for 6 months or more, it may signal a behavioral disorder called oppositional defiant disorder (ODD). About 5 to 15 percent of children experience ODD during their lives.

Symptoms of the disorder include anger, temper tantrums, and mean or hateful language. A child may also argue frequently, refuse to comply with adult requests or rules, and blame others for his or her mistakes. While experts aren't sure of the exact cause of ODD, they believe that a number of genetic, psychological, and social factors may contribute to the condition's development.

ODD often occurs along with other mental or behavioral problems, such as attention-deficit/hyperactivity disorder (ADHD), anxiety disorders, and depression. What's more, studies have shown that children with ODD have abnormal amounts of brain chemicals called neurotransmitters, which suggests a biological factor. Social issues, such as child abuse, exposure to violence, or a lack of supervision, may also play a role in ODD.

Both medical treatment and psychological counseling can help a child with ODD. A physician can help treat a mental issue related to ODD, such as depression or ADHD, with a prescription medication. Meanwhile, a therapist can teach parents how to manage their child's behavior and can aid the child in coming to terms with his or her emotions.

ADDITIONAL FACT

1. *Research suggests that defects in or injuries to certain areas of the brain can lead to behavioral problems such as ODD in children.*

✦✦✦

Asthma

Since at least ancient Greece, there are records of healers treating the chronic lung disorder asthma. Throughout the centuries, remedies have included breathing in herbs and animal feces steamed over hot stones, eating large quantities of chicken soup, and simply praying. Although modern scientists have yet to unearth a cure for the disease, they've developed far more effective medicines.

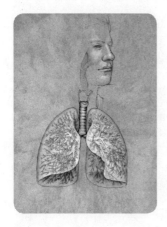

Afflicting some 22 million Americans, asthma is caused by inflamed bronchial airways, the tubes that transport air in and out of the lungs. These airways constrict as mucus clogs the passageways, causing episodes of wheezing, coughing, chest tightness, and shortness of breath. About half of all asthma cases develop before age 10 and are typically linked to a genetic sensitivity to allergens, such as pollen and dust mites. In fact, experts estimate that a child with one asthmatic parent has roughly a one-in-four chance of inheriting the disease; having two parents raises those odds to nearly three in four. But allergies, viral infections, and chronic exposure to pollutants can also lead to the onset of asthma in adults.

A variety of triggers, including allergens, cigarette smoke, and respiratory infections, can bring on an asthma attack. These bouts are treated with a fast-acting bronchodilator, which relaxes the airway muscles. This medicine is administered through a handheld inhaler or, for more severe cases, a mouthpiece or mask called a nebulizer. People with asthma may also often take a daily corticosteroid to control inflammation and prevent the onset of symptoms.

ADDITIONAL FACTS

1. *In the late 1800s, manufacturers marketed asthma cigarettes, which contained herbs.*

2. *The word* asthma *is derived from a Greek word meaning "to gasp."*

3. *Children with asthma often outgrow it by adulthood.*

✦✦✦

Dilantin

Phenytoin, sold in the United States under the brand names Dilantin and Phenytek, is an antiepileptic, or anticonvulsant, drug. It works by slowing down impulses in the brain that cause convulsions (fits or seizures), and may be prescribed to people with epilepsy or other seizure disorders.

Despite its widespread use today, however, the drug's original discovery was accidental. Diphenylhydantoin was developed by scientists who were seeking to invent a new sedative. The drug's powerful antiseizure effects were only noticed in 1938 after it failed to work as they had originally hoped.

Specifically. the scientists realized that the drug could be used to treat tonic-clonic (or grand mal) seizures (it is not effective for myoclonic, atonic, or absence seizures). It was marketed as Dilantin, and its generic name was later changed to phenytoin sodium. While Dilantin and generic phenytoin pills are available only in strengths of up to 100 milligrams, a newer brand called Phenytek comes in timed-release 300-milligram doses (each capsule containing three "mini-tabs" that release medication in stages), allowing patients to take one pill a day instead of two or three. Phenytoin is also available in chewable tablet form or as liquid medicine.

The drug can have numerous harmful side effects, including nausea and difficulty concentrating in the short term and rashes or excessive hair growth in the long term. Dilantin can also interact with other drugs, including antidepressants and antacids.

An overdose of phenytoin can be very dangerous or even fatal. Overdose symptoms may include twitching eyes; slurred speech; loss of balance; muscle stiffness, weakness, or tremor; nausea and vomiting; and slow or shallow breathing. Allergic reactions can be severe as well and may be indicated by fever, sore throat, a blistering skin rash, confusion, hallucinations, extreme thirst, or easy bruising or bleeding. Less-serious side effects are more likely to occur, such as twitching, a mild skin rash or itching, headache, joint pain, and swollen or tender gums.

ADDITIONAL FACTS

1. *Anyone taking an antiseizure medication should wear a medical alert bracelet or carry an ID card to alert doctors or medical workers in case of an emergency.*

2. *The medication can lower blood sugar, so people with diabetes who take it should monitor their levels regularly.*

3. *Phenytoin increases the risk of gum disease, so anyone taking it should brush and floss regularly.*

◆◆◆

Learning

The old expression "You learn something new every day" may very well be true: Research shows that the brain continues to form new neurons throughout life, especially if it's kept healthy and stimulated with mental exercise. Learning is indeed a lifelong process, beginning even before you're born and occurring every time you acquire and store a new piece of knowledge.

Many parts of the brain work together when you learn new information: First, a stimulus must be registered through the senses—whether it's reading a statistic, hearing a song, tasting a strange food, or touching a hot stove for the first time. The brain then must decide how to react and adapt. Finally, this situation is stored as a long-term memory so you can recall that knowledge when needed.

Learning occurs when something is repeated over and over—this is why review is such an important component of classroom education. When you first try to ride a bike or memorize a new math formula, it's difficult because your brain hasn't formed new pathways between the neurons on which the information will be stored. But with practice and repetition, you get better as these connections grow stronger—and eventually you can perform the task or apply the formula without much conscious thought at all. The ability of the brain to form new connections and physically change shape in response to new experiences is called neuroplasticity.

Learning also seems to work best when several senses are involved; scent especially has been shown to help reinforce the process. In one study, when students inhaled a rose-scented odor first while playing a memory game and again later while they slept, they were better able to recall those memories the next day.

The simplest type of learning is nonassociative, in which a person or animal learns simply through repetition. Associative learning, also known as conditioning, occurs when the brain makes a lasting connection between two stimuli—an example is the classic experiment of Ivan Pavlov, who trained dogs to salivate and expect food every time he rang a bell.

ADDITIONAL FACTS

1. *Rote learning is an often-criticized technique that focuses on memorizing material so that it can be recalled exactly the way it was read or heard, while avoiding any complexities or actual understanding of the content.*

2. *Although physical connections are made between neurons within the brain when new information is learned, new visible "wrinkles" in the brain are not formed. The folds that can be seen on the outside of the cerebral cortex are there only so the brain can fit inside the head.*

3. *Many methods have been suggested is to better retain memories. One herbal supplement said to increase retention, ginkgo biloba, is a tree native to Asia. Evidence is mixed, with many scientific studies showing it has no effect.*

◆◆◆

Mitosis

The secret of how human life works can be traced back to the lowly salamander. In the 1880s, a German biologist named Walther Flemming (1843–1905) began studying the larvae of these amphibians. After staining the organisms with a special dye that made them easier to see under a microscope, Flemming tracked how a threadlike material in the nucleus shortened and split in half during different phases of cell division. He named this process of cell reproduction mitosis, after the Greek word for "thread."

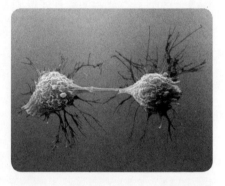

The importance of this discovery, however, wasn't fully acknowledged until decades later, when scientists identified those threads: They were chromosomes, structures that contain each individual's genetic information. When a human cell cleaves into two identical structures, it undergoes a series of steps that stretch over 24 hours. The process begins with a division in the cell's command center, or nucleus: During the step called prophase, the chromatids (a set of two chromosomes joined by a buttonlike centromere) condense into tightly coiled packages. At the same time, two bundles of tubes called centrioles migrate to opposite ends of the nucleus and grow long tubules that stretch toward each other, forming what's called the mitotic spindle.

In the next stage, metaphase, the chromatids line up neatly along the mitotic spindle. Then, during anaphase, the centromeres release, splitting each chromatid in two; the halves are dragged toward opposite ends of the cell. At that point, telophase commences, and the chromosomes begin to set up a new home: They unfurl, and a nuclear membrane grows around them. Finally, in a process called cytokinesis, the cell pinches in the middle and splits in two, each part having a full complement of chromosomes.

ADDITIONAL FACTS

1. *Before mitosis occurs, cells undergo a process called interphase, in which their DNA replicates to form a second set in preparation for the onset of mitosis.*

2. *Mitosis can take anywhere from a few minutes to more than an hour, depending on the kind of cells and the type of organism.*

✦✦✦

Fitness

Being physically fit is extremely important for maintaining good health. People who are active live longer and are more likely to maintain a healthy weight. And exercise can improve or even prevent medical conditions such as diabetes, heart disease, high blood pressure, stroke, and some cancers.

There are many definitions of *fitness,* but the simplest is cardiovascular fitness. This means that with vigorous activity, your heart rate (pulse) does not exceed the expected maximum for your age. A common formula: Subtract your age from 220 and take 80 percent of that as your maximum. For example, for a 40-year-old, $220 - 40 = 180$, and $180 \times 0.8 = 144$, the maximum pulse rate.

Most adults should engage in moderate physical activity for at least 30 minutes five times a week in order to be physically fit. Moderate-intensity physical activity should make you breathe harder, but you should still have enough breath to carry on a conversation. Examples of moderate physical activity include walking briskly, dancing, swimming, or bicycling. Weight training and stretching can also improve your fitness level.

It can be difficult to get enough exercise. However, it's important to make physical activity a priority. Some people schedule exercise into their days, including waking up early, arranging for lunchtime workouts, or taking an evening class. You can also add physical movement to your regular activities, such as housework, by doing them more energetically. Another way of incorporating exercise into your routine is to spend your free time with family and friends doing activities you enjoy, such as hiking, playing sports, or going for a walk after dinner.

To be successful at an exercise program, it is also important to have concrete goals. Begin with short-term goals, such as walking for 10 minutes a day, 3 days a week. Then try to build up to at least 30 minutes of moderate-intensity physical activity at least five times a week. Tracking your progress by writing down your goals and activities will help keep you motivated.

ADDITIONAL FACTS

1. *In order to lose weight and keep off extra weight, you will probably need to be physically active for more than 30 minutes a day.*

2. *Regular physical activity increases your energy level and enhances your mood.*

3. *Men over 40, women over 50, and people with chronic health problems should discuss a physical activity program with their health care provides before starting.*

4. *Studies show that vigorous exercise is associated with a 30 percent reduction in a woman's risk of breast cancer.*

◆◆◆

The First Ambulance, Bellevue Hospital, New York City

One of the first and most influential hospitals in the United States, Bellevue was founded in 1736 in lower Manhattan as a six-bed infirmary and almshouse for the indigent of New York City. Over the next 200 years, the hospital launched the nation's first maternity ward, its first children's clinic, and, interestingly, its first urban ambulance service.

The idea for a hospital ambulance system stemmed from the Civil War, during which army ambulance service was common. The physician Edward B. Dalton (1834–1872) had been in charge of the field ambulance corps of the Army of the Potomac during the war, and when he was put in charge of transportation and organization at Bellevue Hospital, he drew largely from his battlefield experience. The methods he installed served as a pattern widely copied throughout the country.

Beginning in 1869, ambulances were dispatched by telegraph from Bellevue Hospital's Centre Street branch; in the first year alone, they responded to more than 1,800 calls for help throughout the city. The horse-drawn carriages were typically staffed by highly trained doctors or surgeons from the hospital; however, if a doctor was not available, the hospital would send an orderly or even a janitor or cook to the scene. Often these ambulances arrived hours late and with attendants with little or no training or equipment to treat the patient. Because of this, the majority of the more seriously injured patients died before reaching the hospital.

As the city's population grew rapidly and industrial accidents became more and more common, the city realized it needed a larger, more efficient ambulance system. (In 1929, the city had only 45 ambulances available to handle 343,000 emergency calls per year.) Today, ambulances in New York City are operated by the Ambulance and Transportation Division of the Department of Hospitals.

In 1999, a retired physician from New York University named Morton Galdston (c. 1913–2003) published a collection of notes he had taken as an intern on 1-month ambulance duty at Bellevue 60 years earlier. His observations provide a description of the economic, social, and public health factors that led to the establishment of an urban ambulance system, and a glimpse of what emergency medical treatment was like at the time.

ADDITIONAL FACTS

1. *Originally, all traffic in New York City was required to yield to an ambulance—except firefighting equipment and the postal service.*

2. *For Bellevue Hospital, the Ambulance Board authorized two ambulances of the type recommended by Dalton. Furthermore, they specified, "Each ambulance shall have a box beneath the driver's seat, containing a quart flask of brandy, two tourniquets, a half-dozen bandages, a half-dozen small sponges, some splint material, pieces of old blankets for padding, strips of various lengths with buckles, and a two-ounce vial of persulphate of iron."*

◆◆◆

Vaccination

The idea of injecting a healthy person with a disease as defense against more severe illness can be traced back to China around 200 BC. Ancient healers blew smallpox scabs into patients' noses in order to protect them from the disease. In 1796, the English physician Edward Jenner (1749–1823) took this technique a step further by injecting a boy with cowpox (a relatively harmless disease related to smallpox) and then, after the boy had healed, exposing him to the smallpox virus. The boy remained healthy. Based on this discovery, Jenner coined the word *vaccine* from the Latin word *vacca,* or "cow."

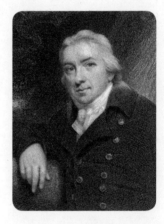

Although Jenner didn't understand the science behind it at the time, researchers have since uncovered how immunization works. Vaccines cause the immune system to ready itself for future attacks. Immunizations made from weakened, harmless strains of viruses are introduced into the body, causing the B and T white blood cells to activate and produce memory cells. These cells reproduce in the body for decades, so that when a person again encounters that specific virus, an arsenal of specialized white blood cells is on hand to destroy it.

Currently, the Centers for Disease Control and Prevention advises that all infants and children receive a number of vaccinations. These shots may be a onetime occurrence or require a number of injections. The diphtheria and tetanus immunization, for instance, consists of a series of five inoculations spread over 5 or 6 years. Since booster shots are required to refresh the body's memory cells every several years, adults need immunizations, too. Because viruses like those that cause the flu constantly mutate and change, a different flu vaccine is needed every year.

ADDITIONAL FACTS

1. *The boy whom Edward Jenner inoculated was the son of a nearby farmer. Jenner asked if he could perform his experiment on the child; surprisingly, the father agreed.*

2. *Some parents have questioned whether preservatives and heavy metals, such as thimerosal and mercury, in vaccines can cause autism in young children. Currently, the Centers for Disease Control and Prevention says that there's no scientific evidence to support this claim.*

◆◆◆

Autoimmune Disease

The body's immune system is necessary for fending off illness. But for the 5 percent of people with autoimmune diseases, this natural defense system turns on itself and attacks body cells as if they were dangerous foreign invaders. There are more than 80 types of these diseases, including rheumatoid arthritis, multiple sclerosis, and lupus. Women are twice as likely to be affected as men are.

Normally, the immune system's attack cells—white blood cells called lymphocytes (B and T cells)—recognize the body's major histocompatibility complex (MCH), a type of personal bar code that every cell contains. But a genetic defect, virus, or induced mutation can produce faulty versions of these cells that ignore this safety feature and instead home in on some of the body's own cells. The body may also grow new cells with different MCHs that the immune system doesn't recognize.

There are two types of autoimmune diseases. One is organ specific, in which the immune system targets antigens in one particular organ. (An example of this is type 1 diabetes, which attacks the insulin-producing cells in the pancreas.) The more common type is systemic, in which several organs or the connective tissues are affected. Symptoms of autoimmune diseases vary, but early signs often include fatigue, muscle aches, and low fever; cycles of flare-ups and remission are common. Treatments depend on the specific disease, but drugs that relieve the inflammatory response are frequently prescribed.

ADDITIONAL FACTS

1. *The autoimmune disease lupus is named after the Latin word for "wolf" because of its skin rash and lesions that resemble wolf bites.*

2. *The holy grail of treating autoimmune disease is being able to suppress the harmful immune mechanisms without affecting the entire system. For example, some multiple sclerosis patients may benefit from injections of antibodies that neutralize the overactive B and T cells.*

3. *Autoimmune diseases often run in families.*

✦✦✦

Antihistamines

Most common allergy symptoms—sneezing, itchy eyes, runny nose—are caused by chemicals called histamines, which the body produces to fight off allergens. Drugs that can counteract these chemicals and relieve symptoms are called antihistamines.

Antihistamines are the most commonly used medications to reduce symptoms caused by pollen, ragweed, dust mites, mold, animal dander, and cockroaches, to name a few. If a person is allergic to any of these triggers, the body produces histamines to fight off the allergens by attaching to cells called histamine receptors, causing inflammation and mucus production. Antihistamines can bond to these receptors instead, preventing histamines from causing symptoms.

Some antihistamines are sold over-the-counter, while others require a prescription. They can be taken as tablets, capsules, or liquids, or, less frequently, by injection or suppository. The most common side effect of antihistamines is drowsiness—it's so common, in fact, that the drug is also used in nighttime cough and cold formulas and over-the-counter sleep medications. Other possible side effects, especially in older people with other health conditions, may include upset stomach, constipation, headache, and dry mouth. These medications should not be given to anyone under the age of 4, as side effects for young children can be life threatening.

Over-the-counter antihistamines include brompheniramine, diphenhydramine, and loratadine, among others. These are the active ingredients in the Dimetapp, Benadryl, and Claritin brand products, respectively. They are often mixed with other drugs, such as pain relievers or decongestants, to treat many symptoms of a cold, the flu, or allergies at once. Prescription antihistamines include fexofenadine (Allegra), cetirizine (Zyrtec), and desloratadine (Clarinex). Prescription nasal sprays such as azelastine (Astelin) are also available. Studies have found these medications to be no more effective than the over-the-counter versions, although they are much less likely to cause drowsiness.

Because antihistamines can cause drowsiness, people taking the drugs are warned to be especially careful while driving a car or operating machinery. Sleeping pills, sedatives, muscle relaxants, blood pressure medications, and alcohol can increase drowsiness caused by antihistamines.

ADDITIONAL FACTS

1. *People with asthma can have more-severe allergic symptoms because their airways are more sensitive. Antihistamines may help keep the airways from closing up during an allergic reaction.*

2. *Antihistamines are sometimes used to treat a chronic hivelike rash called urticaria; they're also prescribed to combat nausea, headaches, anxiety, stiffness, and tremors in patients with Parkinson's disease.*

3. *Antihistamines can also relieve itchiness caused by insect bites and stings, poison ivy, and poison oak.*

✦✦✦

Intelligence

There are many ways to describe a person's way of thinking: He can be artistic, creative, clever, or knowledgeable, or she can have a good memory. But to explain how well people can solve problems and understand the world around them, we use the term *intelligence*.

One widely accepted definition of intelligence was published in 1994 in an article called "Mainstream Science on Intelligence":

> *A very general mental capability that, among other things, involves the ability to reason, plan, solve problems, think abstractly, comprehend complex ideas, learn quickly, and learn from experience. It is not merely book learning, a narrow academic skill, or test-taking smarts. Rather, it reflects a broader and deeper capability for comprehending our surroundings—"catching on," "making sense" of things, or "figuring out" what to do.*

Researchers have argued about whether it's possible to quantify intelligence. The most accepted way to do this is with an intelligence quotient (IQ) test that includes math and logic problems, memory and visual exercises, and questions about rearranged words or sentences. An average IQ score is 90 to 110, a score above 130 is considered superior intelligence, and a score below 70 indicates mental retardation. These tests have faced criticism, however, for being culturally biased and not allowing for multiple correct answers on subjective questions.

Because IQ tests measure not just the quantity of a person's knowledge but also the ability to understand ideas, learning new information doesn't necessarily increase your IQ. It may exercise your mind, however, which could help you develop greater cognitive skills. Overall, a person's IQ does not tend to change much over the years.

High intelligence seems to run in families, although studies have not found specific genes that make much of an impact. It's also been suggested that the ratio of body weight to brain volume, and the location of gray matter in the brain, might affect intelligence levels. Family upbringing seems to affect childhood IQ, but by late adolescence, this factor is less important: Adoptive siblings, once they're grown, tend to show vastly different intelligence levels, while twins and other full siblings seem to be much closer in IQ.

ADDITIONAL FACTS

1. *In 1983, the psychologist Howard Gardner (1943–) defined several types of intelligence, including verbal, visual, physical, musical, mathematical, introspective, and interpersonal. Most standard definitions of intelligence do not factor in many of these traits.*

2. *After the death of Albert Einstein (1879–1955), his brain was measured and found to be 15 percent wider than most human brains. It also contained abnormal-looking parietal lobes, which some theorize may have aided his mathematics skills.*

3. *American Mensa, an "organization for smart people," requires a score of 130 on the Stanford-Binet 5th edition IQ test to qualify for membership.*

✦ ✦ ✦

Meiosis

While the overwhelming majority of cells in the body regenerate through mitosis, the sperm and egg cells reproduce through another series of events called meiosis. This process is critical for reproduction, because that's how chromosomes from each parent combine to create a new, unique individual.

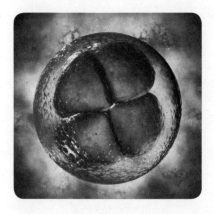

In mitosis, a cell takes four steps to divide and produces two identical cells with 46 (diploid) chromosomes. In meiosis, this cycle occurs twice and forms four daughter cells that each contain one (haploid) set of 23 chromosomes. But before the cycle even starts, each of the chromosomes duplicates to become a pair of chromatids joined by a connecting centromere; at first glance, it looks something like the letter X. During prophase, these chromatids shorten and join up with a pair from the other parent. At this point, the chromatids begin crossing over, or swapping genetic material. This process explains why you may have your mom's eyes and your dad's curly hair, for instance.

After metaphase, anaphase, and telophase, two daughter cells, each with one diploid set of chromatids, are left. Now a second meiotic division occurs to split each of these in two. These chromatids do not duplicate; instead, they're split, reducing the number of chromosomes per cell to half. That leaves four daughter cells, each with a haploid set of new chromosomes—23 per cell instead of 46. Then fertilization combines two cells, each with half the number of chromosomes needed to produce a unique person.

ADDITIONAL FACTS

1. *The word* meiosis, *which is pronounced* "my-OH-sis," *is derived from the Greek* meioun, *which means "to diminish."*

2. *The chromatids' process of crossing over is called recombination.*

♦♦♦

Cardiovascular Training

Cardiovascular training is a type of aerobic exercise that causes you to breathe more deeply and forces your heart to work harder to pump blood. It improves your health in many ways, including reducing the risk of early death, coronary heart disease, stroke, high blood pressure, type 2 diabetes, colon and breast cancers, and depression. Some examples of cardiovascular exercise are walking, running, aerobic dance, bicycling, rowing, and swimming.

For true cardiovascular training, you need to be sure to reach your target heart rate. You can check this by measuring your heart rate (in beats per minute). If you count your pulse for 15 seconds and multiply the number of beats by 4, you'll get an accurate measurement in beats per minute.

Your target heart rate depends on your age. Generally, your maximum heart rate is about 220 minus your age. When you're just beginning an exercise program, it's best to aim for the lowest target heart rate, which is about 60 percent of your maximum. As your fitness improves, you can exercise harder to drive your heart rate closer to the top target number, which is about 85 percent of your maximum heart rate.

Generally, a desirable goal to work up to is four to six 30- to 60-minute workouts a week. You should start by speaking with your doctor about developing an appropriate program for you. It's always a good idea to start slowly.

To prevent injuries, it's best to begin every workout with a 5- to 10-minute warmup, including light activity at an easy pace and stretching to help make your muscles and joints more flexible. You should do the same thing at the end of your workout to cool down and return your heart rate to normal. Stop exercising at any time if you have pain or feel dizzy, faint, or nauseated.

ADDITIONAL FACTS

1. *People sometimes find it difficult to stick to an exercise plan. It helps if you choose an activity that you enjoy, work out with a friend, and vary the kind of exercise you do. This keeps workouts from becoming boring and helps prevent injury.*

2. *Avoid working out after you eat or when it's too hot or cold outside.*

3. *Walking 1 mile at least three times a week is the minimum necessary to improve your cardiovascular health.*

◆◆◆

Vitamin C and Scurvy

Scurvy, a fatal vitamin C deficiency that ravaged the British navy in the eighteenth century, caused extensive suffering and death for sailors at sea. But one valuable thing did come out of the epidemic: the world's first controlled clinical trial.

Military hygiene in the 1700s was deplorable; the Scottish naval surgeon James Lind (1716–1794) once noted that for centuries, armies had lost "more of their men by sickness than by sword." Even as Britain neared the pinnacle of its naval power, its expeditions sometimes lost more than half their crews to disease.

A grisly and painful disease, scurvy causes huge black-and-blue marks and reddish spots on the body, bleeding gums, loss of teeth, and, eventually, heart failure and death. Unsanitary conditions onboard ships contributed to the high death rate at sea.

Lind suspected that the illness arose from the military's diet, which consisted of only nonperishable items and insufficient fresh fruits and vegetables. To prove his hypothesis, he devised one of the first controlled clinical trials in history.

In his seminal *Treatise on the Scurvy,* published in 1754, Lind summarized the experiment. He selected 12 sailors with scurvy, divided them into six groups, and fed each group a different diet. The two sailors who received oranges and lemons speedily recovered; the rest did not. Lind concluded that the citrus fruits cured scurvy, but it was later discovered that it was the vitamin C contained in these fruits that treated the illness.

General hygiene on ships gradually improved in the late eighteenth century, allowing the British to expand their empire unimpeded by scurvy. By the 1790s, all British naval ships were required to carry citrus fruits. Limes were often used in place of oranges and lemons—and British sailors subsequently became known as Limeys.

ADDITIONAL FACTS

1. *Ascorbic acid, the chemical form of vitamin C, was discovered by Hungarian researcher Albert Szent-Györgyi (1893–1986) in 1928—an achievement among many for which he garnered the Nobel Prize in Physiology or Medicine in 1937.*

2. *Ascorbic acid supplements are widely used across the world. They have been lauded (although not definitively proven) as a cure for and deterrent to the common cold, an antiaging remedy, and a preventive against cancer and heart disease.*

3. *Most other mammals produce their own vitamin C, making them immune from scurvy. Guinea pigs, some types of bats, and our fellow primates are the only other animals that lack the enzymes needed to produce vitamin C.*

◆◆◆

Rash

Your skin is your body's first line of defense against injury, germs, and other potential harm. Throughout a lifetime, it takes quite a beating, weathering countless scrapes, cuts, and injuries. As if that weren't enough, nearly every person suffers from a handful of rashes—bouts of irritated, puffy skin.

Rashes can come in many shapes and sizes, depending on the trigger. Viruses, fungi, parasites, medications, chemicals, allergies, and heat can cause the skin to become red, lumpy, dry, cracked, itchy, blistered, or tender. Most rashes are mild and go away on their own, but some require medical treatment, and a few may be signs of more serious diseases, such as Lyme disease.

One of the most common rashes, contact dermatitis, causes patches of raised, red bumps. It occurs when the skin comes into contact with an irritating or allergy-causing substance, such as soap, laundry detergent, poison ivy, rubber products, and metals in jewelry. Dermatitis usually disappears on its own after exposure to the irritant ceases. Another frequent skin condition is eczema, which leads to dry, itchy, scaly, and blistered skin. Although scientists aren't sure of the exact cause, the ailment tends to affect those with a family history of allergies or asthma. Over-the-counter or prescription cortisone creams treat eczema.

Hives, or urticaria, is another type of rash that's brought on by stress, allergies, perspiration, or extreme heat or cold. The skin responds to these factors by producing the chemical histamine, which causes inflammation of the skin. Most frequently, outbreaks appear as pale bumps surrounded by redness. Since there are a variety of other potential causes of rashes, it's best to see a dermatologist, who'll try to pinpoint the exact reason and prescribe the appropriate treatment.

ADDITIONAL FACTS

1. *Why does scratching an itch feel so good? Neurobiologists say that scratching creates a slight pain, which overrides the itchy sensation.*

2. *For people with very sensitive skin, vigorous touching can trigger the release of histamine, causing swelling at the site. In one such condition, called dermatographia, lightly scratching the skin results in a pattern of raised, red lines that look like writing.*

✦✦✦

Pneumonia

Until 1936, pneumonia was the number one cause of death in the United States. In most cases, an infection spreads to the lungs, causing them to become inflamed. As a result, pus fills the air sacs, and oxygen levels fall. This oxygen shortage coupled with a spreading infection can have a lethal effect. But, thanks to the advent of infection-stopping antibiotics, pneumonia is now usually an easily curable condition, taking the lives of only 60,000 people a year.

Although most cases start off as a cough and fever, symptoms can vary depending on what type of infection causes the illness. Viral infections, with their flulike symptoms and clear or white phlegm, lead to half of all cases of pneumonia. Viruses lead to an excess of fluid in the respiratory system, creating an environment where bacteria can grow. As a result, secondary bacterial pneumonia can develop, causing a high fever, chills, sweating, and a cough with yellow- or green-tinted phlegm. One strain in particular, *Streptococcus pneumoniae,* is the most common cause of bacterial pneumonia. In 1977, a vaccine that protects against this bacteria was released; it's now recommended for at-risk groups, such as the chronically ill and the elderly.

In mycoplasmal pneumonia, tiny pathogen called mycoplasma leads to mild flulike symptoms. Because some people with these symptoms feel well enough to go about their daily lives, this type is often called walking pneumonia. Less common are fungal pneumonia, which causes mild to serious symptoms, and *Pneumocystis carinii* pneumonia, which strikes people with compromised immune systems and leads to cough, fever, and shortness of breath.

To diagnose the condition, a physician will use a stethoscope to listen to your breathing. He or she may also request a chest x-ray to diagnose and determine the extent of the infection. Bacterial pneumonias are often confined to one lobe of the lung and are called lobar, while cases that affect both lungs are called double pneumonia.

ADDITIONAL FACTS

1. *An allergic response to certain kinds of dust, such as that produced by moldy room humidifiers or rat droppings, can lead to hypersensitivity pneumonia. Symptoms include chills, cough, muscle pain, and headache.*

2. *The dancer and actor Fred Astaire (1899–1987), the Russian author Leo Tolstoy (1828–1910), and the American president William Henry Harrison (1773–1841) all died of pneumonia.*

◆ ◆ ◆

Cortisone

A corticosteroid is a hormone released by the body in times of stress. Medicines made from synthetic versions of this hormone, such as cortisone and cortisol, are widely used to treat allergies, skin conditions, arthritis, and breathing disorders. Cortisone also suppresses the immune system, a phenomenon that may help explain the connection between stress and illness. This can be an unwanted side effect, but it can also be helpful in treating autoimmune conditions in which the body's natural defenses overreact.

In the 1930s at the Mayo Clinic in Rochester, Minnesota, the biochemist Edward Kendall (1886–1972) and the rheumatologist Philip Hench (1896–1965) noticed that some of the clinic's arthritis patients experienced temporary pain relief after stressful events like illness, childbirth, or surgery. This observation lead them to theorize that the experience had triggered the creation of a substance in the body that acted as a natural antirheumatic. They identified a hormone, called compound E, which they believed was responsible for this reaction, but were not able to begin testing until 1948. The results were amazing: the first patient to receive an injection of compound E reported less pain within 3 days. Today, compound E is known as cortisone, and injections are a common treatment for arthritis, joint and tendon inflammation, and sports overuse injuries.

Similar compounds, including cortisol, can be taken orally or inhaled to treat autoimmune disorders such as allergies, asthma, Crohn's disease, lupus, rheumatoid arthritis, and ulcerative colitis and to help prevent the rejection of transplanted organs. One of the most common oral corticosteroids is the drug prednisone. Topical cortisone creams are also available in prescription and nonprescription strengths for the treatment of eczema, psoriasis, and other skin irritations.

Corticosteroids can suppress fever and the entire immune system, making people more susceptible to serious illness and infection. Anyone receiving corticosteroid treatment should avoid people who have chicken pox or measles and should not receive vaccines made from live viruses. People who take other medications or who have liver or kidney disease, diabetes, a thyroid disorder, osteoporosis, glaucoma, cataracts, stomach ulcers, mental illness, or high blood pressure may need special tests to determine whether they can safely take cortisone. Cortisone usually should be avoided during pregnancy and breastfeeding, and it can affect growth in children.

ADDITIONAL FACTS

1. *In the body, most naturally occurring corticosteroids are produced in the morning hours.*

2. *Edward Kendall and Philip Hench were awarded the Nobel Prize in Physiology or Medicine in 1950 for their discovery of cortisone.*

3. *Natural cortisone is produced in the adrenal cortex. It is also known as hydrocortisone.*

❖❖❖

Sleep

When we close our eyes and rest our bodies for the night, our brains do not stop working. In ways that scientists are just beginning to understand, sleep is an important part of learning, memorization, and physical restoration that is as vital to the body as air, water, and food.

The transition to sleep is a multistep process that involves many changes to the body. A chemical, adenosine, builds up in the blood and creates a feeling of drowsiness. Once the lights go down, the brain begins producing melatonin—a hormone that helps us doze in the dark and wake up in the presence of light. Sleep involves a cycle of four incremental stages progressing from shallow to deep, followed by a rapid eye movement (REM) stage that includes accelerated breathing, back-and-forth eye twitching, and temporary limb paralysis. REM sleep seems to produce dreams, aid in overnight memorization, and contribute to restoration and alertness the next day.

Most people need 7 to 8 hours of sleep a night to function optimally the next day. Periods of prolonged sleep deprivation can cause fatigue and impairment and raise a person's risk of diabetes, heart disease, and depression. Lack of sleep also alters levels of appetite and satiety hormones, leading sleepy people to eat more.

Episodes of insomnia—the inability to sleep—are often triggered by stress, distraction, pain, or illness. If insomnia lasts for more than a few weeks, the body may become used to its new sleep pattern and need to be retrained to get back to a normal schedule. Over-the-counter antihistamines or prescription hypnotic drugs can be used to induce sleep, although experts agree that cognitive behavioral therapy—working with a doctor to discover what behaviors keep you awake and learn better sleep habits—is the best way to beat chronic insomnia. Other sleep disorders include sleep apnea, in which a person's airway becomes obstructed and he or she repeatedly stops breathing at night; restless legs syndrome, a condition that keeps people awake with a constant urge to move their legs; and parasomnias, including sleepwalking and very bad nightmares.

ADDITIONAL FACTS

1. *Leonardo da Vinci (1452–1519) was said to have slept for only 15 minutes out of every 4 hours—or a total of only 1½ hours per day. Sleep researchers have since proved that this schedule is possible to follow, but only temporarily.*

2. *In the first and lightest stage of sleep, many people experience sudden involuntary muscle contractions called hypnic myoclonia, or "sleep starts," often preceded by a sensation of falling.*

3. *The first REM sleep period occurs about 70 to 90 minutes after a person falls asleep, and a complete cycle takes 90 to 110 minutes, on average.*

4. *Limbs become temporarily paralyzed during REM sleep, so our dreams are only in our heads. But in a rare condition called REM sleep behavior disorder, paralysis doesn't kick in and people may act out their dreams—often with dangerous consequences, such as wrestling with their bed partner or running into walls.*

◆◆◆

Chromosome

Chromosomes are another testament to our bodies' amazing engineering. Because human DNA is too long to fit into a cell's nucleus—the entire strand of DNA consists of 20,000 to 25,000 genes and stretches up to 6 feet in length—the genes are efficiently packaged into a microscopic structure, the chromosome. Like thread around a spool, DNA coils tightly around itself in a spiral ladder shape called a double helix, and sequences of DNA line up to form a chromosome. Each cell contains 46 of these chromosomes, one set of 23 from the mother and one set of 23 from the father.

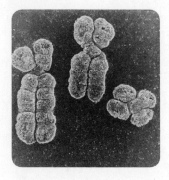

Each chromosome has a cinched waist called a centromere that divides it into two sections, or arms. The shorter arm is known as the p arm, while the longer one is the q arm. At the ends of each arm are protective stretches of DNA called telomeres. Like the tips on shoelaces, telomeres prevent chromosomes from unraveling.

Because cells reproduce to replace themselves, chromosomes must divide to ensure that each new cell receives a full set of genes. Any changes to their number or structure can lead to serious health problems. Some cancers, such as a type of leukemia, are caused by defective genes, while extra chromosomes can lead to genetic disorders, such as Down syndrome.

To study a person's chromosome set, scientists often treat cells with chemicals to define and stain the chromosomes. Then they take a picture of the stained chromosomes, called a karyotype. This process of staining gave the structure its name: *Chromosome* is derived from the Greek words for "color" (*chroma*) and "body" (*soma*).

ADDITIONAL FACTS

1. *Scientists first discovered chromosomes in the late 1800s but did not understand their function. In the early 1900s, the American geneticist Thomas Hunt Morgan (1866–1945) ascertained the link between chromosomes and inherited traits through studies of fruit flies.*

2. *When not dividing, chromosomes are not visible under the microscope; they remain curled up in the ·nucleus of the cell.*

3. *In some cells, telomeres lose a tiny part of their DNA each time the cell replicates; when the telomere becomes completely depleted, cell division cycles may stop, which is part of the aging process.*

◆◆◆

Weight-Bearing Exercise

Weight-bearing, or load-bearing, exercise is exercise you do on your feet that requires you to work against gravity. It is the best type of exercise for building and maintaining bone mass, which is important for preventing bone fractures and the form of bone loss known as osteoporosis. Examples of weight-bearing exercise include aerobics, dancing, gardening, hiking, jogging, stairclimbing, tennis, walking, and weight training. Generally, athletes have a bone density that is 13 percent higher than that of nonathletes. Conversely, complete bed rest leads to serious bone loss.

Bones are living tissues that respond to exercise by becoming stronger, just like muscles. Physical activity early in life helps you develop higher peak bone mass. The more bone mass you have before age 25 to 30, the healthier you will be in later years, when your body gradually loses bone.

As you get older, the benefits of activity for augmenting bone mass are not as great, but doing weight-bearing exercise is still important. A program that builds muscle and improves balance and coordination can generally maintain bone density and help prevent falling, which is a major concern in older people. Falls raise the probability of fracturing a bone in the hip, spine, wrist, or another part of the skeleton. Fractures affect quality of life, result in loss of independence, and can even lead to premature death.

Older adults should engage in at least 30 minutes of moderate physical activity daily and include a mix of weight-bearing exercise, strength training, and balance training. Exercise combined with adequate calcium and vitamin D intake can help reduce age-related bone loss. However, excessive exercise can be bad for bones and especially harmful to joints.

ADDITIONAL FACTS

1. *Certain exercise machines, such as treadmills, stairclimbers, ski machines, and resistance devices, provide some weight-bearing exercise. Bicycling and swimming are not weight-bearing exercises, although they have other health benefits.*

2. *People who already have osteoporosis generally should continue to exercise to preserve bone and strengthen the back and hips. You should avoid high-impact exercise and check with your doctor to determine what kind of exercise is safe.*

3. *Exercise alone can prevent or cure osteoporosis.*

✦✦✦

Edward Jenner and Smallpox

The British scientist Edward Jenner (1749–1823), as a boy in the mid-1700s, reportedly overheard a dairymaid mention that because she'd lived through a case of cowpox, she was safe from the smallpox epidemic ravaging Europe. Today, we have that chance encounter to thank for the eradication of the deadly smallpox virus.

Smallpox probably originated in Africa, spreading to India and then to Europe around AD 700. By the 18th century in Europe, 400,000 people died of smallpox annually, and many survivors went blind or were left with disfiguring scars. The disease was called variola—or small pox, to distinguish the illness from syphilis, which was called "the Great Pox."

Because those who did survive smallpox became immune to later exposure, a procedure called variolation—known today as inoculation—became popular: A sample of body fluid taken from a pustule of someone who was sick with smallpox was injected under the skin of an uninfected person. Although a small percentage of patients developed full-blown smallpox (or another blood-transmitted disease), most came down with only a milder case and survived.

Variolated as a young boy, Edward Jenner grew up to become a renowned biologist in England. He had always been curious about how cowpox could protect against smallpox, and in 1796, he injected pus from the arm of a dairymaid sick with cowpox into an 8-year-old boy. The boy came down with a fever and mild cold, but when Jenner later injected him with smallpox, the boy developed no infection. Jenner called the procedure *vaccination,* a word he coined from the Latin *vaca,* for "cow."

The practice of vaccination spread to most European countries and reached America by 1800, while variolation was phased out. The mid-1900s saw the development of more stable, freeze-dried vaccines, and smallpox was declared extinct worldwide in 1980. Vaccinations work by tricking the immune system into producing immune cells that protect against the real disease-causing organism. Since Jenner's discovery, vaccines for influenza, pneumonia, rabies, meningitis, and other serious conditions have been developed.

ADDITIONAL FACTS

1. *It's now recognized that Benjamin Jesty (1737–1816) was probably the first person to use cowpox to vaccinate against smallpox, performing the procedure on himself and his family in 1774. Jenner gets credit, however, for popularizing the technique throughout the world.*

2. *Jenner was also interested in hot-air balloons, and he built and launched a successful model in 1784.*

3. *Smallpox has been identified as a possible agent of bioterrorism, especially since the September 11, 2001, terrorist attacks. Some doctors have gone so far as to suggest preemptive vaccinations.*

✦✦✦

Chicken Pox

Most of us remember chicken pox as a very itchy rite of passage in childhood. After all, the illness affected about 4 million children a year until 1995. That's when a vaccine for the illness was approved for use in the United States. Although chicken pox is still a common occurrence, the number of cases has plummeted as a result.

Caused by the varicella-zoster virus, chicken pox is spread by coming into close contact with an infected person. Once the virus enters the body, it takes about 2 weeks for it to multiply and spread. The first symptoms include fever, headache, and a cough, followed by those hallmark pink bumps. They turn into fluid-filled blisters and eventually crust over and scab before healing.

In children, chicken pox is a mild—though uncomfortable—condition. In adults, it can be more severe, particularly among pregnant women and those with compromised immune systems. Complications include a bacterial infection of the skin, inflammation of the brain (encephalitis), and pneumonia. What's more, the varicella-zoster virus can remain in the nerve cells and then, years later, reactivate and resurface as shingles, a condition that causes painful blisters. About 10 percent of people who have experienced chicken pox develop shingles.

Today, however, the chicken pox vaccine is administered to all children about the time they turn 1 year old and again between the ages of 4 and 6. Experts say the vaccine is effective 90 percent of the time; if a case does occur in an immunized person, it's extremely mild. Still, some parents are wary of administering the vaccine, preferring to send their children to "pox parties." These gatherings are held purposely to expose children to an already-infected child, in the hope that they'll also come down with a case of chicken pox to build immunity against it.

ADDITIONAL FACTS

1. *Chicken pox gets its name from its trademark bumps, although experts debate how. Some say that it's because the marks resemble chickpeas, which in Latin are called* cicer. *Others say it's because they look like peck marks made by a chicken.*

2. *People over 65 years of age may have severe shingles and should be revaccinated, according to medical authorities.*

✦✦✦

Bronchitis

A tight chest. Hacking cough. Yellowish or greenish phlegm. These symptoms are all telltale signs of bronchitis, an inflammation of the bronchi, the main air passageways that lead to the lungs. When these tubes swell, thick mucus forms inside them, making it difficult for you to breathe. This common condition can be triggered by a number of causes, including viral or bacterial infections and inhalation of cigarette smoke or irritating chemicals.

There are two main types of bronchitis: acute and chronic. Acute bronchitis is the fleeting version, lasting for anywhere from a few days to several weeks. It often comes hand in hand with the viruses and bacteria that cause colds, flu, and strep throat. Most often, it's treated with expectorants, cough suppressants, or a broncho-dilator (a medicine that helps open the air passageways); if bacteria are to blame, a course of antibiotics is in order.

Chronic bronchitis, or a case that lasts longer than 3 months, is a persistent condi-tion. Most frequently, it's due to cigarette smoke or chemical substances that irritate the bronchi. Gastroesophageal reflux disease, or GERD, which causes stomach acids to back up into the esophagus, is another culprit. Although experts estimate that as many as 14 million Americans suffer from chronic bronchitis, about half of those cases go undiagnosed. The illness is treated in much the same way as acute bronchi-tisis.

If you suspect that you have bronchitis, a physician can screen for the disease by using a stethoscope to listen to your breathing. He or she may also request a chest x-ray or a sputum test, which checks for bacteria in your phlegm. Other screenings may be administered to rule out other breathing disorders, such as asthma and emphysema.

ADDITIONAL FACTS

1. *Chronic bronchitis is one form of chronic obstructive pulmonary disease, a cluster of lung problems that make it difficult to breathe.*

2. *Smoking accounts for 80 percent of chronic bronchitis cases.*

✦✦✦

Prozac

Prescribed so commonly that it has become a staple of popular culture, the antidepressant Prozac was introduced in the United States in 1987. The drug was the first selective serotonin reuptake inhibitor (SSRI) on the market, a class of medications that have helped millions of people overcome depression by increasing the amount of serotonin, a chemical that regulates mood, in the brain.

Prozac—along with its generic version, fluoxetine hydrochloride—is used today to treat clinical depression, obsessive-compulsive disorder, bulimia, and panic disorder. Because of its popularity over the past 20 years, Prozac has been the subject of movies and books, including Elizabeth Wurtzel's (1967–) 1994 autobiography *Prozac Nation*. The drug is available by prescription only, and the recommended length of treatment is 6 to 12 months. Patients who stop taking the medication as soon as they start to feel better often see depressive symptoms return.

Side effects of Prozac can include nausea, difficulty sleeping, drowsiness, anxiety, tremors, loss of appetite, or decreased sex drive. These tend to occur early in treatment and go away within a few weeks. A rash can be a sign of a serious medical condition. All antidepressants carry a black box warning about their potential to cause increased suicidal thoughts and actions; patients need to balance this risk and any others associated with the medication against the potential risks of depression itself—which include suicide. Because of these risks, people should be monitored closely while taking any antidepressant.

As with most antidepressants, it can take 4 or more weeks to begin to experience the full benefits of treatment. Not all antidepressants work for all patients, and many people must go through a period of trial and error with different drugs in order to find one that's effective. A 2008 study concluded that no antidepressant is more effective overall than another, although costs and side effects vary. A specific formulation of Prozac called Prozac Weekly is the first antidepressant designed to be taken just once a week. Prozac is also approved for use in children with major depressive disorder or obsessive-compulsive disorder.

ADDITIONAL FACTS

1. *Legal cases have suggested there is a link between antidepressant use and violence. In 1989, a man in Kentucky who had taken Prozac for 4 weeks shot and killed eight people and then himself, resulting in a lawsuit against the manufacturer.*

2. *Other SSRIs include sertraline (Zoloft) and paroxetine (Paxil).*

3. *More than 22.2 million prescriptions for generic formulations of fluoxetine were filled in the United States in 2007, making it the third-most-prescribed antidepressant.*

◆◆◆

Dreaming

"To sleep: perchance to dream: ay, there's the rub"
—William Shakespeare, *Hamlet*

Everyone dreams, and our nightly hallucinations have fascinated artists and poets for millennia. But only recently has science begun to unravel some of the mysteries of dreaming, and oneirologists—reseachers who study dreams—continue to explore the exact role that dreams play in the human mind.

For centuries, dreams were believed to be caused by supernatural forces, and dream sequences appear in many religious traditions. A key event in the scientific understanding of dreams came in 1953, when researchers established that most dreams take place during a phase of sleep called REM, for rapid eye movement.

This link provided a clue to the mental function dreaming may play. REM sleep is associated with learning and memory, and some scientists believe that dreams may be, too. When a person enters REM sleep, the body also temporarily shuts off motion in the limbs. This state enables the brain to dream about activities without directing the body to act them out. There is also activity during this sleep stage in the cerebral cortex, the outer layer of the brain that is responsible for learning, thinking, and organizing information—and where dream story lines are created.

Much is uncertain about dreams, but researchers do know that most last from 5 to 20 minutes, and people with normal sleep cycles usually dream for about 2 hours a night—even if they don't remember it. The brain may incorporate an external stimulus, such as music that is playing or a conversation that's going on in the background, into a dream during REM sleep. Personal experiences from the past day or week also frequently work their way into dreams.

The average person has thousands of dreams every year, and research suggests that most people dream about the same things. In 1966, researchers at Western Reserve University (now Case Western Reserve University) in Cleveland studied reports from people all over the world and compiled a list of the most common themes. Being chased, falling, having one's teeth fall out, experiencing embarrassing moments, enduring the deaths of loved ones, and falling in love with random people are among the top dreams across nations and cultures. Relatively few—10 percent of respondents—dreamed about sex. Other research has claimed that 12 percent of people dream only in black-and-white, although that finding has been debated.

ADDITIONAL FACTS

1. *Paul McCartney (1942–) claimed that the music to the hit Beatles song "Yesterday" came to him during a dream in May 1965.*

2. *Somnambulism—better known as sleepwalking—is a rare, unrelated phenomenon in which people get out of bed, move around, and sometimes talk out loud before returning to sleep.*

3. *Many animals, including rats, dogs, and chimpanzees, are also believed to have dreams.*

◆ ◆ ◆

Sex-Linked Disease

What do calico cat fur, color blindness, and the bleeding disorder hemophilia have in common? These conditions are all results of a gene on the X chromosome. Illnesses caused by this type of genetic blip, passed on through one of the sex chromosomes, are known as sex-linked diseases.

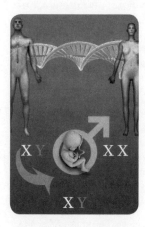

The majority of these diseases, such as Duchenne muscular dystrophy and fragile X syndrome, are the result of an X chromosome gene. As a result, they are much more common in men than in women. That's because women are defined by an XX pair of sex chromosomes, while men have an XY set. In order for a female to have a sex-linked disease, she would have to inherit two affected X chromosomes—one from the mother and one from the father. If only one parent passes down a gene for the disease, the woman becomes a carrier of a recessive gene and can pass it on to her offspring.

Males, on the other hand, have only one X chromosome. If it has the abnormal gene, they get the disease. The Y does not contain nearly as many genes as the X chromosome, so it can't override the recessive gene. However, the Y chromosome does have genetic details about the formation and function of the testes, so it's necessary for development of a normal male body.

ADDITIONAL FACTS

1. *Queen Victoria of England (1837–1901) was a carrier of the sex-linked disease hemophilia, a condition in which the blood does not clot properly. Her great-grandson, Alexei (1904–1918), an heir to the Russian throne, developed the disease. His parents employed the mystic healer Rasputin (1872–1916) to help relieve Alexei's pain and stem the bleeding; the power they yielded to the fame-hungry monk led to the Russian Revolution in 1917.*

2. *Females who are carriers of a sex-linked disease have a normal X chromosome, which usually protects them so that they have no symptoms of the disease they carry. But in rare instances, it's the normal X that is inactivated, and symptoms may occur.*

✦✦✦

Pilates

Pilates is a type of exercise that uses controlled movements to tone and strengthen the body. The exercises may be done with equipment or on a mat on the floor. Pilates improves your flexibility and mental and physical well-being; strengthens your muscles, including those of your core (torso); and increases your circulation. The regimen is also thought to improve your posture, make you less prone to injury, and lead to better overall health.

Pilates' founder, Joseph H. Pilates (1880–1967), was a frail child and took up many sports to grow stronger. As a nurse in World War I, he originally used the techniques of Pilates to rehabilitate immobile patients. He based his exercise methods on yoga and Chinese martial arts, incorporating elements of concentration, precision, control, breathing, and flowing movements.

Pilates is an excellent form of exercise whether you are just beginning an exercise program or you exercise all the time. There are many centers that offer Pilates classes. To avoid injury if you take up Pilates, make sure that you're supervised by a qualified instructor who has completed several hundred hours of training in Pilates techniques and instruction.

Most people beginning a Pilates program focus on the mat exercises, which are designed so that you use your own body weight as resistance. The moves follow a set sequence, with exercises proceeding from one to another in a progression. Pilates machines use resistance to strengthen and tone the body. Pilates does not add muscle bulk.

Beginners should start with basic exercises and build up to advanced moves. It's important to wear comfortable clothing and no shoes, stay focused on combining your breathing and your body motion, and use flowing movements. You can do the exercises quickly to increase your heart rate. Be sure to speak with your doctor before beginning any workout program.

ADDITIONAL FACTS

1. *Pilates has been a favorite of dancers and gymnasts for decades and is now popular among Hollywood actors.*

2. *A Pilates workout has benefits for the cardiovascular system as well as for flexibility and muscle tone.*

◆◆◆

Edinburgh Medical School and Grave Robbers

A major problem facing human anatomy researchers in the early days of medicine was that doctors and students needed human cadavers to dissect and study, but society and religion were opposed to defiling the human body. When sufficient numbers of bodies weren't available in 19th-century Scotland, scientists had to rely on grave robbing—and even murder.

In the 1700s and early 1800s, Parliament allowed only the bodies of executed criminals to be donated to science, creating a shortage of supplies for the professors and students at the elite Edinburgh Medical School. Doctors and medical researchers asked Parliament to pass an Anatomy Act, that would allow scientists access to the unclaimed remains of people who died in poorhouses and hospitals, but the idea was hotly disputed by the lower class and by the Roman Catholic Church. So instead, scientists turned to a shadowy network of grave robbers that developed across Britain to fill the demand for corpses. These "resurrection men" ransacked graveyards for recently interred bodies and sold them to doctors who turned a blind eye to their provenance. A body might fetch £7, an enormous sum in the early 19th century. The invasion of the body snatchers became so bad that some cemeteries posted sentries or built walls to keep out the thieves.

Two workmen in Edinburgh, William Burke (1792–1829) and William Hare (1792–1870), took the business model a step further. Grasping the enormous profits to be made selling cadavers, the men decided to forgo grave robbing in favor of murder: They operated boardinghouses in town, where they lured poor people, vagrants, and prostitutes who wouldn't be missed—at least not by anyone important. To prevent the doctors who bought the corpses from growing suspicious, Burke and Hare suffocated their victims so there would be no visible injuries or signs of foul play.

It's suspected that the pair killed between 16 and 30 people before being arrested in 1828. Hare testified against Burke and was freed, while Burke was hanged in January 1829, in front of 25,000 people. His body was donated to medicine for dissection, and his skeleton remains on display at the University of Edinburgh's Medical School Museum.

ADDITIONAL FACTS

1. *It was suspected that the head of the Edinburgh Medical School, Robert Knox (1791–1862), was a knowing accomplice in the plot. A popular street song of the day includes the lines "Burke's the butcher, Hare's the thief, Knox the boy who buys the beef."*

2. *Two slang terms coined around this time were* Burking, *meaning "murdering," and* Burkophobia, *referring to the public's hysteria and paranoia that a murderer lurked around every corner.*

3. *In New York City around the same time, grave robbing for the benefit of medical schools was also rampant. Public outcry was strong, leading to occasional street riots when citizens feared that bodies of family members had been stolen.*

◆◆◆

German Measles

Back when America was still a British colony and the candle was the primary lighting fixture, a German physician named Daniel Sennert (1572–1637) noticed a red rash on some of his few patients. He named it *röteln,* or rubella, from a Latin word meaning "red." More than 2 centuries later, German researchers shed more light on the illness, distinguishing it from the more serious version of measles, which also causes a red rash. That's how rubella came to be known as the German measles.

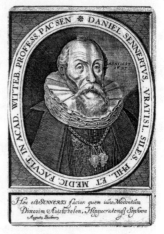

Also called 3-day measles, rubella is a virus that's spread by inhaling the respiratory secretions, such as a cough or sneeze, from an infected person. Symptoms, such as a mild fever, headache, red eyes, and stuffy nose, usually appear about 2 weeks after infection. The telltale sign is a fine pink rash that starts on the face and spreads to the torso, arms, and legs; it lasts for about 3 days. Roughly three out of four adult women who contract German measles experience arthritis-like symptoms in their fingers, wrists, and knees for a month. In rare instances, the virus can lead to an infection of the ear or, more dangerously, the brain.

Because the rubella infection is mild and often requires no treatment, experts believed that it was harmless. But in 1941, an Australian physician discovered that the virus can attack a pregnant woman's fetus, resulting in birth defects, deafness, cataracts, and growth retardation. Fortunately, a vaccine for the virus was developed in 1969. This measles, mumps, and rubella, or MMR, inoculation is given to all children at 12 to 15 months of age, and then again to girls between 4 and 6 years old in an effort to protect future pregnancies. Because of the vaccine, the Centers for Disease Control and Prevention says that rubella has been nearly eliminated in the United States.

ADDITIONAL FACTS

1. *About half of countries worldwide use the rubella vaccine.*

2. *In 1999, there was a rubella outbreak of 12 cases in Arkansas.*

3. *Rubella is contagious about a week before the rash develops, and then for 1 to 2 weeks after it disappears.*

◆◆◆

Meningitis

If you've ever knocked your head into an overhead lamp or doorway, you have the meninges to thank for protecting your brain. This three-layer membrane surrounds the brain and spinal cord. But when the meninges and the cerebrospinal fluid that cushions the brain become infected and inflamed, it can trigger a potentially life-threatening condition called meningitis.

Although viruses, fungi, and protozoa can all cause the infection that brings on meningitis, bacterial meningitis is the most dangerous. Because these cases are contagious and are easily spread in close quarters, such as college dormitories, they often grab newspaper headlines and other media attention. The most common culprits are strains called *Streptococcus pneumoniae* (pneumococcus) and *Neisseria meningitidis* (meningococcus).

One reason why bacterial meningitis is such a threat is because symptoms often come on rapidly—and can be lethal within a few hours. As the bacteria begin to multiply in the bloodstream, the earliest signs are a fever and possibly a rash. When bacteria infect the meninges, inflammation and pus thicken the cerebrospinal fluid, leading to vomiting, severe headache, and a stiffening of the neck. If the fluid blocks a ventricle, it can pool and create harmful pressure in the brain. This can result in coma or even death.

Most forms of viral meningitis, on the other hand, are rarely fatal and usually clear up in about 2 weeks. Symptoms include a rash, a sore throat, joint aches and pains, and a splitting headache. Physicians test for meningitis with a throat culture, chest x-ray, and spinal tap to analyze the cerebrospinal fluid. If a case of bacterial meningitis is diagnosed, it is treated with antibiotics or, rarely, by procedures to drain any accumulation of fluid in the brain.

ADDITIONAL FACTS

1. *Before antibiotics were invented, half of bacterial meningitis cases were deadly.*

2. *The word* meninges *is derived from the Greek word* meninx, *which means "membrane."*

3. *Although meningitis can develop at any time, bacterial types are more likely to occur during the winter, and viral cases are more common in summer.*

✦✦✦

Valium

Easily recognized as a little white pill with a trademark *V,* Valium (along with its generic version, diazepam) has been one of the most frequently prescribed medications in the world for the past half century. The first blockbuster benzo-diazepine medication, Valium proved a safer, stronger, and more effective treat-ment for anxiety disorders than similar drugs in the 1960s, and it is still widely used today.

Benzodiazepines are quieting medications that slow down the central nervous sys-tem and affect chemicals in the brain that may become unbalanced and cause panic, insomnia, or anxiety. Valium was the second such drug to be invented by the Hoffmann–La Roche pharmaceutical company and, once approved in 1963, it quickly outsold its weaker, less effective predecessor. Diazepam was the top-selling pharmaceutical in the United States from 1969 to 1982, with peak sales of 2.3 billion tablets in 1978. In contrast to narcotics and barbiturates, Valium is much less dan-gerous, and relatively few deaths have been attributed to Valium alone.

However, Valium can be abused, and it is habit forming. Prescriptions tapered off as awareness of the drug's dangers grew, although it is still widely prescribed. Benzo-diazepines are also frequently prescribed for insomnia, although a newer class of drugs called nonbenzodiazepines—which tend to cause fewer side effects and less of a hungover feeling in the morning—have become the recommended first line of treatment for sleep-related problems.

Valium may also be used to treat agitation, shakiness, and hallucinations during alcohol withdrawal; to relax patients before surgery; and to relieve certain types of muscle pain. Alcohol and other sedative medications should not be used at the same time as Valium, and people with glaucoma, asthma, or other breathing problems; kidney or liver disease; or a history of depression or drug addiction may need a dos-age adjustment to safely take Valium. Accidental falls are common in older people who take Valium because they may feel the drug's effects more strongly.

ADDITIONAL FACTS

1. *According to the World Health Organization, diazepam is an "essential drug," necessary to meet the needs of a basic health care system.*

2. *Neurologists have begun prescribing diazepam for the treatment of certain types of epilepsy and for a rare disorder called stiff person syndrome.*

3. *Valium has earned the nicknames Executive Excedrin, for its popularity among corporate types, and Mother's Little Helper—after the 1966 Rolling Stones song—for its use by harried middle-class house-wives.*

◆◆◆

Cerebral Angiogram

When doctors suspect a stroke or damage to the arteries in a person's brain has occured, they may perform an MRI or CT scan. Sometimes, a magnetic resonance angiogram (MRA) can make the diagnosis when a CT scan or MRI does not. However, even an MRA may not be specific and may show only that there is an abnormality. If imaging detects an abnormality, the next step in diagnosing the problem is to do a cerebral angiogram, in which dye is injected into the bloodstream so x-rays can determine the flow and shape of the brain's vessels.

Arteries are not normally seen in an x-ray, so a special material called contrast dye is injected into one or both of the carotid arteries—the major blood vessels on either side of your trachea, where you can feel your pulse. The process is monitored by a fluoroscope, a special x-ray that sends the images to a TV monitor.

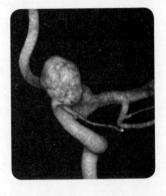

The contrast dye is injected into an artery in the groin or neck through a catheter, which is a piece of thin, soft tubing. Periodically a saline solution containing heparin, a blood thinner, is flushed through the catheter to prevent blood from clotting while the dye moves through the bloodstream. X-rays are taken, with the bones and tissues being filtered out by specialized computer software, leaving a picture of just the vessels and any abnormalities, such as leaks or ruptures where blood might be spilling out into other areas. These pictures can help doctors pinpoint a problem in the brain or evaluate the arteries of the head and neck before surgery.

The entire procedure takes 1 to 3 hours, and the patient must rest for 6 to 8 hours after the test. If no complications arise, the patient can leave the hospital the same day.

ADDITIONAL FACTS

1. *Patients remain conscious during a cerebral angiogram, and a nurse may occasionally ask questions or request that the patient do simple tasks in order to monitor how he or she is feeling.*

2. *There is a slight sensation of pressure as the catheter moves through the artery and a hot, rushing feeling as the dye is injected.*

◆◆◆

Fragile X Syndrome

Every human being possesses more than 20,000 genes, the DNA instructions for our own individual blueprint. Each of them plays a crucial role in our formation, and any malfunction in that sequence can have major consequences. Case in point: A single misstep on the X chromosome is the most common cause of inherited mental retardation, also known as fragile X syndrome. This genetic disorder, which affects 1 in 4,000 males and 1 in 6,000 females, can cause developmental delays, learning disabilities, and speech and behavioral problems. Physical symptoms are subtle and include a long, narrow face and large ears.

The genetic smoking gun for the syndrome was first discovered in 1991 by three March of Dimes researchers, who named it FMR1 (fragile X mental retardation-1). The gene, which is located on a long arm of the X chromosome, may repeat in what's called a permutation. But if this duplication occurs too many times, the gene shuts off completely. As a result, it doesn't make the protein that it's assigned to produce; scientists believe that this specific protein regulates communication between the nerve cells in the brain.

Because the FMR1 gene is located on the X chromosome, it's easier for men, who have only one X chromosome, to be affected. Women must get two of the genes, one from each parent, in order to develop the syndrome. If a female inherits only one FMR1 gene, she becomes a carrier and can pass the condition on to her child. (About 1 in 259 women are carriers.) Blood tests that screen for the gene can diagnose fragile X syndrome.

ADDITIONAL FACTS

1. *Fragile X syndrome is the cause of about 5 percent of autism cases.*

2. *Females with the syndrome usually have milder symptoms than men.*

3. *People with fragile X syndrome may be more sensitive to light, sounds, touch, and textures.*

❖❖❖

Stretching

Stretching is the process of extending the length of the muscles in your body. It is an important part of any exercise program because it increases your flexibility. Greater flexibility improves your daily performance, making all activities easier and less tiring. Stretching also reduces injuries, increases the range of motion of the joints, relaxes tense muscles, corrects exercise posture, and leads to better coordination.

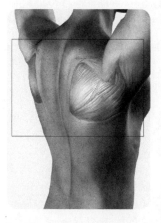

It's beneficial to stretch your muscles before you work out, but only if you have warmed up first for at least 5 to 10 minutes. Warming up should consist of light aerobic exercise, usually a lower-intensity version of the movements you do during the rest of your workout. Stretching cold muscles can lead to pulled or torn muscles. You should also stretch after your workout. If you stretch only afterward, you should increase the intensity of your exercise more slowly than if you had stretched early in the workout.

It's important to do your stretching properly. Stretching should not hurt. If it does hurt, you should relax your muscles or alter your position to the point where the stretch is comfortable. Do not bounce during stretching. Hold each stretch for 10 to 30 seconds, and do each stretch two or three times. Remember to breathe. Stretch both sides of your body equally.

You should target all the major muscle groups, including the calves, thighs, hips, lower back, shoulders, and neck. If you play a particular sport or engage in a specific type of exercise, do stretches that are designed to target the muscles used in those activities. For example, if you play tennis, be sure to stretch your arm muscles.

ADDITIONAL FACTS

1. *You should discuss stretching with your doctor or physical therapist if you have an injury or a chronic condition. Under those circumstances, typical stretches may cause further harm, and an altered approach may be necessary.*

2. *Certain types of massage, such as Japanese shiatsu, utilize stretching techniques.*

3. *Tai chi (from China) and yoga (from India) employ stretching as a form of exercise in itself.*

◆◆◆

Chloroform

"What a blessing she has chloroform," Queen Victoria (1819–1901) is rumored to have said in 1859, when her oldest daughter gave birth with the help of the popular anesthetic; the Queen herself had used chloroform, years earlier. But while chloroform saved many patients a great deal of pain over the years, it also caused much death and suffering during its controversial history.

Chloroform was first prepared in 1831 by the American chemist Samuel Guthrie (1782–1848), who was attempting to create an inexpensive pesticide by mixing whiskey with chlorinated lime. The mysterious chemical—estimated to be 40 times sweeter than table sugar—became known as Guthrie's sweet whiskey. In 1847, the Scottish physician Sir James Young Simpson (1811–1870) began using a chloroform solution to induce unconsciousness before surgery. Chloroform was nonflammable and put people to sleep relatively quickly, both advantages that allowed it to replace ether as the most commonly used anesthetic.

Doctors noted that the effects of chloroform were divided into five stages, depending on the dose or the length of time spent inhaling it:

1. The patient became insensible but retained consciousness.
2. The patient entered a lethargic state in which some pain could be felt.
3. The patient was physically incapable and could feel no pain.
4. The patient exhibited stertorous breathing and complete muscle relaxation.
5. The patient suffered an often fatal paralysis of the chest muscles.

Stage 3 was recommended for most surgical procedures—but the amount of chloroform required to send a patient from stage 3 to stage 5 was very small. Fatalities soon began to occur, along with liver damage and other permanent health problems from "delayed chloroform poisoning." In 1911, Alfred Goodman Levy (1866–1954) proved in animal experiments that chloroform caused cardiac fibrillation, an irregular heart rhythm. But even with its dangers, chloroform became a popular form of anesthesia in Europe and, with lesser enthusiasm, in America. Between 1865 and 1920, chloroform was used in 80 to 95 percent of all anesthesia procedures performed in English- and German-speaking European countries, even though it greatly increased the mortality rate. With the introduction of safer and easier gas anesthesia, which used agents such as nitrous oxide, the use of chloroform declined in the 1930s.

ADDITIONAL FACTS

1. *Today, chloroform is regarded as a possible cause of cancer.*

2. *Chlorinated tap water often contains small traces of chloroform.*

3. *Women in the late 1800s used chloroform for labor, although physicians heavily debated the safety of this practice. Childbirth was a natural phenomenon, they reasoned, and many assumed that pain was a necessary part of the process.*

✦✦✦

Measles

It used to be that everyone came down with a case of measles sometime during his or her life. Some 90 percent of the American population suffered through a bout of the virus, also called rubeola, by the time they celebrated their 15th birthdays. But that all changed in 1963, when the measles vaccine was invented. Cases of the illness in the United States have dwindled from between 3 million and 4 million a year to a paltry 60 or so.

The measles virus is spread through close contact and is highly contagious. The virus first multiplies in the throat and lungs and then spreads throughout the body. At first, a sufferer experiences inflamed eyes, a cough, a mild fever, a sore throat, and a runny nose. About 2 days later, the fever spikes as high as 104°F and tiny white spots with bluish centers, called Koplik's spots, appear on the inside of the mouth. A red, slightly itchy rash also spreads over the body. These symptoms last for about a week and disappear on their own.

Measles can be serious and life threatening, especially in young children. Across the globe, nearly 1 million people die of the illness every year, because measles can lead to dehydration, bronchitis, pneumonia, and encephalitis (an inflammation of the brain). Due to the severity of the condition, experts recommend that all children receive a measles, mumps, and rubella, or MMR, vaccination. The first is administered to all children at 12 to 15 months of age, and the second to girls between the ages of 4 and 6.

ADDITIONAL FACTS

1. *In the 10th century, the Persian physician Rhazes (860–932) declared measles more dreaded than smallpox.*

2. *Koplik's spots are named after the American pediatrician Henry Koplik (1859–1927), who discovered them.*

3. *Each year, there are 30 million to 40 million cases of measles around the globe.*

◆◆◆

Tuberculosis

At the age of 5, Robert Koch (1843–1910) announced to his astonished parents that he had taught himself to read with the newspaper. This was the first sign of the young German boy's precocious nature. Koch later went on to become a renowned physician and scientist. In 1882, he presented a lecture on the discovery of the bacterium *Mycobacterium tuberculosis,* the cause of the disease tuberculosis (TB). The audience sat stunned—and, one by one, went to look at the stained slides as evidence.

M. tuberculosis is spread when someone with the disease coughs, speaks, or sneezes, diffusing microscopic droplets in the air. TB is fairly difficult to contract; in most cases, long-term contact with an infected person, such as a family member, is required. About a month after infection, the body's immune system kicks in and surrounds the bacteria in the lungs. This can lead to latent TB, which isn't contagious and won't cause symptoms. In fact, although one-third of the world's population has come in contact with the TB bacterium, 90 percent have this harmless form of the disease or have walled it off to a point where the bacteria die from lack of nutrients.

For the other group of sufferers, TB can be deadly. When the immune system fails, the TB bacteria attack the lungs and enter the bloodstream, through which the organisms can spread to other areas of the body. Symptoms include a cough lasting more than 3 weeks, bloody phlegm, chest pain, fever, chills, and weight loss. This active form of TB is contagious.

Physicians screen for the infection with the Mantoux test, in which a small amount of a substance called PPD tuberculin is injected into the skin. If a raised bump appears in 2 days, a TB infection is likely. Both the latent and the active forms of TB are treated with medication to destroy the bacteria. Because TB bacteria grow slowly, the course of medication usually lasts for 6 months to a year.

ADDITIONAL FACTS

1. *The Greek physician Hippocrates (c. 460–c. 377 BC) said something that contradicts the oath named in his honor, which binds physicians to treat anyone in need of medical attention. He warned his colleagues against seeing patients with late-stage phthisis (tuberculosis), as the patients' inevitable deaths would stain the doctors' reputations as physicians.*

2. *Worldwide, someone is infected with* M. tuberculosis *every second.*

◆◆◆

Effexor

Although selective serotonin reuptake inhibitors (SSRIs) such as Prozac are a common treatment for depression, not every patient finds relief with them. Often people who don't respond to these medications can be helped with another class of drugs called serotonin-norepinephrine reuptake inhibitors (SNRIs), such as Effexor.

Prescribed for major depression and anxiety disorders, Effexor, whose generic form is venlafaxine, was first released in 1993. Because of significant side effects and suspicions that the drug may increase the risk of suicide, however, it is not recommended as a first-line treatment. It is currently available in standard and extended-release capsule formulas.

Like other SNRIs, Effexor works by blocking the transporter proteins that are supposed to take serotonin and norepinephrine—key neurotransmitters that affect mood—out of the brain and back to their storage vesicles. Because these drugs have also been shown to increase the availability of dopamine, they are sometimes called serotonin-norepinephrine-dopamine reuptake inhibitors.

It usually takes about 3 to 4 weeks for a patient to feel the effects of Effexor and other SNRIs. The half-life of Effexor is relatively short, so patients are advised to adhere to a strict medication routine, taking usually two or three pills a day; missing even one dose can result in withdrawal symptoms. Side effects of Effexor can include high blood pressure, increased heart rate, and increased eye pressure. In addition, patients can develop a potentially fatal syndrome if they take Effexor around the same time they've taken other medications or substances that affect serotonin—migraine drugs, other antidepressants, or St. John's wort, for example. Patients should not begin taking Effexor within 14 days of stopping treatment with any drug known as an MAO—or monoamine oxidase—inhibitor.

Effexor is in the phenethylamine class of chemicals, which includes amphetamine and methamphetamine. It can have stimulatory effects and can cause weight loss in patients with depression and anxiety disorder. Other patients find Effexor highly sedating.

ADDITIONAL FACTS

1. *Effexor is often prescribed off-label—for uses that have not been specifically approved by the Food and Drug Administration—to treat a wide variety of other conditions, including migraines, muscle weakness in narcoleptics, and hot flashes.*

2. *At dosages higher than the recommended maximum of 375 milligrams per day, venlafaxine has been shown to cause memory loss.*

3. *Effexor is perhaps one of the most likely antidepressants to trigger manic states—which include feelings of euphoria and risky behavior—in patients with undiagnosed bipolar disorder.*

❖❖❖

Spinal Tap

To obtain samples of cerebrospinal fluid (CSF), the substance that surrounds the brain and spine, doctors perform a procedure called a lumbar puncture, better known as a spinal tap. The test involves inserting a needle into the space between two vertebrae of the lower back and into the CSF-filled space surrounding the spinal cord and withdrawing fluid for testing. To avoid injuring the spinal cord, the patient must lie still, in a fetal position, during the half-hour procedure. Although often uncomfortable, spinal taps are rarely as painful as they sound, and they provide important information that helps doctors detect a variety of serious diseases.

Lumbar punctures are performed to diagnose meningitis, an infection of the membrane that surrounds the brain. They can also be used to test for neurological disorders such as multiple sclerosis, neurosyphilis, or a type of neuropathy called Guillain-Barré syndrome. A local anesthetic is used, although mild discomfort or pain may still occur.

CSF is usually clear, so a cloudy or colored sample can indicate infection, bleeding, or a buildup of protein or cells. Higher-than-normal CSF pressure may result from increased pressure within the skull; low CSF pressure may be a sign of shock, fainting, or a diabetic coma.

Basic results from a lumbar puncture are available within an hour of the test, but bacteria cultures generally take about 2 days for analysis.

In many cases, doctors will recommend that patients lie down after a spinal tap. Headaches occur in 5 to 10 percent of patients, while bleeding or infections after the procedure occur rarely. However, the test is more risky for people who take blood thinners or are particularly susceptible to infection.

ADDITIONAL FACTS

1. *The lumbar puncture procedure was brought to the United States by the Harvard Medical School professor Arthur Wentworth. His career was nearly destroyed when he was prosecuted (although he was later acquitted) for having obtained spinal fluid from children.*

2. *During a procedure called a myelogram, dye is injected into the CSF and then x-rays or CT scans are performed.*

3. *Syphilis involving the brain is usually diagnosed by performing a lumbar puncture and testing the CSF.*

◆◆◆

Krafft-Ebing

When it comes to sex, the German neuropsychiatrist Richard Baron von Krafft-Ebing (1840–1902) wrote the book—literally. In 1886, he published *Psychopathia Sexualis,* a groundbreaking study of sexual deviance. Intending the work as a reference for physicians and forensic scientists, Krafft-Ebing documented the most sordid details in Latin to discourage lay readers. Still, the book became commercially popular, going on to publish 12 editions.

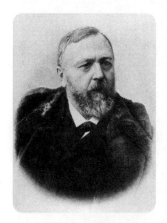

In his work, Krafft-Ebing detailed 45 case studies of sexual aberrations ranging from impotence to necrophilia and grouped them into three categories: hyperaesthesia (an abnormally exaggerated sexual instinct), anaesthesia (an absence of sexual instinct), and paraesthesia (perversion of the sexual instinct). In describing the patients, Krafft-Ebing introduced to the general public numerous terms that have lasted until today, such as *heterosexual, homosexual,* and *fetishism.* He also coined the words *sadism,* after the libertine French author Marquis de Sade (1740–1814), and *masochism,* after the Austrian novelist Leopold von Sacher-Masoch (1836–1895), whose characters often gained sexual pleasure from experiencing pain and humiliation.

Besides introducing society to these titillating topics, *Psychopathia Sexualis* also established a connection between sexuality and biology. Although the main line of thinking at the time was that sexual deviance was due to insanity or the devil's work, Krafft-Ebing suggested that sexual behavior was governed by the brain and spine and that genetics played a role.

Beyond the study of sex, Krafft-Ebing made many contributions to the field of psychiatry. He popularized forensics and hypnosis, among other disciplines. Krafft-Ebing also made psychiatric treatments more palatable to the middle and upper classes, by founding a suburban sanatorium for the "nervous."

ADDITIONAL FACTS

1. *At the age of 32, Krafft-Ebing became a professor of psychology at the Universities of Strasbourg in France.*

2. *The famed psychologist Carl Jung (1875–1961) was near the end of his studies in archaeology when he read* Psychopathia Sexualis, *which inspired him to switch to psychology.*

3. *Krafft-Ebing earned a medical degree from the University of Heidelberg in Germany.*

◆◆◆

Yoga

Yoga is a lifestyle practice whose main goal is to train your mind, body, and breathing. This helps you relax and manage stress and anxiety. Yoga includes physical exercise, but movement is just one component of this lifestyle philosophy.

Yoga began more than 3,000 years ago in India. The word *yoga* is Sanskrit and means to "yoke," or unite, the mind, body, and spirit. Traditionally, yoga students are required to adhere to a strict regimen of behavior, diet, and meditation. However, you do not have to strictly follow yoga in order to derive some of its stress-reducing benefits.

The physical part of yoga is called hatha yoga. It focuses on poses, which are often named after animals. When practicing hatha yoga, a person goes through a series of poses while controlling his or her breathing.

Yoga is easy to learn and does not require any equipment. In addition to being relaxing, it tones your body, stretches your muscles, and strengthens your cardiovascular system. There are many different types of hatha yoga. In the United States, the fast-paced form known as Vinyasa, or power, yoga is very popular. Other types of hatha yoga include Bikram yoga, which is practiced in rooms that have been heated above 100°F, and gentle yoga, which is performed at a much slower pace.

Yoga classes are offered at many centers and feature instruction in poses, breathing, meditation, and, in some cases, chanting. There are classes for people of all abilities. You should speak with your doctor before starting any exercise program.

In a typical hatha yoga class, you will learn 10 to 30 poses, ranging from easy to hard. For example, the easier Corpse Pose involves lying on the floor while completely relaxed. There are also very difficult poses that take years of practice to master.

ADDITIONAL FACTS

1. *Before taking a yoga class, you should make sure that the instructor is certified and has had at least 200 hours of training in yoga techniques.*

2. *To practice yoga, you should dress comfortably. You do not need shoes, as yoga is done barefoot.*

◆◆◆

Semmelweis and Childbed Fever

The "savior of mothers," as Ignaz Semmelweis (1818–1865) is often called, was a Hungarian physician who drastically reduced the death rate in 19th-century Austrian birth clinics by implementing a simple procedure: hand washing.

In 1844, Semmelweis was put in charge of a teaching hospital in Vienna that had two maternity wards—one attended by midwives and one attended by doctors and medical students. He noticed that the mortality rate of women in the midwife clinic was much lower than in the physician clinic, about 2 percent versus 16 percent, and that most of the deaths resulted from a mysterious sepsis (infection) known as puerperal fever, or childbed fever. When he requested that the staffs of the two wards be switched, he determined that it was the personnel, not the wards themselves, that were associated with the high mortality rates. Women who gave birth at home, he noticed, also had a much lower risk of developing childbed fever.

While all birth attendants followed the same routine, Semmelweis did recognize one difference: The physicians and students also performed daily autopsies on women who had died the day before, the medics often traveling directly between cadavers and women in labor and seldom washing their hands. In 1847, a fellow professor at the hospital cut his hand during an autopsy and subsequently died of a condition resembling childbed fever. Semmelweis determined that it must have been the same illness—which was clearly contagious, being transmitted from dead women's bodies to living women's exposed genital areas (and to this one unfortunate doctor) via the physicians' hands.

Semmelweis experimented with various cleansing agents and mandated that all birth attendants wash their hands in a chlorinated lime solution before each vaginal examination. The mortality rate fell to less than 3 percent almost immediately, but his theories were widely rejected and he was ridiculed by a society that did not believe that disease could be caused by germs. By the end of the 19th century, however, germ theory had been proven by Louis Pasteur (1822–1895), and the need for antibacterial agents during childbirth was well appreciated. Today it is understood that most childbed fever was caused by *Streptococcus*, bacteria introduced into the genital tract during delivery.

ADDITIONAL FACTS

1. *After the medical community dismissed Semmelweis's observations, he wrote a series of angry and embittered letters to his former professors and colleagues, accusing them of being "medical Neros" and "murderers."*

2. *It is rumored that Semmelweis became mentally ill in his later years. He died in a psychiatric institution in Vienna, ironically from what was rumored to be sepsis from a self-inflicted wound.*

3. *Ancient Hindu and Greek texts offered advice on hygiene for birth attendants, and the Hippocratic Corpus mentioned childbed fever. But no physician before Semmelweis seemed to grasp the true cause.*

◆◆◆

Mumps

Whenever a delicious dessert makes your mouth water, your salivary glands are at work. The largest of these glands, called the parotids, are located between your ears and your upper jaw. When the parotid glands become infected with the mumps virus, they swell, giving the illness its telltale symptom of chipmunk cheeks.

Named for an old word meaning either "lump" or "mumble," mumps is spread through infected saliva by inhaling a sneeze or sharing utensils or beverages. In 15 percent of cases, there are no signs. But, for the unlucky majority, symptoms appear about 2 to 3 weeks after infection; they include a fever, headache, fatigue, loss of appetite, swollen salivary glands, and pain when chewing or swallowing. Although most people fully recover within 2 weeks, mumps can lead to potentially dangerous complications. If the virus spreads, it can cause encephalitis (inflammation of the brain) and even hearing loss. Other complications include orchitis (inflammation of the testicles) in men, oophoritis (inflammation of the ovaries) in women, and miscarriage in pregnant women.

Although the majority of cases occur in children younger than 15, young adults who get mumps are at serious risk for sterility. Thanks to the invention of the mumps vaccine in 1967, the average number of people affected by mumps each year has dwindled from 200,000 to less than 1,000. Still, outbreaks of the disease occur: In 2006, more than 1,100 people in the Midwest were infected with the virus.

ADDITIONAL FACTS

1. *According to Irish lore, rubbing the head of a child with mumps against the back of a pig could cause the illness to transfer to the animal and cure the child.*

2. *The mumps vaccine, a series of two inoculations, is usually given in combination with those for measles and rubella.*

✦✦✦

Shingles

For the vast majority of us, chicken pox is a once-in-a-lifetime occurrence. But for roughly 1 million unlucky people, it can resurface as a painful skin rash called shingles, also known as herpes zoster.

When you get infected with chicken pox, the virus—varicella-zoster—never completely leaves the body, even after you heal. It lies dormant in nerve cells for years and even decades until, for reasons experts aren't exactly sure of, it reactivates. People age 50 or older or those with compromised immune systems, such as those with cancer or AIDS, are most vulnerable.

The virus travels across nerve pathways to the skin, where it manifests as reddish bumps. Because shingles follows the nerve, this rash usually appears on only one side of the body, in the area of a skin nerve. After a few days, it develops into fluid-filled blisters and may be accompanied by fever, chills, nausea, and diarrhea. Although the blisters break open and crust over every week, a case of shingles can last for a few weeks. In some 15 percent of cases, pain can linger for 1 to 3 months, a condition called postherpetic neuralgia.

Shingles typically goes away on its own, but a physician can prescribe antiviral medication to speed recovery and pain relievers and anti-inflammatory drugs to ease the pain. If the condition spreads to the eye, it can leave scars that can damage vision and lead to glaucoma.

ADDITIONAL FACTS

1. *In Italy, shingles is called Saint Anthony's fire* (fuoco di Sant'Antonio).

2. *In 2006, a vaccine to prevent shingles was introduced on the market. Two years later, the Centers for Disease Control and Prevention recommended that all people ages 60 and older receive the vaccine.*

◆◆◆

Epinephrine

Some people have serious allergies to things that don't bother other people: A bee sting or a bite of shellfish, for example, can cause people allergic to them to have trouble breathing and even die. But a drug known as epinephrine, or adrenaline, which mimics natural fight-or-flight hormones in the body, may be used to open airways and treat sudden allergic reactions.

Delivered by injection, epinephrine jump-starts the heart and relaxes airway muscles. It can also help treat the anaphylactic shock, wheezing, shortness of breath, and swollen or closed lungs that result from allergic reactions. In addition, it tightens blood vessels, which raises dangerously low blood pressure. Epinephrine is also used to treat people who go into cardiac arrest.

People who suffer severe allergic reactions often carry prefilled, single-use, automatic epinephrine injection devices with them (brand names include EpiPen and Twinject) that can be stuck into the thigh if a reaction occurs. After injecting themselves, people should go to the hospital and avoid physical activity. Injections can cause side effects such as upset stomach, sweating, dizziness, weakness, paleness, headache, and uncontrollable shaking.

Epinephrine may also be prescribed as a liquid eyedrop formula to treat glaucoma or administered during eye surgery to reduce pressure in the vessels around the eyes. These eyedrops may cause temporarily blurred or decreased vision, stinging or irritated eyes, and headache. Symptoms of too much medicine being absorbed into the body include fast or irregular heartbeat, faintness, increased swelling, paleness, and trembling.

People with asthma, diabetes, eye disease, heart or blood vessel disease, high blood pressure, sulfite allergies, or an overactive thyroid may not be able to take epinephrine.

ADDITIONAL FACTS

1. *Both the Latin word* ad *and the Greek word* epi *mean "near" or "around." The Latin* ren *and Greek* nephros *both mean "kidney." Thus we have the adrenal gland, which sits on top of the kidney and secretes epinephrine.*

2. *The term* adrenaline junkie *is often used to describe someone who seems to be addicted to thrilling or stressful behavior that releases natural adrenaline, such as extreme sports and risk taking.*

3. *For as many as 35 percent of people, a single dose from an EpiPen is not enough to stop a severe allergic reaction, and they may require a second injection.*

✦✦✦

Psychiatrists and Psychologists

When someone experiences mental or emotional distress and feels he needs professional help, he may visit a psychiatrist or psychologist. Both types of doctors can provide counseling and coping solutions for problems such as family tension, workplace stress, substance abuse, rehabilitation from a brain injury, or mental illness. The main difference between the two is that psychiatrists can prescribe medications, while most psychologists cannot.

Psychiatrists are licensed physicians (MDs) and often achieve board certification in neurology and psychiatry. They may have trained less in talk therapy and counseling sessions, instead focusing on the biological causes of and solutions for behavioral issues—such as chemical imbalances and pharmaceuticals. As medical doctors, psychiatrists can order or perform the full range of physical and mental tests that might be needed to evaluate a patient and can prescribe medication or medical procedures, such as electroconvulsive therapy, if needed. There are numerous specialties within psychiatry focusing, for example, on children, substance abuse, and geriatric psychology.

Psychologists, on the other hand, hold doctoral degrees (PhD, PsyD, or EdD) but are not medical physicians. They may be licensed in two ways: Clinical psychologists deal directly with patients in hospitals, private practice, or educational or community settings, while research psychologists conduct experiments on the physical, cognitive, or social aspects of human behavior, often in university or government laboratories. While psychologists are required to know the basics of human biology, their approach tends to focus on holistic treatments that include questioning, observing, and talking through problems with their patients. Psychologists are typically focused on behavior—including the effects of medication on behavior—so they often collaborate with medical doctors who do prescribe drugs. Psychologists may also choose to work as consultants or researchers in the industrial, sports, law, or school sectors, evaluating programs and suggesting more efficient ways to organize and execute goals.

ADDITIONAL FACTS

1. *Appropriately trained psychologists in Louisiana, New Mexico, and certain government health care settings can legally prescribe medications.*

2. *The number of years of education and training is different for psychiatrists than for psychologists: 6 to 7 years, following an undergraduate degree, for psychiatrists, versus 3 to 4 for psychologists.*

3. *There are about 42,000 psychiatrists and 166,000 psychologists in the United States. Counseling sessions are gradually becoming more affordable for the general public as employee healthcare programs begin to recognize the need for mental health coverage.*

◆◆◆

Libido

In the simplest terms, libido is sexual desire. But although the definition is fairly easy to grasp, the inner workings of this drive are less tangible and far more complex.

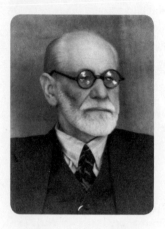

In psychology, there are a few prevalent theories about what, exactly, libido is. The founder of psychoanalysis, Sigmund Freud (1856–1939), originally coined the term. He believed that a human's libido was the driving force of existence. He theorized that in each individual there is a struggle between three functions: The ego drives the achievement of libidinous desires in a socially acceptable way, the superego internalizes social behaviors and can cause a person to feel shame or guilt about their sexual urges, and the id is the libido and aggression in its rawest form. Later, the psychologist Carl Jung (1875–1961) viewed the libido in a more general sense, as psychic energy.

In addition to this pondering, scientists bring up another point: They say that the libido is influenced by the combination of sex hormones, such as testosterone and estrogen, and mental state. Stress, depression, and other emotions can hamper libido, and some prescription drugs, such alcohol and antianxiety pills, can do the same.

ADDITIONAL FACTS

1. *The antonym of* libido *is* destrudo, *which, in Freudian psychology, is the destructive impulse.*

2. *The term* obsolagnium *describes a waning sexual desire due to age. But many experts argue that the cause isn't physical; rather, many older adults stop seeing themselves as sexual beings.*

3. *Low libido affects about 15 percent of men and 30 percent of women.*

◆◆◆

Heart-Healthy Diet

A heart-healthy diet will reduce your blood cholesterol and decrease your risk of coronary artery disease, heart attack, and stroke. Maintaining a heart-healthy diet calls for limiting unhealthy fats and cholesterol, selecting low-fat protein sources, increasing the amounts of fruits and vegetables you eat, choosing products made from whole grains rather than refined flour, reducing your salt intake, and limiting yourself to moderate portion sizes. People who create meal plans ahead of time and incorporate these concepts are the most successful at sticking to a heart-healthy diet.

The most important step you can take toward achieving heart healthy nutrition is to limit how much saturated and trans fats you eat. Saturated fats should make up less than 10 percent of your daily calories, trans fats should account for less than 1 percent, and cholesterol should be limited to less than 300 milligrams daily if you are a healthy adult and less than 200 milligrams a day if you have high cholesterol. You should limit the quantity of solid fats in your diet, such as butter, margarine, and shortening, and use low-fat substitutions. When you do use fats, choose monounsaturated fats, such as canola oil and olive oil. The polyunsaturated fats found in avocados, nuts, olives, and seeds are also good choices for a heart-healthy diet. However, all fats should be eaten in moderation.

When you look for low-fat protein sources, your best options are fish, lean meats, and skinless poultry; low-fat dairy products; and egg whites or egg substitutes. Certain types of fish, such as herring, mackerel, and salmon, are particularly heart healthy because they have high amounts of omega-3 fatty acids, which can lower blood fats. Legumes such as beans, lentils, and peas, as well as soy protein, are also good sources of protein.

ADDITIONAL FACTS

1. *To reduce fat and cholesterol, eat no more than 6 ounces (cooked) of meat, poultry, or fish daily. Make sure you eat fish at least twice a week.*

2. *To lower your salt intake, do not use table salt and do pay attention to the nutrition labels of packaged foods to check their sodium content.*

◆ ◆ ◆

Louis Pasteur and Pasteurization

Virtually all the milk and cheese you buy in grocery stores today has undergone a sterilization process called pasteurization, which kills germs and makes dairy products safe to eat. This process was developed by the French microbiologist Louis Pasteur (1822–1895), who was instrumental in proving where germs come from and what they do.

Trained as a chemist, Pasteur went to work in 1854 researching solutions for the production problems of French manufacturers of alcoholic drinks. He invented pasteurization—the process of heating and then cooling liquids to kill bacteria—as a way of preventing wine and beer from going sour, an invaluable discovery for France's brewers and vintners. Pasteur also did much to disprove the ancient theory of spontaneous generation. In a famous experiment, he monitored soup in three groups of flasks: one that was open to the air, another that was sealed tightly with cotton, and a third that was fitted with a swan-necked spout that kept air out. Only the soup in the swan-necked flask was unexposed to air and did not grow bacteria, proving that microbes must be introduced from the environment.

Applying pasteurization to dairy products sharply reduced foodborne illnesses in France. Before the advent of pasteurization, many diseases were transmitted through raw milk. Straight from the cow may seem like the best way to drink milk, but in fact bacteria from within an animal's body can make people fatally ill. Animals also collect foreign organisms on and around their udders, and these organisms end up in raw milk as well.

Traditionally, the process of pasteurization involved heating milk to a temperature just short of a boil and keeping it there long enough to ensure that the bacteria were dead. Commercial cartons of milk today, however, are usually heated to 285°F for 1 to 2 seconds in a process called ultrahigh-temperature pasteurization. This method of treating dairy products has the added benefit of extending the amount of time before they will spoil in the fridge.

Some people today claim that unpasteurized milk is healthier and better tasting, but scientists warn against the danger of foodborne illnesses caused by pathogens such as *Escherichia coli, Listeria,* and *Salmonella.* It is illegal to sell raw milk across state lines and in more than 20 states.

ADDITIONAL FACTS

1. *Pasteur saved a troubled silk industry in southern France—where silkworms were dying at an alarming rate—by identifying parasitic infections among the silkworms and advocating that only disease-free eggs should be selected.*

2. *Pasteur also enhanced the practice of vaccination by helping to explain the causes of anthrax, cholera, smallpox, and tuberculosis and developing a vaccine for rabies.*

3. *Milk today goes through another process called homogenization, which prevents it from separating into fat-free milk and full-fat cream. The procedure breaks up molecules of fat into such small particles that they remain suspended throughout the liquid and create a smooth, uniform texture.*

◆ ◆ ◆

Fifth Disease

About half of people worldwide have been infected with parvovirus B19, but the majority of them don't realize it because of its mild symptoms. Parvovirus is better known as fifth disease, because it's the fifth in a group of childhood illnesses that causes similar rashes: measles, rubella (German measles), chicken pox, and roseola (exanthem subitum).

Most common in the late winter and early spring, fifth disease is spread like a cold— by touching infected surfaces or breathing in the germs. At first, the sickness may seem like a cold, causing a fever, headache, fatigue, slightly upset stomach, and stuffy or runny nose. But after about a week, a bright red rash appears on both cheeks. (That's why fifth disease is also called slapped cheek disease.) After another few days, the rash can spread to the arms, torso, buttocks, and thighs and take on a pink, weblike appearance. This rash may come and go for up to 3 weeks, but the virus usually goes away on its own without medical intervention.

Although fifth disease is generally thought of as a childhood ailment, it can affect adults who haven't already experienced it; but after an initial exposure, a person has lifetime immunity. In adults, parvovirus can lead to joint pain, especially in the hands, wrists, knees, and ankles. Moms-to-be should pay close attention; a small percentage of women, particularly those infected during the first trimester of pregnancy, have babies with serious complications as a result of the virus. The most common problem is fetal anemia, which can cause congestive heart failure in a newborn. As a result, doctors closely monitor the fetuses of women infected with parvovirus.

ADDITIONAL FACTS

1. *Parvovirus B19 is also called erythema infectiosum.*

2. *Parvovirus can infect pets, particularly dogs, but that's not the same strain as parvovirus B19. The latter virus can't be spread from animals to humans.*

3. *People with sickle-cell disease or those with weakened immune systems, such as chemotherapy patients, may experience complications due to fifth disease.*

◆◆◆

Leukemia

The majority of the blood cells that circulate through the body are grown in the bone marrow, the soft tissue that lies inside bones. Since blood cells live for only a few days to 3 months, the marrow generates billions of blood cells every day. But when the bone marrow produces cancerous white blood cells that don't function properly, the condition is called leukemia. Since these cells don't die when they normally should, they crowd out healthy blood cells and prevent them from fighting infection throughout the body.

Every year, some 40,000 Americans develop this cancer of the bone marrow and blood, and it takes the lives of 21,000. How dangerous the disease is depends on whether it's the chronic type, which spreads slowly, or the acute variety, which worsens rapidly. The categories of leukemia are further divided by which types of cells they affect: Lymphocytic (or lymphoid) leukemias involve cells that grow into B or T cells, while myeloid leukemias alter the cells that develop into red blood cells, platelets, or several types of white blood cells. Acute myeloid (or myelogenous) leukemia is the most common form that affects both children and adults, while the acute lymphocytic type accounts for 75 percent of childhood leukemias. People with chronic lymphocytic and myeloid forms can have the disease for years before they experience symptoms.

Symptoms of leukemia include fever, chills, fatigue, swollen lymph nodes, weight loss, and bone pain, among others. Physicians screen for leukemia by testing the blood cells and bone marrow for cancerous cells. Treatments for the disease include chemotherapy, radiation therapy, and bone marrow or stem cell transplants. Because of scientific advances, 5-year survival rates for the disease have quadrupled over the past 5 decades. In the early 1960s, a person had a 14 percent chance of living 5 years after a diagnosis; today, the odds are about 51 percent.

ADDITIONAL FACTS

1. *Being exposed to radiation or certain toxic chemicals, smoking cigarettes, or having a family history of the disease raises the risk of leukemia.*

2. *The ancient Chinese, Greeks, and Romans all treated leukemia with arsenic. Researchers today believe that the poison may actually have some benefit against the disease by inducing the death of the cancerous cells.*

❖❖❖

Anticholinergics and Acetylcholine

The brain and nerves release a chemical neurotransmitter called acetylcholine, which helps regulate muscle movement, sweat gland function, and intestinal function. Medications that block this chemical are called anticholinergics. Because they relax muscles and open up airways, anticholinergics are used to treat stomach cramps and irritable bowel syndrome, uncontrollable movements and muscle spasms, asthma and other breathing disorders, and urinary incontinence.

When used for the treatment of asthma or chronic obstructive pulmonary disease often called COPD, the muscle-relaxing properties of anticholinergics open up the pathways to the lungs, making it easier to breath. There are both long- and short-acting anticholinergics, which can be delivered by either an inhaler or a nebulizer.

Anticholinergics (also called antispasmodics) are sometimes used to prevent nausea or vomiting or are given by injection before surgery to help relax patients and decrease saliva secretion. During an operation, they can be used to keep the heartbeat normal.

Anticholinergics were the first medications approved for the treatment of Parkinson's disease, a condition caused in part by lower-than-normal dopamine levels in the brain. They are used to block nerve impulses and help control the muscles of the limbs and the rest of the body, as well as to decrease levels of acetylcholine so that they achieve a closer balance with dopamine levels.

Other commonly used anticholinergics include atropine, belladonna, dicyclomine, and scopolamine. Side effects of any anticholinergic medication can include fast or irregular heartbeat, dry nose and mouth, constipation, decreased sweating and increased body temperature, blurred vision, dizziness, and drowsiness.

ADDITIONAL FACTS

1. *Acetylcholine was the first neurotransmitter identified. It was discovered in 1914 and was originally named vagusstoff because it was released from the vagus nerve.*

2. *A 2008 study found that the use of anticholinergic drugs is associated with a more rapid decline in cognitive performance in older adults.*

3. *Many drugs that are not specifically advertised or described as anticholinergics do in fact have milder anticholinergic properties. These include drugs such as warfarin, furosemide, hydrochlorothiazide, and ranitidine.*

❖❖❖

Hydrocephalus

An excessive accumulation of fluid in the brain is known as hydrocephalus or hydrocephaly, from the Greek words *hydro* (meaning "water") and *cephalus* (meaning "head"). The term is something of a misnomer, however, since the fluid in question is not actually water, as was once believed, but a combination of brain chemicals called cerebrospinal fluid. The brain needs cerebrospinal fluid, but too much of it can cause brain swelling, illness, blurred vision, and disorientation.

Normally, the fluid in the skull keeps the brain buoyant, serves as a shock-absorbing cushion, delivers nutrients, and carries away wastes. The fluid is produced continuously, so any condition that blocks absorption back into the bloodstream will result in overaccumulation in the ventricles. Babies can be born with a congenital form of hydrocephalus, of which the most telling sign is a rapidly expanding head circumference. Other types of hydrocephalus can be acquired at any age as a result of head trauma, infection, a complication of surgery, and other, unknown reasons. When a person's skull cannot expand to accommodate the fluid buildup, symptoms such as nausea, vomiting, drowsiness, irritability, or coordination problems occur.

Hydrocephalus is diagnosed through ultrasonography, CT scans, or MRIs. The most common treatment involves inserting a shunt with an adjustable valve into the brain's ventricles, which diverts the flow of fluid down into the abdomen or chest, where it can be absorbed into the bloodstream. These shunts aren't perfect; they typically require regular monitoring to correct over- or underdrainage. Proper treatment, however, can often help patients recover completely and lead normal lives with few limitations.

ADDITIONAL FACTS

1. *Normal pressure hydrocephalus, a condition most common in elderly people, is sometimes misdiagnosed as untreatable Alzheimer's disease or dementia. Symptoms include disorientation and clumsiness, memory loss, urinary incontinence, and a shuffling gait.*

2. *One of the most common causes of hydrocephalus is aqueductal stenosis, a narrowing of the aqueduct of Sylvius—a small passage between the third and fourth ventricles, in the middle of the brain.*

3. *In 2007, French scientists discussed the remarkable case of a 44-year-old man with hydrocephalus whose brain had been reduced to little more than a thin sheet of tissue due to the buildup of fluid in his skull. Doctors were amazed that the married father of two, who was examined after reporting weakness in his left leg, still had an IQ of 75 and led a normal life, despite having so little brain tissue left.*

4. *One or 2 of every 1,000 babies is born with hydrocephalus, making the condition as common as Down syndrome and more common than spina bifida or brain tumors.*

◆◆◆

Orgasm

Orgasms vary from person to person, but they all have one thing in common: They are sudden, pleasurable discharges of sexual tension that result in muscular contractions in the genital region. The effects are felt throughout the entire body as muscles contract, heart rate speeds up, brain wave patterns shift, and pupils dilate.

Although the end result is pretty similar, men and women are stimulated in different ways. In men, stimulation of nerve endings on the penis—particularly the glans, or tip—leads to ejaculation. During orgasm, nerves going to the prostate trigger the ejaculation. This feeling of enjoyment, say evolutionary biologists, is a built-in reward system that promotes human reproduction. (However, it *is* possible for a man to have an orgasm without ejaculation, and ejaculation may occur without orgasm by direct stimulation of the prostatic nerves.)

In women, stimulation of nerves in the clitoris, the nipples, and possibly the labia minora and the G-spot (an area on the front wall of the vagina that's the female prostate gland) builds up to orgasm. Signals are transmitted to an area of the brain called the hypothalamus, which then secretes a hormone called oxytocin. It's spread to the blood, brain, and spinal cord, triggering those pleasurable feelings and muscle contractions. Unlike in men, female orgasms don't play a role in reproduction. This may explain why some 30 percent of women report rarely experiencing an orgasm during sex. However, it's physically possible for women to experience more than one orgasm during sexual intercourse. In both men and women, the brain participates, and the orgasm is often described as a reflex.

Along with the enjoyable effects, orgasms may also help protect health. Studies show that orgasms can lower stress levels, improve sleep quality, and, in men, reduce the risk of prostate cancer.

ADDITIONAL FACTS

1. *A woman named Xaviera Hollander (1943–), author of* The Happy Hooker, *reportedly experienced an orgasm when a police officer placed a hand on her shoulder.*

2. *In French, orgasms are described as* la petite mort, *or "the little death."*

3. *Until the 1930s, doctors stimulated orgasms in women to treat "hysteria." This clinical procedure was called a medical massage.*

✦✦✦

Mediterranean Diet

A Mediterranean diet is generally rich in olive oil, grains, fruits, nuts, vegetables, and fish. It also includes a moderate amount of red wine and restricts meats, high-fat dairy products, and other types of alcohol. It is called a Mediterranean diet because these are the general dietary patterns of the 16 countries that border the Mediterranean Sea. People who follow a Mediterranean diet consume less saturated fat and more fiber than do people who eat an average American diet. Research has shown that people who maintained a Mediterranean-style diet lost more weight over a 2-year period than people who followed either a high-protein or a low-fat diet.

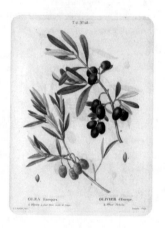

However, the Mediterranean diet still contains a high percentage of calories from fat, which contributes to a growing problem of obesity in Mediterranean countries. The good news is that the majority of these calories come from monounsaturated fats, the kind found in olive oil. This is a better option for fat intake, since monounsaturated fats do not raise cholesterol as much as saturated fats (from animal products) do. As a result, the occurrence of heart disease in Mediterranean countries is lower than in the United States. There is also evidence that eating a Mediterranean diet may reduce your risk of cancer, Parkinson's disease, and Alzheimer's disease. Further studies are needed to determine whether the Mediterranean diet leads to a lower number of deaths from heart disease.

ADDITIONAL FACTS

1. *The American Heart Association currently recommends that most people consume 25 to 35 percent of their calories from fat, whether or not they are trying to lose weight. Saturated fats, found in meat products and tropical oils, should be limited to 7 percent of your daily calories, and trans fat, found in commercially baked goods, should make up no more than 1 percent of your daily calorie intake.*

2. *People who have heart disease should minimize their consumption of foods high in saturated or trans fats.*

◆◆◆

Gregor Mendel and Genetics

The "Father of Genetics," Gregor Mendel (1822–1884), is responsible for our understanding of hereditary traits such as green eyes and brown hair. By cross-breeding plants that had different traits, he discovered the basic laws of genetics still observed today.

Mendel was a Czech priest and biology professor at the University of Vienna. Through his experiments with pea pod plants, he discovered guidelines about how hereditary traits pass from one generation to another. Mendel's law of segregation states that the sex cells of a plant may contain two different traits, but not both of those traits—a plant can have white flowers or purple flowers, but not both. His law of independent assortment (later known as Mendel's law of inheritance) states that characteristics are inherited independently of each other—some people with blond hair have blue eyes, but not all people with blond hair have blue eyes. He also ascertained that each inherited characteristic is determined by two hereditary factors (known today as alleles), one from each parent. These factors decide whether a trait is dominant or recessive—or, in other words, whether it will be expressed visibly.

Between 1856 and 1863, Mendel worked in an experimental garden, breeding different combinations of pea pod plants and carefully recording the outcomes. He worked with seven characteristics: plant height, pod shape and color, seed shape and color, and flower position and color. His results showed that when a yellow pea and a green pea were bred together, for example, their offspring plant was always yellow—but in the next generation, green peas appeared in a ratio of one to three. He determined that green was a recessive trait and yellow a dominant one, meaning that green plants could occur only when an offspring received a green trait from *each* parent, not from just one.

Mendel published his research in 1866, but it wasn't until 1900, after his death, that his work was rediscovered and his findings built upon. William Bateson (1861–1926), a British geneticist who followed up on Mendel's previous work, coined the terms *gene, genetics,* and *allele* in the early 1900s. In the next several decades, thanks to Mendel's early research, genes and chromosomes were better defined.

ADDITIONAL FACTS

1. *The rediscovery of Mendel's work led to the descriptions of genotype (the set of genes an organism carries) and phenotype (an organism's observable characteristics, influenced both by the genotype and by the environment).*

2. *The terms* homozygous *and* heterozygous *were later coined to describe genes that, respectively, contained two of the same alleles (two yellow dominant traits or two green recessives, for example) or one of each (such as one green recessive and one yellow dominant).*

3. *In the 1950s, Arthur Kornberg (1918–2007) and Severo Ochoa (1905–1993) described DNA, the molecule of which genes are made, and James Watson (1928–) and Francis Crick (1916–2004) showed that DNA's structure was a double helix.*

4. *Humans and chimpanzees share 98 percent of their genes.*

✦ ✦ ✦

Chills

Chills are the feeling of cold—often accompanied by shivering or paleness—that comes after exposure to frigid temperatures or during a viral or bacterial infection. In an effort to generate heat in the body, the muscles contract and relax rapidly, sometimes causing visible shaking.

When someone comes down with an infection, the body often combats it by raising core temperature. This fever resets the internal thermostat in the hypothalamus, a control center of sorts that resides in the middle of the base of the brain. In response to this resetting of its temperature, the body automatically reacts with a number of mechanisms. The autonomic nervous system is triggered to release stress hormones, which often causes sweating. Since it is primarily the brain that's causing the chill, a scary situation or a strong emotion may set off a chill as well. When the chill is accompanied by a cold sweat and hair standing on end, it results from this activation of the autonomic nervous system. What's more, the hypothalamus resets the hunger hormones, so you experience a dip in appetite. That's why children often don't feel hungry when they're sick.

If your child experiences a chill due to sickness, try to monitor his or her body temperature, and consult your doctor if the child is feverish. A dose of over-the-counter acetaminophen or ibuprofen can help lower a fever. Chills are sometimes associated with more serious illnesses, such as malaria, infections of the bloodstream, leukemia, and cancerous tumors called lymphomas.

ADDITIONAL FACT

1. *In ancient Chinese medicine, herbalists prescribed ginger to "warm up" organs, thereby treating the chills.*

✦✦✦

Hodgkin's Disease

The British physician Thomas Hodgkin's life (1798–1866) is the stuff that movies are made of: Born a Quaker, he was forbidden by his religion from marrying his love, a first cousin. He pursued a career in medicine, introducing the stethoscope to England and working as a professor of medicine. In his later years, he embarked on a second career studying geography and philosophy, traveling through the Middle East. But despite all these dramas and accomplishments, Hodgkin is best known for identifying a type of cancer in the lymphatic system, a part of the immune system.

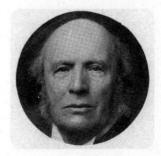

This network of vessels and nodes stores and produces white blood cells; the tonsils, thymus, bone marrow, and spleen are also parts of the lymphatic system. When certain white blood cells called B cells mutate and become cancerous, that's called Hodgkin's lymphoma, or Hodgkin's disease. The other types of lymphoma, which are more common, are known as non-Hodgkin's lymphoma. The symptoms and diagnostic testing procedures are similar for all of them, but the prognosis is much better for Hodgkin's disease.

Symptoms include swelling of the lymph nodes, fever, fatigue, weight loss, and itching. Depending on the severity of the disease, treatments include radiation and chemotherapy. If the cancer has spread throughout the body, a bone marrow transplant may be required. Each year, some 8,000 Americans develop non-Hodgkin's lymphoma, and 1,350 die of it. If caught early enough, the disease can be cured.

ADDITIONAL FACTS

1. *Abnormal, cancerous B cells are known as Reed-Sternberg cells, named after the two scientists who discovered them.*

2. *Men, people between the ages of 15 and 40 or over the age of 55, and those who have had illnesses caused by the Epstein-Barr virus, such as mononucleosis, are more likely to develop Hodgkin's disease.*

❖❖❖

Nexium

Used to treat heartburn, Nexium (esomeprazole) is one of the mostly commonly prescribed treatments for the irritating disorder also known as acid reflux or gastroesophageal reflux disease (GERD). The drug treats symptoms of the disease and also helps reverse damage that may have been caused when stomach acid rose into the throat.

Heartburn occurs when acid from the stomach travels up the esophagus, the pipeline that brings food from the mouth down into the stomach. Over the long term, the presence of stomach acid in the esophagus can produce more serious diseases.

Marketed as the "healing purple pill," Nexium has been prescribed more than 147 million times since it was approved by the Food and Drug Administration in 2001. It is available in delayed-release capsule form and is usually taken once a day for 4 to 8 weeks to relieve persistent heartburn and to prevent or heal damage to the esophagus.

Esomeprazole, the active ingredient in Nexium, works by turning off the acid-producing pumps in the stomach. The drug may be prescribed (sometimes along with antibiotics) to prevent ulcer formation caused by infection with *Helicobacter pylori* bacteria or by the use of nonsteroidal anti-inflammatory drugs. Possible side effects include headache, diarrhea, and abdominal pain. Confusion, drowsiness, fast heartbeat, seizures, and blurred vision may be signs of an overdose. Some medications, such as Reyataz (atazanavir), Valium (diazepam), blood thinners, and iron supplements, may interact with Nexium and may require a dosage adjustment or special tests during treatment.

Nexium is chemically very similar to Prilosec, a heartburn drug that became an over-the-counter medication in 2001 when its manufacturer's exclusivity patent expired. Prilosec's active ingredient, omeprazole, is a combination of esomeprazole and romeprazole molecules. Independent studies have shown that both molecules convert to the same ingredient in the stomach and that there is little difference between the two drugs, and critics have suggested that the maker of both medications, AstraZeneca, introduced Nexium solely to reap more profits following the expiration of Prilosec's patent.

ADDITIONAL FACTS

1. *Nexium capsules can either be swallowed whole or broken open and mixed into food or consumed through a feeding tube.*

2. *Esomeprazole is also used for long-term treatment of conditions (such as Zollinger-Ellison syndrome) in which the stomach makes too much acid.*

◆◆◆

Epilepsy

Epilepsy is a disorder in which clusters of brain cells send out the wrong electrical signals, causing people to have recurring seizures. About 2.3 million people in the United States, or just under 1 percent of the population, have some form of epilepsy.

The causes of epilepsy are unknown in many cases, although some triggers include illness, high fever, brain injury, chemical imbalance, and abnormal brain development.

During an epileptic seizure, people may feel strange sensations and emotions, exhibit unusual behaviors, lose consciousness or appear to be in a trancelike state, or have violent muscle spasms. A seizure can last from a few seconds to a few minutes, and people may recover right away or remain dazed and sleepy for some time afterward.

While there is no cure, epilepsy sometimes goes away on its own. When it doesn't, antiseizure medications can control symptoms, and surgery or implanted devices such as nerve stimulators may help treat severe cases. A meal plan called the ketogenic diet, which calls for high fat, low carbohydrate food, may help some children with epilepsy.

Epilepsy often takes an emotional toll on its victims, especially children who may suffer from taunting and bullying as a result of seizures at school. Additionally, epilepsy can impose unwanted limits on adults with the disorder, who are, for instance, denied driver's licenses in some states. But, in about 80 percent of cases, epilepsy can be treated and people with the disorder can lead normal lives, holding the same jobs and performing the same tasks as anyone else.

ADDITIONAL FACTS

1. *Though epilepsy itself is not life threatening, people with epilepsy are at higher-than-normal risk of drowning, status epilepticus (30 minutes or more of uninterrupted seizure), and sudden death with no obvious medical explanation.*

2. *Before having a seizure, some people experience warning sensations—a perceived change in sound, light, or temperature, for example—called an aura. The African folk singer Vusi Mahlasela (1965–) described his aura as a smell of bananas: "Whenever I smelt that, I'd just sit down wherever I was until the blackness came," he once said.*

3. *Scientists are currently experimenting with treatments by transplanting fetal pig neurons into the brains of epilepsy patients to learn whether stem cell transplants might help control seizures.*

✦ ✦ ✦

Priapism

Today, many farmers place a straw-stuffed scarecrow in their fields to guard their crops. But in ancient Rome, the figure of choice was Priapus, the god of virility and animal and vegetable fertility. He was represented as a misshapen character of a man—a gnomelike frame with an enormous phallus. It's after this figure that priapism, a condition involving an erection lasting at least 4 hours and up to a few days, is named. But unlike the comical deity, priapism is no laughing matter: The condition is painful and, if not treated promptly, can lead to permanent scarring or erectile dysfunction.

During a normal erection, the penis fills with blood, which drains back into the body after orgasm. But in priapism, which isn't associated with sexual desire or orgasm, blood becomes trapped in the erectile tissue of the penis. (The tip of the penis remains soft.) In many cases, narcotics, such as cocaine, or prescription drugs, such as antidepressants, antianxiety pills, blood thinners, and erectile dysfunction treatments, are the culprit. Other causes include sickle-cell disease, blood clots, tumors, or spinal cord injuries. And in a few instances, there is simply no discernible reason.

There are two types of priapism. The most common is ischemic, or low flow, in which bloodflow is impaired or obstructed. This form usually goes away on its own; ice packs and compression can help alleviate it. But in about 10 percent of cases, the erection is triggered by a ruptured artery or an injury to the penis, called nonischemic, or high-flow, priapism. A medical emergency, this type of priapism is treated by draining the blood, injecting the penis with an agent that reduces bloodflow, or performing surgery.

ADDITIONAL FACTS

1. *Priapism most often affects males between the ages of 5 and 10, and 20 and 50.*

2. *More than 40 percent of men with sickle-cell disease experience priapism at some point.*

3. *In rare cases, black widow spider bites and carbon monoxide poisoning can also cause priapism.*

❖❖❖

Fiber

Dietary fiber is an important component of a healthy diet. It is recommended that men under the age of 50 eat at least 38 grams of fiber daily and women under 50 eat at least 25 grams daily. Fiber is found in beans, fruits, nuts, vegetables, and whole grains.

Even though your body cannot digest it, fiber has many health benefits. Foods that are high in fiber add bulk, making you feel full faster, which helps with weight control. Fiber also aids in digestion and the absorption of nutrients. Additionally, high-fiber foods can help with treating constipation, hemorrhoids, diverticulitis (inflammation of pouches in the digestive tract), and irritable bowel syndrome. There is also evidence that high-fiber foods help lower your cholesterol and reduce your risk of coronary heart disease, type 2 diabetes, and some kinds of cancers.

You can increase the fiber in your diet by eating at least 2 cups of fruit and 2½ cups of vegetables daily, replacing refined white bread with whole grain breads, and eating brown rice instead of white. Additionally, check nutrition information labels for the amounts of dietary fiber in store-bought products and aim for 5 grams of fiber per serving. You can also add ¼ cup of wheat bran to foods such as applesauce, cooked cereal, or meat loaf.

When you add fiber to your diet, you should increase it gradually to avoid gas, bloating, and cramps. Try making one change to your diet at a time and then waiting at least several days to implement another change. Additionally, you need to drink more fluids when you increase the amount of fiber you eat, as liquids help your body process fiber. Aim for eight glasses of water or unsweetened beverages daily.

ADDITIONAL FACTS

1. *There is no evidence that fiber supplements are harmful.*

2. *Doctors frequently recommend high-fiber diets for people with digestive disorders such as irritable bowel syndrome or chronic constipation.*

3. *You should consult your doctor before taking fiber supplements, as they can alter the absorption of medications and may have other undesirable effects, such as bloating.*

❖ ❖ ❖

Lister and Antisepsis

For as long as mankind has performed surgery, there have been methods of preventing infection and promoting healing. Ancient civilizations used vinegar and wine to dress wounds, iodine became popular in France, and hand washing was instituted in Austrian maternity wards in the 1800s. But it was the British surgeon Joseph Lister (1827–1912) who made antiseptic practices standard in operating rooms throughout the Western world.

When Lister became chair of surgery at Glasgow University in Scotland, survival rates from operations were abysmal. From reading the works of Louis Pasteur (1822–1895), Lister knew that gangrene—the rotting of organic tissue—was the result of airborne bacteria entering an open wound. He also knew that carbolic acid was effective in reducing infection among cattle on farms fertilized with raw sewage, so he experimented with it as a wound covering. He began dressing surgery sites in carbolic-soaked fabric, spraying the operating room with a carbolic mist, and rinsing his hands with the solution before operating. His postsurgery mortality rates plummeted.

Grim outcomes during the Franco-Prussian War of 1870 further drove home the importance of antisepsis: More than half of the French soldiers who had limbs amputated eventually died of gangrene or fever. Lister's methods began to spread to other countries. In Munich, one surgeon reduced the rate of infection in his ward from four out of five patients in 1872 to zero in 1875. Many doctors continued to deny the existence of microscopic bacteria, however, and argued that a clean operating room was all they needed. The pioneering surgeon William Halsted (1852–1922) adopted the technique but was forced to operate in the garden of New York City's Bellevue Hospital because his colleagues complained about carbolic fumes.

Newer ways to reduce infection—such as face masks, surgical gowns, sterilization with heat, and the elimination of large operating theaters—were gaining in popularity, however, while criticism of the irritating carbolic spray mounted. Though "Listerism" succeeded in hammering home the importance of antisepsis during surgery, the practice was largely abandoned by 1900.

ADDITIONAL FACTS

1. *Among the many honors he acquired in his lifetime, Lister became Lord Lister of Lyme Regis in 1897 when he was made a baron by Queen Victoria (1819–1901). He has also been immortalized as the namesake for the mouthwash Listerine—though he played no role in its invention.*

2. *To help spray his operating room with carbolic acid, Lister developed a "donkey engine," a 3-foot-high, steam-driven pump that vaporized the liquid.*

3. *Lister's father, Joseph Jackson Lister (1786–1869), was a well-known optical researcher and played an important role in perfecting complex microscopes by eliminating chromatic and spherical aberration.*

◆◆◆

Fever

A fever, or uptick in a person's internal thermostat, is one of the ways the body fights off infection and illness. Researchers believe that this warming may help destroy bacteria and viruses that are sensitive to temperature changes. Most of the time, fevers go away on their own within a few days.

The hypothalamus, a section of the brain located in the middle of the brain's base, controls the body's temperature. It's normally set at around 98.6°F, although it tends to be a degree lower in the morning and higher in the afternoon. But when viruses or bacteria invade the body, the hypothalamus resets the baseline at a higher number, such as 102°F. As a result, you may experience sweating, chills, muscle aches, and a loss of appetite as the body attempts to cool itself. The old wives' tale stating "feed a cold, starve a fever" is untrue. The body requires calories to fight off an infection; experts recommend trying to keep up normal food intake and replenishing fluid levels by drinking plenty of liquids. A sunburn or heat exhaustion may also trigger a fever.

Although they make us feel miserable, fevers aren't usually dangerous in adolescents unless they're higher than 103°F. In young children and infants, however, even a mild fever may indicate a serious infection; you should call a physician if a baby or young child has one. To check for a fever, you can use a thermometer inserted into the mouth, armpit, or rectum. (Armpit, forehead, and mouth readings are typically about 1 degree lower than a temperature taken in the rectum.) Ask your doctor for advice about when to call and what to do.

Drinking plenty of fluids and taking a lukewarm sponge bath may provide some relief from a fever. Although a cold bath may seem tempting, by lowering the skin temperature, it can actually cause a fever to rise. To help lower a fever, acetaminophen or ibuprofen is often effective. But avoid giving aspirin to children, as it can cause Reye's syndrome, a rare but serious condition.

ADDITIONAL FACTS

1. *The Italian astronomer and physicist Galileo (1564–1642) invented a water thermometer in 1593. In 1714, Daniel Gabriel Fahrenheit (1686–1736) made the first mercury thermometer.*

2. *A much-lower-than-normal temperature may indicate neurological impairment, severe bacterial infection, or a suppressed immune system.*

◆ ◆ ◆

Colon Cancer

In many ways, the colon is the body's trash compactor. This 5-foot-long, muscular organ, also called the large intestine, absorbs water from food and readies waste for elimination through a final 6-inch stretch called the rectum. The colon is also the third-most-common site for cancer to take hold: Cancers of the colon or rectum (called colorectal cancer) strike 1 in 20 people, with more than 155,000 new cases in the United States every year.

Like all other tissues, colon cells constantly grow and divide in an orderly fashion to replace old and worn-out cells. But in some cases, this process can veer off track, and cells can multiply even when new ones aren't necessary. This unchecked growth most commonly develops into a polyp, a tissue mass attached to the intestinal lining. Once a polyp forms, it often takes several years for these irregular cells to mutate and become cancerous. In its later stages, the cancer can spread to other organs in the body and to the lymph nodes; as a result, colorectal cancer is the second-most-frequent cause of cancer death (after lung cancer).

Fortunately, if caught early on, colorectal cancers are highly treatable with surgery. For more advanced cancers, chemotherapy is necessary. Symptoms of the disease include abdominal pain, bloody stools, fatigue, and unexplained weight loss. To diagnose colorectal cancer, physicians can administer a stool test and perform a barium enema, which uses an x-ray to screen for polyps or cancerous growths. A colonoscopy, in which a physician inserts a flexible tube attached to tiny camera to examine the inside of the colon, is recommended every 10 years starting at age 50. The television news anchor Katie Couric (1957–), whose husband died of colon cancer, publicized this routine screening in a *Today* show segment in 2000. In the months after the segment aired, the number of colonoscopies jumped by more than 20 percent—something experts dubbed the Katie Couric effect.

ADDITIONAL FACTS

1. *As with most other cancers, lifestyle changes can lower the risk of developing colon cancer. Research shows that eating a diet high in whole grains, fruits, and vegetables and low in saturated fats slashes the risk of the disease.*

2. *Scientists have uncovered cancers in the remains of dinosaurs that lived more than 200 million years ago.*

3. *The first successful surgery for colon cancer was performed in 1829 by the Parisian surgeon Jacques Lisfranc (1790–1847).*

◆◆◆

Endorphins

Released when the body encounters stress or pain, endorphins are a natural brain chemical that can provide a "rush" of pleasure similar to that experienced with opioid drug use. Endorphin rushes are often reported by athletes after long, intense exercise sessions or in the wake of a physical injury.

The discovery of endorphins dates to the 1970s, when researchers were puzzled to discover that the brain had a special set of receptors that responded to opiate drugs like morphine. They thought it was odd that brains from all over the world were equipped to deal with a drug originally found only in the Middle East. The existence of the receptors provided a clue that the body manufactured its own natural painkillers. These chemicals, sometimes known as endogenous opioids, were soon discovered in the body.

Unlike opioids, the body's natural endorphins are not addicting—at least not physically. The chemicals are short-lived and disappear before the body can develop any form of dependency on them. Additionally, people feel no withdrawal symptoms when endorphins aren't produced.

Some people claim to be addicted to endorphins, however, in the form of a "runner's high" achieved during prolonged, intense running. The idea of runner's high had been hypothesized for years, but because it wasn't possible to look inside someone's brain before and after exercise, it remained unproven until 2008. German researchers used positron emission tomography (PET) scans combined with psychological mood tests to prove that running did indeed provide a flood of endorphins to the limbic and prefrontal areas of the brain—the parts associated with emotion and euphoria. It's believed that endorphins are released into the blood when oxygen flow to the muscles decreases and lactic acid accumulates in a process called acidosis, which may cause cramps and physical exhaustion.

ADDITIONAL FACTS

1. *Studies have shown that people who experience chronic pain have lower-than-normal levels of endorphins in their spinal fluid. Some medications and procedures, such as acupuncture, may activate endorphin systems in these patients.*

2. *Endorphins also stimulate the immune system by activating natural killer cells in the blood and can postpone the effects of aging.*

3. *There are four different types of endorphins: alpha, beta, gamma, and sigma. Beta-endorphins consist of 30 amino acid subunits and show the greatest increase during exercise.*

◆◆◆

Deafness

Some people are born deaf. Others lose their hearing through injury, infection, or long-term exposure to loud noise. For others, deafness develops slowly with age. Whatever the reason, a diagnosis of hearing loss or deafness may require learning to communicate in a whole new way.

Hearing occurs when sound waves enter the outer ear and are converted into vibrations by the eardrum. These vibrations are amplified by three tiny bones (the stirrup, hammer, and anvil in Latin) in the middle ear, which respond to the eardrum and transmit the impulses to the inner ear. In the inner ear, nerve centers process those vibrations into electrical impulses and send them to the brain, where they are recognized as sounds.

Most hearing loss occurs when the inner ear or auditory nerves are damaged. In particular, loud music or noises, meningitis, or high fever may damage the cochlea, a structure in the inner ear. Certain antibiotics, chemotherapy drugs, and very high doses of anti-inflammatory drugs such as aspirin can also damage the inner ear, leading to hearing loss or ringing in the ear (called tinnitus). Temporary loss of hearing can also happen when sound waves cannot reach your inner ear because of fluid buildup, excessive earwax, or a punctured eardrum.

Diminished hearing can often be improved with hearing aids that amplify sound waves. A recently developed surgical procedure called a cochlear implant may restore hearing in some people with severe deafness by replacing damaged parts of the inner ear.

For people who are born deaf or lose their hearing completely, however, learning sign language often provides the best way to communicate. American Sign Language, developed in the 19th century, is understood by millions of people in the United States and in many other countries that have adopted the language.

ADDITIONAL FACTS

1. *Many schools and colleges have been established especially for the deaf, including Gallaudet University in Washington, DC, founded in 1857.*

2. *Presbycusis, or hearing loss in old age, affects about three-quarters of people over age 75.*

3. *Exposure to any sound above 85 to 90 decibels—the volume of a motorcycle, snowmobile, or lawn mower—puts a person at risk for hearing damage. The pain threshold, at which ears might actually hurt from the noise, is 140 decibels, or the volume of a jet engine during takeoff.*

✦✦✦

Kinsey

When Alfred Kinsey (1894–1956) was 44 years old, the administration at Indiana University asked him to teach a marriage course. Although his specialty was biology—specifically, the study of wasps—he agreed. It was this decision that forever altered his career, and the study of human sexuality. During his 18 years of studing sexual behavior, Kinsey interviewed more than 18,500 men and women to gather research for his two books, *Sexual Behavior in the Human Male* and *Sexual Behavior in the Human Female*. Together, these works sold more than half a million copies and were translated into 12 languages.

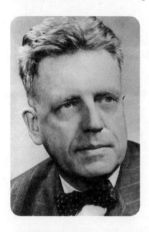

It's easy to understand why Kinsey's research shocked the world. He argued that some 30 percent of men and 13 percent of women had a same-sex orgasmic experience by age 45. Challenging the predominant view at the time that homosexuality was a mental illness or aberrant behavior, Kinsey wrote that homosexuality and heterosexuality were not mutually exclusive behaviors. Instead, he claimed, they existed on a sliding continuum, and people could shift from one side to the other throughout their lives.

Another notion that Kinsey turned on its head was the idea that women were not interested in sex, partaking in it mainly to please their partners and for procreation. He reported that half of the females he'd interviewed had had premarital intercourse and one in four had engaged in an extramarital affair. What's more, Kinsey found that masturbation was a widespread act that the majority of men and women engaged in regularly. Throughout his life—and after his death—experts went on to challenge Kinsey's findings, making the point that his interview process wasn't scientifically sound and that he had studied only well-to-do, white adults under the age of 35. Still, Kinsey's work made an indelible mark on the way the medical community and society as a whole thought about sex.

ADDITIONAL FACTS

1. *In 2004, a biopic entitled* Kinsey *was released in theaters. The actor Liam Neeson (1952–) played the title role.*

2. *Kinsey's works later became known as simply the Kinsey Report.*

3. *Kinsey later headed Indiana University's Institute for Sex Research, which was renamed the Kinsey Institute for Research in Sex, Gender, and Reproduction in 1982, decades after his passing.*

✦✦✦

Body Mass Index

Your body mass index (BMI) results from a formula used to estimate a healthy weight for you, based on your height. Being overweight or having a BMI that is too high can lead to major health problems, including type 2 diabetes, heart disease, high blood pressure, sleep apnea, arthritis, and varicose veins.

To calculate your BMI, start by multiplying your weight in pounds by 703. Divide the answer by your height in inches. Divide that result by your height in inches again. A woman or man who is 5 feet 4 inches (64 inches) tall and weighs 120 pounds has a BMI of 20.6: $[(120 \times 703) \div 64] \div 64 = 20.6$.

There are five standard BMI categories. Someone with a BMI of below 18.5 is underweight, 18.5 to 24.9 is considered healthy, 25.0 to 29.9 qualifies as overweight, 30.0 to 39.9 is categorized as obese, and 40.0 or higher is considered morbidly obese. These ranges should not be used to assess the BMIs of children.

Your BMI is partially determined by heredity. People from different ethnic backgrounds tend to have different body fat distribution (they build up fat in different parts of their bodies) or body composition (proportions of bone, muscle, and fat). However, no matter what your genetic predisposition, you can have a healthy body and keep your weight in control by eating a balanced, reduced-calorie diet and exercising. Simple forms of exercise, such as walking for 20 minutes daily, can have positive effects on your health and help control your BMI.

ADDITIONAL FACTS

1. *It's estimated that 300,000 deaths a year in the United States could be prevented if everyone maintained a healthy BMI.*

2. *Studies show that the average age of a first heart attack for people with BMIs of 18.5 and under is 75. For people with BMIs of 40 and over, the average age is 59.*

3. *Sometimes your BMI is not the best way to tell whether you need to lose weight. For example, very muscular individuals may have higher BMIs, because muscle weighs more than fat. And people over 65 may benefit from having a BMI between 25 and 27, rather than under 25.*

✦✦✦

Ultrasound

The theory behind ultrasound technology—using sound echoes to determine the distance of an object—has been around for centuries. The further away a canyon wall is, the longer it takes for your voice to echo off it and return to you. It wasn't until mankind started to apply this concept to probing the depths of the sea, however, that scientists awakened to its potential for medical use.

The discovery of piezoelectricity in 1877 by the French physicist Pierre Curie (1859–1906) is often considered the founding of ultrasonics. Piezoelectricity is the ability certain substances have to give off pulses of energy when force is applied to them. One of the first practical applications of the new discovery came during World War I, when Paul Langevin (1872–1946), a former student of Curie's, realized that piezoelectric crystals might give off sound waves that could be used to measure distances and detect enemy vessels at sea. He used this knowledge to develop the first sonographic imaging tool and helped scientists in France and Britain develop the first primitive sonar system for use against German U-boats.

In the 1920s, ultrasound technology was popularly embraced as a wonder treatment, wrongly believed to have amazing curative powers. It was used unsuccessfully against a host of illnesses, including cancer. (In reality, ultrasound waves are among the least intrusive waves that can be directed at the body.)

Indeed, ultrasonics' real contribution to medicine was its diagnostic capabilities, not its treatment potential. In the 1940s, the Austrian neurologist Karl Dussik (1908–1968) first tried to beam ultrasound waves at a patient in an effort to pinpoint the location of a brain tumor. A few years later, the American naval doctor George Ludwig (1922–1973) used ultrasound to diagnose gallstones; ultrasonic detection of breast and colon cancer followed. And the most well known application of ultrasound today, the detection of a fetal heartbeat and monitoring of fetal growth, was first described in 1959 in Glasgow, Scotland, by the physician and professor Ian Donald (1910–1987).

A modern ultrasound machine is a relatively simple device, firing out ultrasonic pulses that progress through the body until they collide with a tissue boundary, at which point the waves bounce back to the machine. A computer calculates the distance , shape, and speed at which the waves traveled forward and back, forming a two-dimensional—or, thanks to advancements in computer processing, a three-dimensional—image of the area.

ADDITIONAL FACTS

1. *Before the development of sonar echolocation, people used long ropes, with knots tied at regular intervals and a heavy piece of lead tied to one end, to measure the depth (in "knots") of water. Although it's not clear why, this process was called sounding.*

2. *Langevin first noted the therapeutic (and dangerous) qualities of high-intensity ultrasound in the 1920s, when he felt pain in his hand while placing it in a water tank being hit with an ultrasound beam.*

✦✦✦

Dehydration

Water makes up, on average, 60 percent of a person's body weight. This simple substance plays many roles: It helps flush out toxins, transport nutrients to cells, and regulate body temperature, among other essential functions. Since you lose about 10 cups of water a day through breathing, perspiration, urination, and sometimes diarrhea, fever, or vomiting, you must replenish that amount of fluid daily. But when you lose more water than you take in, that leads to a deficit called dehydration.

The first signs of dehydration include a dry mouth, fatigue, thirst, headache, dark-colored urine, and dizziness or light-headedness. These mild or moderate cases can be reversed by simply taking in more fluid. Severe dehydration is much more serious and can cause the body to go into life-threatening shock. Symptoms include low blood pressure, rapid heartbeat, fever, sunken eyes, extreme thirst and confusion, and shriveled or dry skin. An oral rehydration solution or, in more serious cases, an intravenous solution may be necessary.

To prevent dehydration, experts recommend drinking at least 8 cups of water a day. Solid food supplies about 20 percent of your water intake; a rare steak, for instance, is about 70 percent water, while some fruits and vegetables, such as watermelon and tomatoes, are more than 90 percent water. Certain situations require additional water intake. Hot or humid weather; pregnancy or breastfeeding; and illnesses that cause fever, diarrhea, or nausea all lead to additional fluid loss. Sweat-inducing exercise may also raise the risk of dehydration; for short workouts, take in an additional 1 to 3 cups of water. Intense exercise that lasts for longer than an hour may require drinks that contain additional sodium to replace what's lost in sweat.

ADDITIONAL FACTS

1. *Beer, wine, colas, and coffee can contribute to overall fluid intake, although they shouldn't make up a significant portion.*

2. *When people are removed from life support, they usually pass away from dehydration.*

♦♦♦

Cyst

The word *cyst* comes from the Greek word meaning "pouch." In medicine, the term describes a membrane-enclosed sac that usually contains air, fluid, or a semisolid material. Several organs, including the kidneys, breasts, and liver, are susceptible to cyst formation. In some instances, these cystic conditions and diseases may be harmful or painful; in others, they can be harmless.

Cysts arise from an assortment of causes and vary in size, often manifesting as an abnormal lump. One common culprit is an infection, such as the bacterial infection that can lead to under-the-skin acne bumps. Cysts may also be the result of an inherited condition, such as cystic fibrosis. In this disease of the mucous glands, a buildup of abnormally thick mucus can lead to scar tissue and cysts in the lungs, making it difficult to breathe.

Blockages in the body are another cause. For instance, when an overgrowth of glands and tissues in a breast blocks milk ducts, a cyst forms. Because a lump in a breast can also signal cancer, physicians often recommend checking the lump with an ultrasound or needle aspiration (in which a sample of the fluid inside the lump is taken) to confirm whether it's benign.

Cysts also occur in the ovaries. When a follicle in one of the ovaries fails to break open and produce an egg, it can grow into a cyst. Although most ovarian cysts go away on their own within a few months, some may rupture, leading to sudden, severe pelvic pain.

Because any number of conditions can lead to a cyst, experts recommend seeing a physician if you notice an abnormal lump anywhere in the body.

ADDITIONAL FACTS

1. *About 10 percent of women have polycystic ovarian syndrome, a condition involving multiple cysts on the ovaries.*

2. *In 2007, an Oklahoma woman had a 93-pound ovarian cyst surgically removed. The cyst was about the size of a beach ball.*

3. *Cysts in the breasts often vary in size according to the phases of the woman's menstrual cycle.*

❖❖❖

Homeopathy

Homeopathy is an alternative medicine practice that seeks to help the body fend off disease by treating illnesses with very small amounts of a substance that, in larger doses, would cause the same symptoms—a concept known as formally as the similia principle and popularly as "like cures like."

In the late 1700s, common medical treatments included bloodletting, purging, blistering, and the use of sulfur and mercury as medications. A German physician and chemist named Samuel Hahnemann (1755–1843) proposed a less-threatening approach to treating illness after reading an old herbal remedy that used cinchona bark to treat malaria. Hahnemann observed that cinchona bark, in large quantities, caused malaria-like symptoms in healthy people. The idea that smaller quantities might jump-start the immune system in those already sick became the basis of homeopathy.

The practice was imported to the United States in 1835, and dozens of homeopathic hospitals opened. Medical advances such as Louis Pasteur's (1822–1895) germ theory, the development of antiseptic techniques, and the discovery of ether anesthesia, however, diminished the popularity of homeopathy as a first-line medical therapy. Most homeopathic institutions closed down by the 1930s.

Homeopathy has experienced a bit of a revival in the United States and other countries. People all over the world seek homeopathic remedies as complementary or alternative forms of treatment for chronic medical conditions. According to a 1999 survey, more than 6 million Americans had used homeopathy in the preceding year.

Plants and other natural sources provide many homeopathic treatments, although the key ingredients are usually highly diluted by a process called potentization—sometimes so much that not one molecule of the original substance remains. Homeopaths believe that dilution extracts the vital essence of the substance and actually makes a formula more effective. These products are marketed as dietary supplements and do not undergo testing or regulation by the Food and Drug Administration.

ADDITIONAL FACTS

1. *The similia principle can be traced back to Hippocrates (c. 460–c. 377 BC) in ancient Greece, who noted that recurrent vomiting could be treated with an emetic (such as ipecacuanha), which would be expected to make the condition worse.*

2. *In the United States, most homeopathy is practiced along with another health care practice for which the practitioner is licensed, such as conventional medicine, dentistry, chiropractic, naturopathy, acupuncture, or (when used to treat animals) veterinary medicine. Arizona, Connecticut, and Nevada license medical doctors specifically for homeopathy.*

3. *Homeopathic treatment is tailored to individual patients, with practitioners selecting remedies according to a person's symptoms, lifestyle, emotional and mental states, and other factors. In fact, two people with the same symptoms may receive different treatments.*

❖❖❖

Paralysis

Paralysis, or the inability to move, occurs when nerve cells in the brain or spinal cord are damaged and muscles cannot function properly. A person may become paralyzed because of illness or injury, and paralysis can be temporary or permanent. Paralysis takes many forms and may strike almost any part of the body, ranging from paralysis on one side of the body (hemiplegia) to paralysis in all four limbs (quadriplegia).

Severe trauma to the head, neck, or back—a spinal fracture in a car crash, for example, or a heavy blow to the head—is a common cause of paralysis. Many diseases can also leave victims paralyzed, including cerebral palsy, multiple sclerosis, muscular dystrophy, Guillain-Barré syndrome, and peripheral neuropathy. Brain tumors and strokes can also cause paralysis.

In rare circumstances, paralysis can also be triggered by allergies; drugs; poisons such as botulinum toxin; or mussels, clams, or oysters contaminated with a specific shellfish toxin.

Typically, damage to the left side of the brain causes the right side of the body to become paralyzed, and vice versa. Injuries to the spinal cord in the lower back may result in paralysis of the legs, while an injury higher up in the neck region can result in paralysis of all four limbs. The degree of paralysis depends on which nerve cells are damaged and how much of the brain or spinal cord is involved, how quickly the blood supply returns to the area, and how soon the disease causing the problem is treated. In severe cases, feeding tubes or intravenous feeding may be required. Frequent position changes and good skin care can help maintain muscle tone and prevent complications and tissue atrophy in people who are paralyzed.

ADDITIONAL FACTS

1. *One form of paralysis is called spasticity. People with spasticity can still move, but have reduced control over their muscles and posture and may suffer from spasms.*

2. *Polio was a major cause of paralysis in the United States until a vaccine was developed in 1955.*

3. *Temporary paralysis may occur when people are transitioning into or out of REM sleep, the stage of sleep in which dreams occur. People experiencing sleep paralysis may be aware of things going on around them but are unable to move or speak.*

◆◆◆

Masters and Johnson

Virginia Johnson (1925–) was an aspiring opera singer when she applied for a research assistant position with William Masters (1915–2001), a gynecologist at Indiana University, in 1957. Neither of them knew it at the time, but it was the start of a lifelong partnership, both personal and professional. Not only did they marry in 1971, but the duo, who later became widely known as Masters and Johnson, went on to publish numerous books and papers that helped change the way society views sex. Without them, today's *Sex and the City* television show— and lifestyle—would never have existed.

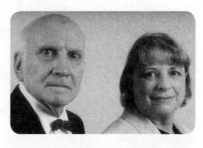

When Masters and Johnson first began their research on human sexuality, it was still viewed as a taboo topic. Their groundbreaking work helped shift that concept of sex to one that viewed the act as a source of great pleasure and intimacy. To conduct their research, the team used polygraph-like tools to measure individuals' responses to sexual activities. Using these devices, they observed more than 700 men and women while the participants had intercourse or masturbated. Masters and Johnson published these results in their 1966 book *Human Sexual Response,* which detailed the four stages of sex: excitement, plateau, orgasm, and resolution. When released, the book created a furor and went on to become a bestseller.

In their later works, Masters and Johnson tackled the subjects of impotence and premature ejaculation in *Human Sexual Inadequacy,* in which they argued that 90 percent of cases stemmed from emotional, not physical, reasons. This caused a shift in the way impotence was treated. They also made the case that homosexuality was not a mental illness but a personal preference, in their 1979 tome *Homosexuality in Perspective*. Although Masters and Johnson divorced in the early 1990s, they remained close friends and associates.

ADDITIONAL FACT

1. *Johnson went on to earn two honorary doctorate of science degrees.*

✦ ✦ ✦

Obesity

Obesity means having too much body fat, and it is unhealthy. Obesity usually occurs when you eat more calories than you use over time and store the extra calories as body fat. People who are obese have increased risks of diabetes, heart disease, stroke, arthritis, and some cancers.

Each person has a different balance between the number of calories he or she needs to take in and the number to burn to maintain a healthy weight. There are a variety of factors that can influence this balance, including your genetic makeup, overeating, consuming high-fat foods, and not being physically active. If you are obese, losing as little as 5 to 10 percent of your weight can decrease your risk of disease.

Typically, body fat levels are measured by using your weight and height to calculate your body mass index (BMI). Your BMI usually correlates with the amount of body fat you have. An adult who has a BMI of 30 or higher is deemed obese, while one who has a BMI of 25 to 29.9 is considered overweight. BMI is not an actual measurement of your body fat and can be inaccurate for certain people, such as athletes, who may have high weights for their heights because of their muscular builds.

Body fat levels can be assessed using other methods, including measuring skin fold thickness and waist circumference, calculating waist-to-hip circumference ratios (abdominal fat is a predictor of risk of obesity-related diseases), and other techniques, such as ultrasound, computed tomography, and MRI. Additionally, besides looking at body fat levels, risk of obesity-related disease should be determined by considering other factors, such as blood pressure and level of activity.

ADDITIONAL FACTS

1. *Adult BMI parameters should not be used for children. For children and teenagers, BMI ranges take into account normal differences in body fat between boys and girls and normal differences at various ages.*

2. *Studies suggest that getting enough sleep helps adults avoid from becoming obese and may even protect children from becoming obese as adults.*

3. *Current information estimates that 30 percent of Americans are obese.*

✦✦✦

William Halsted and Modern Surgery

Surgery as we know it today is generally safe, effective, and as noninvasive as possible. For this, we have the American surgeon William Halsted to thank.

A giant in the history of American science, Halsted (1852–1922) was born in New York City to a wealthy family and earned a medical degree from Columbia University College of Physicians and Surgeons. He toured Europe after leaving medical school, absorbing new ideas about surgical practices. When he returned, he became an attending doctor and surgeon at Bellevue Hospital Medical School in New York. He also emerged as one of the city's leading proponents of using cocaine as a painkiller. Many of his experiments with the drug were conducted on himself and other doctors; as a result, Halsted became addicted to the drug for 2 years, and several of his colleagues died. The addiction seriously threatened Halsted's career, and he was invited to leave New York in 1886 and referred to the new department of pathology at the recently opened Johns Hopkins Hospital in Baltimore, where he could work without having contact with patients.

Settling in Baltimore, Halsted beat his cocaine addiction (by switching to morphine) and revived his career at the newly formed Johns Hopkins University, where he became chief surgeon in 1890. He began developing a set of surgical techniques that would be known as Halstead School of Surgery. Halsted emphasized keeping a hygienic operating environment, using small stitches and high-quality sutures, and handling body tissues as gently as possible. His recommendations influenced a generation of American doctors who trained at Johns Hopkins and spread his ideas throughout the medical community.

Although shy and reclusive—he hated leaving Baltimore—Halsted became one of the nation's most sought-after surgeons. He also contributed to advances in the treatment of many diseases, including breast cancer, gallstones, and thyroid disorders. Halstead's method for treating breast cancer, for instance, became the treatment of choice for more than half a century, although it is not commonly used today. He died, ironically, from an infection following gallbladder surgery.

ADDITIONAL FACTS

1. *Halsted is also credited with the invention of mosquito clamps (small clamps used to hold a blood vessel closed) and rubber surgical gloves, which he ordered custom-made from the Goodyear Rubber Company.*

2. *Chicago's Halsted Street is named for the surgeon's grandfather, an early investor in Windy City real estate.*

3. *Two of Halsted's most well known students were the neurosurgeons Harvey Cushing (1869–1939) and Walter Dandy (1886–1946).*

◆ ◆ ◆

Tonsillitis

At the very back of your throat, above and behind the tongue, are two fleshy pads called tonsils. These balls of tissue are part of the immune system, filtering out bacteria and viruses and generating illness-fighting antibodies. But when an infection causes the tonsils to become red and inflamed, that's called tonsillitis. This condition is particularly common among children.

The usual signs of tonsillitis include a sore throat, fever, chills, loss of voice, and tender lymph glands in the jaw and neck. The tonsils also become swollen and covered in white patches; children may suffer from a stomachache as well. In the majority of cases, a virus is the culprit, and the infection will go away on its own in 4 days to 2 weeks. Gargling with warm salt water and taking ibuprofen can help ease the pain and soothe the throat.

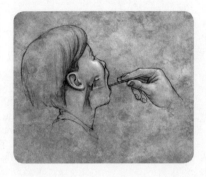

If you suspect that your child has tonsillitis, he or she should see a physician for an examination and a throat culture to rule out strep throat and to determine whether the illness was brought on by another type of bacterial infection. In either case, a course of antibiotics is required. The surgical removal of the tonsils—called tonsillectomy—is seldom done in adults. But in children and adolescents, it may be recommended if the swollen tonsils interfere with breathing, the illness doesn't improve with antibiotics, or the infections recur frequently (at least seven throat infections in a year; five or more per year over 2 years; or three or more serious cases per year over a 3-year span). It takes about 2 weeks to recover from the outpatient procedure. Tonsillectomy formerly was very common but now is less so, because the immune function of the tonsils is better appreciated.

ADDITIONAL FACTS

1. *The first tonsillectomy was reportedly performed in AD 30 by the Roman medical writer Celsus.*

2. *To make a saltwater solution, mix ¼ teaspoon of salt with a cup of warm water.*

◆◆◆

Breast Cancer

In this era of pink-ribbon advocacy and mammogram reminders, it's easy to forget that breast cancer used to be a difficult-to-treat and little-discussed disease. The condition was shrouded in secrecy until the 1970s and 1980s, when a number of brave women—including first ladies Betty Ford (1918–) and Nancy Reagan (1921–)—stepped forward to discuss their personal experiences, starting a public discourse about the disease. Because of the increase in research and screening the survival rate for breast cancer has jumped over the past few decades.

Still, one in eight women who lives to the age of 80 will develop the disease sometime in their lives. Breast cancer strikes mainly women; men make up 1 percent of cases, or about 1,500 a year. Cancer is the result of abnormal cells that don't die when they're programmed to. Instead, they grow out of control, eventually clustering into tumors. About 85 percent of breast cancers originate in the mammary ducts, while the rest begin in the lobules (the sacs where milk is produced). Although it was once thought that tumors grew before the cancer spread to other areas of the body, scientists are finding that cancerous cells can spread early on in certain variants of the disease.

In order to detect breast cancer as early as possible, public health organizations recommend that women perform breast self-exams to check for lumps and undergo yearly mammograms beginning at age 40. Because genes play a role in breast cancer, some women with a strong family history of the disease may opt to undergo genetic testing for BRCA1 and BRCA2 mutations. Women with these genes are three to seven times more likely to develop breast cancer.

Warning signs of the disease include a change in breast size or shape, an irregular or sunken nipple, a hard lump, and bloody discharge from the nipple. Treatment often involves a combination of treatments, including surgery, radiation, chemotherapy, and hormonal or targeted therapies. If the cancer is detected early enough, the chances of recovery are excellent: Today, the 5-year survival rate (the likelihood of being alive 5 years after diagnosis) is 86 percent.

ADDITIONAL FACTS

1. *Studies show that women who are overweight have a slightly greater risk of developing breast cancer.*

2. *Drinking more than one alcoholic beverage a day can raise estrogen levels in the body and increase the odds of having breast cancer.*

✦✦✦

Viagra

Sometimes when men want to have sex, they have difficulty achieving or maintaining an erection—a condition called erectile dysfunction (ED). This is common in older men, or it may be caused by health issues such as depression, diabetes, or high blood pressure. In 1998, the Food and Drug Administration approved Viagra—the first oral medication to treat most types of ED.

Viagra (sildenafil), which was originally tested as a heart medication and whose true value was discovered accidentally, was a vast improvement over earlier injection treatments for ED: Instead of an immediate and uncontrollable erection, Viagra causes an erection only when a man is sexually aroused. Today, 9 Viagra pills are dispensed every second—that's nearly 300 million tablets a year.

To understand how Viagra works, it's important first to understand how an erection forms. When a man becomes sexually aroused, nitric oxide is released into the blood. The nitric oxide stimulates the production of a chemical called cyclic guanosine monophosphate (cGMP), which relaxes the smooth muscles that line the penis. Blood can then flow in freely, inflating it like a water balloon.

At the same time, another enzyme called phosphodiesterase (PDE) works to deactivate the cGMP. The body should produce enough nitric oxide to maintain levels of cGMP until ejaculation occurs, but when a person has ED, this doesn't always happen. Viagra works by attaching to and disabling PDE in the penis so that the cGMP can build up. The larger the amount of cGMP, the greater the bloodflow and the greater the degree of erection.

Viagra targets one specific enzyme, called PDE-5, that is found primarily in the penis. However, the drug also has an effect on PDE-6—an enzyme in the retina. This can cause people who take Viagra to temporarily see with a bluish tinge. Viagra can also cause headaches and, infrequently, painful erections lasting as long as 24 hours (called priapism). There is also concern that younger men who take Viagra recreationally may become dependent and unable to have sex without it.

Drugs that contain nitrates, such as nitroglycerin for chest pain, can interact with Viagra. While Viagra is safe to take along with medications for heart disease, high blood pressure, and depression, there have been several cases of patients dying of heart attacks, sometimes during sex, after taking Viagra. One hypothesis is that these elderly patients are just not prepared for the physical exertion of sexual activity.

ADDITIONAL FACTS

1. *In 2008, a Google search for Viagra listed more than 17 million Web pages. In comparison, a search for aspirin listed only 3.3 million.*

2. *Texas A&M University, in a state that is one of the nation's top producers of watermelons, announced in 2008 that researchers had identified in watermelon rind a Viagra-like compound called citrulline, which helps relax the body's blood vessels.*

◆◆◆

Headaches

One of the most common types of pain that virtually everyone experiences at one point or another is a headache. Headaches usually are not serious, but they may occur frequently—and are sometimes an indicator of a more dangerous injury or health condition.

Tension headaches are the most common type of headache, often caused by stress or emotional strain. They may last for a few minutes to a few days and are usually characterized by pain or pressure on both sides of the head. Doctors believe that a change in brain chemicals can trigger tension headaches and that spasms in the muscles of the neck, jaw, face, head, and scalp may also play a role.

Cluster headaches occur in groups or cycles, often several times a day for months, and then disappear for just as long. Their cause is unknown. Severe and debilitating, cluster headaches are usually felt more on one side of the head than the other, and they are more common in men than in women.

About 11 percent of the population experiences **migraines,** a painful, sometimes disabling type of headache that's often accompanied by nausea, vomiting, and sensitivity to light, noise, and smells. These throbbing headaches involve changes in chemicals and blood vessels in the brain and tend to last 6 to 48 hours. Some people have migraines several times a month, while others get them once a year or less. Some migraine sufferers can learn to identify and avoid triggers, such as certain foods or smells. They are more common in women than in men.

Headaches can also be caused by sinus infections; eyestrain; a blow to the head; dehydration; fever or cold; or withdrawal from caffeine, alcohol, or pain-relieving drugs. Severe or unrelenting headaches may signal a more serious problem, such as a brain tumor; an injury; or inflammation, stroke, or internal bleeding in the skull cavity. Treatment for most types of headaches includes over-the-counter pain relievers such as aspirin, acetaminophen, ibuprofen, or naproxen. Resting in a cool, dark room or applying a warm or cool compress to the head may also relieve pain.

ADDITIONAL FACTS

1. *About 15 to 20 percent of migraine sufferers experience a visual signal—such as lights or wavy lines—called an aura. Scientists aren't sure why, but those who experience aura are at higher risk for heart disease and stroke.*

2. *Anyone under the age of 20 should not take aspirin, because it has been linked to Reye's syndrome, a rare but serious disorder that affects only children.*

3. *A technique called biofeedback, in which a person uses signals from monitoring equipment to learn how to mentally control blood pressure, heart rate, skin temperature, and other autonomic functions, has been shown to decrease headache and migraine pain.*

◆◆◆

Gender Identity

Even at as young as 18 months, toddlers are already aware of whether they're boys or girls. This innate sense of yourself—as male or female—is called gender identity. It influences how you dress, how you style your hair, how you carry yourself, and even the way you speak. Some experts say that gender identity is firmly established by the time a child turns 4 years old.

Ultimately, your chromosomes and biological makeup not only determine your sex, but also dictate your gender identity. But in every culture, the way you're treated plays a role, too. Beginning at birth, parents treat babies according to their physical sex. Boys are wrapped up in blue blankets and bounced, while girl infants are wrapped in pink and often handled more gently in Western societies, such as the United States and Europe. As a result, children develop gender-appropriate behaviors. Of course, this doesn't mean that a boy who likes dolls has a gender identity problem, as long as he identifies and feels comfortable with being male. Similarly, a girl who likes sports and climbs trees—behaviors that in the past would have earned her the moniker *tomboy*—is now seen as behaving no differently from the rest of her gender.

But when someone feels trapped in a body that's incompatible with his or her gender identity, that's called transsexualism, a type of gender identity disorder. People in this situation have a strong desire to live as the other sex; they often cross-dress and take on mannerisms that mimic those of the other gender. In some cases, transsexuals undergo hormone therapy and an irreversible genital surgery to transform themselves into the opposite sex.

ADDITIONAL FACTS

1. *Some cultures do not view gender with the same bipolarity as Western cultures do. In Thailand, for instance, there is a third gender in addition to male and female: the kathoey, or a person of indeterminate sex.*

2. *A small-town physician named Stanley H. Biber (1923–2006) performed the first sex reassignment surgery in 1969. He went on to complete some 4,000 of these procedures in Hoehne, Colorado.*

3. *Hermaphrodites—people born with both male and female sex organs—do not have gender identity disorders if they're raised as one specific sex.*

✦✦✦

Weight Loss Drugs

Weight loss drugs suppress the appetite, inhibit the absorption of fat, or act in other ways to help people who are overweight lose weight. However, these drugs are not a good choice for everyone and are prescribed for people who have weight-related health problems and have trouble losing weight. They are not usually for people who just want to shed a few pounds.

Candidates for weight loss drugs usually must meet certain conditions. For example, good candidates include people who have a body mass index (BMI) of greater than 30. Others are individuals who have a BMI of greater than 27, have found that other methods of weight loss have not worked for them, and have medical complications from obesity, such as diabetes, high blood pressure, or sleep apnea.

Some weight loss drugs are approved for long-term use, and others are suitable only for the short term. Sibutramine (Meridia), an appetite suppressant, and orlistat (Xenical), a fat-absorption inhibitor, are acceptable for long-term use. Phentermine (Adipex-P), an appetite suppressant, and Alli, the reduced-strength version of orlistat, have been approved for short-term use. All these drugs have possible side effects, such as increased blood pressure and oily bowel movements.

Most weight loss drugs are modest in their effectiveness, but combining the drugs with a low-calorie diet and exercise can help you drop more weight than lifestyle changes alone can. Losing just 5 to 10 percent of your body weight can have significant benefits for your health, including decreases in blood pressure and levels of blood glucose, insulin, and triglycerides. Because weight loss drugs have not been on the market long enough for long-term studies, their safety is still largely unknown.

ADDITIONAL FACTS

1. *A newer drug called rimonabant is approved for use in some countries but has not been approved in the United States.*

2. *Fenfluramine and dexfenfluramine, two appetite suppressant drugs, were withdrawn from the market in 1997 because their use both alone and in combination with phentermine (fen-phen) was linked to the development of valvular heart disease and primary pulmonary hypertension, a potentially fatal disorder.*

◆◆◆

Radiotherapy

One of the most common treatments for cancer is radiotherapy, a process that involves zapping tumors with a beam of high-energy radiation in an effort to kill cancerous cells. Radiation therapy evolved over the course of the 20th century into a highly effective treatment against many types of cancers, especially when it is coupled with surgery or chemotherapy.

Radiation has been used for healing purposes almost since the discovery of x-rays by German physicist Wilhelm Conrad Röntgen (1845–1923) in 1895. Shortly after Röntgen's discovery, a medical student in Chicago named Emil Grubbe (1875–1960) began studying x-rays and noticed that his neck and hands were peeling after continued exposure. If x-rays could disfigure his skin, Grubbe wondered, could they have the same effect on a tumor? Grubbe put the idea to the test by irradiating a breast cancer patient, who showed great improvement after the treatment. Within a few years, cancer patients throughout the United States and Europe were undergoing radiotherapy.

In the early 1900s, Marie Curie (1867–1934) discovered the radioactive elements polonium and radium, which were also put to use in treating cancer. (Radium was later replaced by the less-toxic cobalt and cesium.) With the invention of CT scans and MRIs, it became possible to view tumors in three dimensions instead of just two, making radiation delivery safer, more efficient, and more effective.

Today, radiotherapy is used on nearly half of cancer patients. Radiation can be administered in several ways: It can be beamed from a machine outside the body; radioactive material, such as isotopes of iodine, strontium 89, phosphate, or cobalt, can be put in capsules and swallowed; or tiny "seeds" can be injected or surgically implanted near the site of the tumor. Healthy cells can also be damaged by radiation—hence the common side effects of swelling, sickness, and exhaustion—but they are generally stronger and more resilient than cancer cells.

ADDITIONAL FACTS

1. *Grubbe, one of the pioneers of radiotherapy, suffered severe health problems as a result of his overexposure to radiation. He lost a hand in 1929, underwent many operations for malignant growths, and ultimately died of cancer.*

2. *Because of its potential side effects, radiation is only used today to treat serious illnesses. Before the dangers of radiation were fully understood, however, it was sometimes used to treat relatively minor ailments like acne.*

3. *Radiotherapy often causes skin problems, and patients are advised to use prescription balms to treat swollen or peeling skin and to avoid scratching or rubbing affected areas.*

❖❖❖

Strep Throat

Strep throat is an infection caused by the bacterium *Streptococcus pyogenes*. Several million people come down with this highly contagious ailment every year, especially during the spring. It's particularly common among children and adolescents.

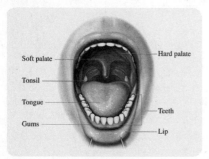

The telltale symptoms of strep throat are severe throat pain, red and swollen tonsils, and tiny red spots on the roof of the mouth. You may have trouble swallowing, and the glands in your neck could be swollen. Fever, headache, stomachache, and rash are all associated with strep throat, but a stuffy nose and cough are more often signs of a cold or flu.

To diagnose the condition, a doctor will check for the presence of *Streptococcus*. She'll swab the back of the throat and perform either a throat culture, in which case it takes up to 2 days to receive the results, or an instant antigen test. If the screening is positive, she'll prescribe antibiotics to kill the bacteria. After antibiotics were first invented in the 1940s, some experts believed that all bacterial infections would be completely eradicated. But within a decade, bacterial strains evolved to be resistant to certain antibiotics. That's why many public health experts discourage physicians from prescribing antibiotics without doing a screening to confirm strep throat.

Although strep throat can go away on its own, untreated cases may lead to more-serious complications. Other infections, such as sinusitis and ear infections, may occur. Kidney inflammation and rheumatic fever, which causes inflammatory deposits in the heart and other body tissues, may lead to permanent damage when strep throat is untreated.

ADDITIONAL FACTS

1. *Strep throat is also called* Streptococcus pharyngitis.

2. *If untreated, about 1 percent of patients develop kidney disease and 3 percent develop heart disease.*

◆◆◆

Prostate Cancer

The prostate is a walnut-size gland in the male reproductive system. Despite its diminutive size, this organ is the target of the second-leading kind of cancer diagnosed in American men. (The first is lung cancer.) Each year, more than 200,000 are diagnosed with prostate cancer—and 40,000 die of it.

Like all other forms of cancer, prostate cancer is caused by abnormal cells that grow more rapidly than regular cells. In this instance, the cancerous cells group together in clumps called tumors. If not treated early on, these tumors can metastasize, or travel to other areas of the body, causing widespread damage. Fortunately, prostate cancer cells usually spread slowly. Early signs include a weakened urine stream; hesitant, slow, frequent, or painful urination; painful ejaculation; and blood or pus in the urine. These effects are similar to those of benign prostatic hyperplasia, or an enlarged prostate, a condition that affects half of men over the age of 60.

Because prostate cancer symptoms are mild and easy to overlook before a tumor spreads, the American Cancer Society recommends that all men ages 50 and above receive a prostate cancer screening every year. This includes a blood test that checks the level of prostate-specific antigen (PSA), a marker of the disease, as well as a digital rectal exam. In this test, a physician inserts a lubricated, gloved finger into the patient's rectum to feel for bumps on the prostate.

If cancer is detected, there are a number of different treatment options, including surgery, radiation, and chemotherapy. Cryotherapy, in which tissue is frozen and destroyed, and hormone therapy are also options. For more serious cases, surgical removal of the prostate may be required.

A number of lifestyle changes can help lower prostate cancer risk. Regular exercise and a low-fat diet have been shown to protect against the disease, as has eating plenty of foods high in lycopene, including tomatoes and watermelon.

ADDITIONAL FACTS

1. *Prostate cancer is more common in African American men than in white, Asian, or Latino men.*

2. *The former South African president Nelson Mandela (1918–), the former New York City mayor Rudy Giuliani (1944–), and the actor Robert De Niro (1943–) are all prostate cancer survivors.*

◆◆◆

Statins

The world's best-selling medicine is Lipitor (atorvastatin), a statin drug that lowers the amount of cholesterol produced by the liver. Statins work by blocking a specific enzyme, hydroxymethylglutaryl-coenzyme A reductase, that is involved in cholesterol synthesis.

High total cholesterol is considered anything greater than 200 milligrams per deciliter. It's also considered problematic if your overall number is below 200 but your LDL, or "bad" cholesterol, is higher than 130. For someone who is overweight or who smokes, doctors may even consider total cholesterol levels as low as 180 to be undesirable.

Some people can control cholesterol levels with exercise and diet. For those who can't, doctors may prescribe statins. These medications are usually taken for life: Once a person stops taking them, his or her cholesterol levels will probably go back up.

Studies have shown that statin drugs can lower LDL cholesterol by 20 to 60 percent, usually within 4 to 6 weeks. They have also been shown to reduce triglycerides and the level of C-reactive protein—a marker of inflammation and heart disease risk—and produce a modest increase in the levels of HDL, or "good" cholesterol. Usually, these results mean large reductions in heart attack and heart disease risk.

Statins also seem to be associated with a lower risk of certain kinds of cancer, blood clots, and other health problems, although long-term studies are still needed to confirm these claims. Dementia, specifically, is an area of much controversy: Some researchers claim that statins appear to prevent the onset of cognitive decline, while others suggest that taking a statin has actually caused confusion or memory loss in patients.

More than 25 million people worldwide take at least one of the following statins: atorvastatin, simvastatin (Zocor), rosuvastatin (Crestor), pravastatin (Pravachol), lovastatin and lovastatin extended release (Mevacor, Altoprev, and Altocor), and fluvastatin (Lescol). These medicines differ in potency and the amount of cholesterol production they inhibit and range from about \$35 to \$140 a month for brand-name drugs. Some medications pair statins with other types of cholesterol-lowering drugs: Vytorin, for example, combines simvastatin with ezetimibe, a cholesterol-absorption inhibitor.

ADDITIONAL FACTS

1. *Statin use can cause a deficiency of the nutrient coenzyme Q_{10}, which can lead to muscle aches, cramping, and, in rare cases, a severe form of muscle fatigue called rhabdomyolysis. In 2001, Bayer HealthCare Pharmaceuticals voluntarily withdrew the statin drug cerivastatin (Baycol) from the market following reports of fatalities due to this condition.*

2. *Eating grapefruit or drinking grapefruit juice while taking many types of statins can cause dangerous complications, and doctors often recommend that people taking statins avoid the fruit.*

3. *People who use statins should not take large amounts of niacin supplements without consulting their doctors.*

◆◆◆

Stroke

A stroke occurs when a vessel in the brain becomes blocked or bursts, preventing blood and oxygen from reaching certain areas. In the deprived parts of the brain, cells can't function properly and begin to die; that's why stroke victims often slur their words or become partially paralyzed. The sooner a person is treated after a stroke, the better the likelihood of recovery—but many people don't know the symptoms and warning signs.

There are two types of strokes: About 80 percent are ischemic, in which a blood clot either forms in or travels to the brain, blocking a blood vessel. Less common (but deadlier) hemorrhagic strokes develop when an artery in the brain leaks or bursts, causing bleeding inside the brain.

Brain damage happens quickly after a stroke, and symptoms may include numbness, weakness, or paralysis of one part or one side of the body; vision problems; trouble understanding and communicating; dizziness; and a severe headache. Less severe symptoms may signal a transient ischemic attack (TIA), sometimes called a ministroke. A TIA is a warning that a more serious, full-blown stroke may happen soon.

To diagnose a stroke, doctors use CT scans or other tests to find the location of the clot or bleeding in the brain. If an ischemic stroke is diagnosed within the first 3 hours, doctors may be able to use antithrombotic (blood-thinning) medications—aspirin, for example—to dissolve the blood clot and improve chances of recovery. A hemorrhagic stroke can be harder to treat. Doctors may perform surgery or use medication to stop bleeding or reduce pressure on the brain. It's important to identify which type of stroke a person's had, because medication to treat one may be fatal to someone who's experienced the other.

After a stroke, patients often start rehabilitation to regain skills that were lost (such as use of one side of the body) or to learn to function with their remaining abilities. However, the rate of recurrence is high—according to the National Institutes of Health, approximately one-quarter of stroke victims will suffer another attack within 5 years. To prevent another stroke, doctors recommend taking preventive measures, such as controlling blood pressure and cholesterol with medications and making healthy lifestyle choices.

ADDITIONAL FACTS

1. *Common disabilities that result from stroke include paralysis (hemiplegia) or weakness (hemiparesis) on one side of the body.*

2. *Smoking cigarettes or using illegal drugs like cocaine are both risk factors for stroke.*

3. *Although less severe than strokes, TIAs can also lead to permanent brain damage or dementia.*

✦✦✦

Homosexuality

One in 10—that's the number of people who are homosexual, according to the famed sex researcher Alfred Kinsey (1894–1956). He was referring to the sexual behavior in which someone is primarily attracted to people of the same sex. But according to more-recent studies, Kinsey's number may be overstated. Three percent of Americans are homosexual, or gay, say scientists.

But whatever the exact number, Kinsey argued that human sexuality is a continuum, with strict heterosexuality at one end and homosexuality at the other. Most people, he said, fall at various points along that line. Published in the 1950s, Kinsey's research introduced a radical notion into an otherwise conservative society. But homosexuality didn't always bear a social stigma: In ancient Greece and Rome, it was a typical occurrence. In the most common coupling, pederasty, an older man had a relationship with a younger one. But with the spread of the Judeo-Christian and Muslim religions, the view that homosexuality is sinful behavior also grew. In the United States, there is an active movement for gay rights and acceptance: States such as Iowa and Massachusetts have passed laws that accept same-sex marriages, although these decisions are controversial. In most cases, they are overturned or caught up in legal red tape.

Underlying this debate over whether homosexuality should be accepted, banned, or even punished is a scientific argument: Is the cause of this sexual orientation choice, nurture, or nature? Some psychologists say that being gay is a result of your environment and how your parents raised you. On the other hand, scientific research on twins shows that identical pairs (two siblings with the same genome) are much more likely to both be homosexual than fraternal twins (two siblings with different genomes) are.

ADDITIONAL FACTS

1. *The term* homosexual *first appeared in an 1869 political pamphlet by Karl Maria Kertbeny (1824–1882).*

2. *Psychologists in the 19th and 20th centuries classified homosexuality as a type of mental illness.*

❖❖❖

Addiction

Addiction usually occurs when someone no longer has control over whether he or she uses a substance such as alcohol or illegal drugs. Addiction can be physical, emotional, or both. In addition to alcohol and illegal drugs, common addictions are to cigarettes, prescription medications, and even glue.

Physical addiction usually occurs when someone's body is dependent on a particular substance. The body develops a tolerance to a substance that it is addicted to, so that it needs more of that substance to achieve the same physical result, such as a "buzz" from cigarettes. People may develop withdrawal symptoms such as diarrhea, shaking, or generally feeling terrible when they stop using a substance to which they're addicted.

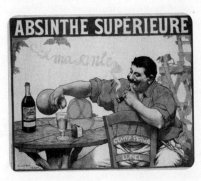

Psychological addiction occurs when the desire for a drug or other substance is emotional. The desire can be so strong that people may resort to lying or stealing in order to obtain the substance. When someone you know has developed an addiction, he may become moody and stop participating in normal activities such as work, hobbies, and socializing.

Overcoming addiction is extremely difficult. Most people need professional help or a treatment program. Additionally, an addict will probably require encouragement and support from friends and family in order to be successful.

ADDITIONAL FACTS

1. *Fifteen percent of Americans will develop an addiction disorder over the courses of their lifetimes.*

2. *Using an illegal substance such as marijuana without the physical or emotional dependency of addiction is merely substance abuse. Substance abuse can lead to the more serious problem of addiction.*

3. *Crack and heroin are so addictive that a user can become addicted after trying them just once.*

4. *It is possible to be addicted to an activity, such as gambling, rather than to a substance. There are medications that can help with compulsive gambling.*

5. *Recent studies indicate that genetics can play a role in addiction. People who carry certain gene variations that are passed on together as a high-risk haplotype may have as much as a 500 percent increased risk of being heavy smokers if they first try cigarettes before the age of 17.*

❖❖❖

Marie Curie and Radium

The discovery of radium changed medicine forever: X-rays, radiation treatment for cancer, and our overall understanding of the atom can all be traced to Marie Curie, who dedicated her life to understanding the mysterious element.

Born in Poland, Curie (1867–1934), née Maria Sklodowska, moved to Paris to study math and physics at the Sorbonne Institute, where she met and shared laboratory space with her future husband, Pierre Curie (1859–1906). In 1897, she began researching spontaneous radiation emitted by uranium compounds, on which the French scientist Henri Becquerel (1852–1908) had recently reported. Together, Marie and Pierre discovered that the mineral pitchblende had the same emission characteristics—a quality she called "radioactive." When they separated out the chemical components of pitchblende, the pair discovered two previously unknown elements: polonium (named for Marie's native country) and radium.

Up to this time, the atom was considered the smallest particle in matter. But the radiation that the Curies observed suggested that the atom was indeed divisible into smaller components, opening the door to a whole new field of physics. The couple, along with Becquerel, was awarded the Nobel Prize in Physics in 1903.

The Curies were unable to accept their award for 2 years, however, because of a mysterious illness that both scientists had begun to suffer from: They were frequently tired, the skin of their fingers always cracked, and they were perpetually sick. They didn't realize—or perhaps didn't want to admit—that their health was being affected by the glowing radiation given off by their laboratory samples.

In 1906, Pierre was struck and killed while crossing the street, leaving Marie with their two young daughters. Marie succeeded Pierre as professor, becoming the first woman to teach at the Sorbonne, and she received a second Nobel Prize in 1911. She volunteered for France during World War I, building portable x-ray machines for use in the trenches. She also distributed radium to kill infections in wounded soldiers. (The element's toxic side effects were realized only in the 1930s, at which point safer substitutes such as cobalt-60 were developed.) Afterward, Curie traveled throughout Europe and the United States, where she became quite a celebrity. She died at 67, of leukemia—probably as a result of her long exposure to radiation.

ADDITIONAL FACTS

1. *For many years Marie's daughter Irène Joliot-Curie (1897–1956) and her husband—also Nobel Prize winners (in chemistry, for advances in nuclear research)—operated the Radium Institute, now renamed the Curie Institute.*

2. *The curie, a measure of radioactivity, is named for Marie Curie.*

3. *In 1921, US president Warren G. Harding (1865–1923) presented Marie Curie with 1 gram of radium on behalf of all women of America, in recognition of her service to science. In 1929, President Herbert Hoover (1874–1964) presented her with $50,000, donated by American friends of science, to purchase radium for use in her laboratory in her native Warsaw.*

✦✦✦

Mononucleosis

Most people think of mononucleosis as the kissing disease. While it's true that the virus that causes the infection is spread through saliva, it can be passed along through coughing, sneezing, or sharing a drink or a food utensil as well. Because symptoms usually don't appear until 6 months after infection, determining the exact culprit may be tricky.

The virus that causes mononucleosis is called Epstein-Barr, named for the two British scientists, Anthony Epstein (1921–) and Yvonne Barr (1932–), who discovered it in 1964. The strain is one of the most common human viruses; by age 35 or 40, it's estimated that up to 95 percent of people have been infected with it. However, only about one in three of those who are exposed during adolescence or young adulthood actually contracts mononucleosis.

Symptoms of the illness include fever; weakness; headache; skin rash; and swollen throat, tonsils, and lymph nodes. A physician can diagnose mononucleosis by performing a test that screens for antibodies for the Epstein-Barr virus. As with the majority of other viruses, there isn't a cure or medication to treat it; the virus will leave the body on its own in about 4 to 8 weeks. Some medications, including antibiotics for an accompanying case of strep throat, may help treat symptoms and secondary infections. In rare cases, mononucleosis can cause the spleen to enlarge and even rupture, which is a medical emergency. Other complications include mild liver inflammation (hepatitis), which may cause jaundice, a yellowing of the skin.

ADDITIONAL FACTS

1. *As with chicken pox, once people are exposed to the Epstein-Barr virus, they build up antibodies to it but are not protected from a later recurrence.*

2. *The Epstein-Barr virus is a type of herpes virus.*

3. *People with mononucleosis are told to avoid exercise and other strenuous activities, because too much physical effort may delay recovery.*

❖ ❖ ❖

Emphysema

The inside of a healthy lung resembles a smooth, pink honeycomb. Attached to the capillaries are 300 million tiny air sacs, or alveoli, where oxygen is exchanged and introduced into the bloodstream. But for emphysema sufferers, these alveoli become damaged and the lungs appear craterous, reminiscent of the moon's surface.

This progressive condition destroys the delicate walls of the alveoli as the lungs become inflamed. As a result, the tiny capillaries collapse, which, over time, can lead to the rupturing of the air sacs. This leaves behind a larger, less elastic space that makes breathing less efficient and more difficult.

Most frequently, emphysema is brought on by smoking cigarettes. That's because smoke interferes with the cilia that line the bronchial tubes, which leads to inflammation over a period of several years. In fact, 91 percent of the 3 million Americans with emphysema are 45 years of age or older. For a small group, a genetic disorder can also raise the risk of this lung disease. These people have chronically low levels of a protein called alpha-1 antitrypsin, an enzyme that protects the lungs from injury caused by cigarette smoke. As a result, smokers with this abnormal gene often develop severe emphysema before the age of 40; nonsmokers with it are largely unaffected.

Unfortunately, the damage caused by emphysema is irreversible. Physicians can only prescribe treatments to control the symptoms, which include trouble breathing, fatigue, and a chronic cough. The treatments include inhaled steroids, bronchodilators that open constricted airways, and supplemental oxygen. Severe cases may lead to heart failure as well as lung failure, and they often require surgery or a lung transplant.

ADDITIONAL FACTS

1. *Smoking cigars and pipes also raises the risk of emphysema.*

2. *The word* emphysema *is derived from a Greek word meaning "to blow into."*

◆◆◆

Tryptophan

Does eating turkey really make people drowsy? This urban legend has been passed down and cited for years, partially thanks to Americans' tendencies to lapse into a food-and-football coma after Thanksgiving dinner. But while turkey does contain the ingredient tryptophan—a chemical known for its sleep-inducing properties—it's no more likely to send you off to dreamland than any other large meal.

Tryptophan is an essential amino acid, which means humans don't produce it internally and must get it from plant and animal sources. It is credited with helping bring about healthy sleep and a stable mood. Tryptophan is found in turkey, chicken, eggs, milk, cheese, fish, soy, nuts, seeds, and legumes—but it works best on an empty stomach, so the type present in food is not a very effective sleep aid.

The dietary supplement L-tryptophan, on the other hand, has been shown to increase levels of serotonin in the brain and help treat insomnia in some patients. L-tryptophan supplements have also been studied for the treatment of premenstrual dysphoric disorder, attention deficit disorder, and seasonal affective disorder, and for smoking cessation, although results have been mixed.

In 1990, contaminated L-tryptophan supplements manufactured in Japan caused an outbreak of eosinophilia-myalgia syndrome, an illness that can cause muscle pain and death, and their sale was banned by the Food and Drug Administration until 2002. Today, tryptophan is available in health food and vitamin stores and is also sold as a prescription drug (Tryptan) often used with antidepressants.

L-tryptophan is considered safe when taken as directed, but it can interact with herbs such as St. John's wort and drugs that induce sleepiness, such as alcohol, cold medicines, pain medications, muscle relaxants, and medications for depression or anxiety.

ADDITIONAL FACTS

1. *In the body, tryptophan is converted into the substances niacin and serotonin.*

2. *The disorder fructose malabsorption syndrome causes improper absorption of tryptophan in the intestine, reduced levels of tryptophan in the blood, and depression.*

3. *There have been no published cases of eosinophilia-myalgia syndrome within the past several years, but people who take L-tryptophan should be aware of its symptoms, including severe muscle pain; weakness, numbness, or burning sensations, especially at night; and dryness, yellowing, or hardening of the skin.*

✦✦✦

Peripheral Neuropathy

A neurological disorder that can cause pain, numbness, tingling, or a burning sensation in the feet and other parts of the body, peripheral neuropathy occurs when the network of nerves that connects the brain with the rest of the body becomes impaired.

This network, known as the peripheral nervous system, carries orders from the brain to the body and also relays sensory perceptions from the body back to the brain. It can be damaged in many different ways, including nutritional deficiencies, alcoholism, inherited disorders, diabetes, or traumatic injuries like car crashes.

In many cases, however, the specific cause of peripheral neuropathy cannot be identified—a condition known as ideopathic neuropathy.

The feet and hands, the body parts farthest from the brain and spinal cord, are affected first; some people with peripheral neuropathy experience muscle weakness and numbness, feeling as if they're wearing gloves and socks all the time. Others may be oversensitive to touch and may feel a burning pain or tingling sensation in their extremities.

There are more than 100 forms of peripheral neuropathy, some of which appear suddenly and aggressively and others that progress very slowly and never seriously affect quality of life. If the autonomic nervous system—which regulates involuntary reactions such as breathing, heart rate, sweating, and digestion—is damaged, the condition can be life threatening.

Inherited peripheral neuropathy cannot be treated, but the pain can be controlled with medications, and mechanical devices can lessen the effects of physical disability. For other forms of damage, nerves can regenerate, as long as the nerve cell itself has not been killed. Treatment and healing can be a slow process, but exercise, a healthful diet, and avoidance of alcohol and cigarette smoke can speed it along.

ADDITIONAL FACTS

1. *The most common inherited form of peripheral neuropathy is Charcot-Marie-Tooth disorder, which damage the protective myelin sheath that surrounds nerves in the brain and spinal cord. Symptoms include gait abnormalities, weakening and wasting of lower-leg and foot muscles, and loss of tendon reflexes—such as the knee-jerk reaction that occurs when a doctor taps your knee with a rubber hammer.*

2. *One relatively simple treatment that provides temporary relief for some people with peripheral neuropathy is the lidocaine patch, an anesthetic that can be applied directly over painful areas.*

3. *People with peripheral neuropathy may not feel a blister or cut on their feet right away and are thus more susceptible to foot infections and sores that won't heal.*

✦✦✦

Lesbianism

The Greek poet Sappho's works are infused with sensuality and passion. Addressing young women preparing themselves for marriage, Sappho (c. 610–c. 580 BC) often invoked the goddess of love, Aphrodite, to seduce a girl she desired. It's from Sappho's home, the island of Lesbos, that the term lesbianism takes its name. Today, the word is used to describe homosexual attraction between two women, or the emotional and sexual attraction of one woman to another. There are an estimated 6 million to 13 million lesbians currently living in the United States.

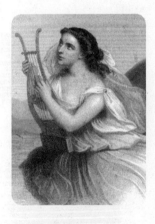

Experts believe that sexual orientation begins to form between middle childhood and early adulthood. For each individual, the experience is different: Some engage in homosexual behavior before they come to terms with their identity, while others recognize they are lesbians before any sexual experience.

Throughout history, lesbians have been sometimes accepted, sometimes penalized, and occasionally even banned. In the late 1800s, the term *Boston marriages* surfaced. It described a romantic union between two women that was not necessarily sexual. The most noted of these involved the writer Sarah Orne Jewett (1849–1909), who wrote about her own relationship in the novel *Deephaven*.

Today, lesbianism has become even more mainstream with the influence of celebrities such as Melissa Etheridge (1961–) and Ellen DeGeneres (1958–), and television shows such as *The L Word*.

ADDITIONAL FACTS

1. *In April 2008, three residents of the Greek isle of Lesbos sued a gay rights organization, the Homosexual and Lesbian Community of Greece, for using the word lesbian in its name.*

2. *One study in the* American Journal of Psychiatry *found that lesbians were three times as likely as other women to have a sister who was also a lesbian, suggesting that there may be a genetic factor in lesbianism.*

♦♦♦

Smoking

Smoking is bad for your health, whether you smoke cigars, cigarettes, or a pipe. It affects every organ in your body and is responsible for lung cancer, lung disease, heart and blood vessel disease, stroke, and cataracts. Women who smoke have a higher risk of developing problems during pregnancy and a greater risk of having a baby die of sudden infant death syndrome. Additionally, inhaling secondhand smoke—the smoke from others nearby who are smoking—results in many of the same problems that smoking does. Even smoking just one to four cigarettes a day will increase your risk of disease and of dying younger than you would otherwise.

To reduce your risk from all of these health problems, you must quit smoking. This is no easy task, because smoking is addictive. Cigarettes contain nicotine, which is an addictive drug. Small amounts of nicotine create pleasant feelings that make the smoker want to smoke more. These sensations wear off in a few minutes, which usually causes the smoker to crave another cigarette. Unless another cigarette is smoked, withdrawal symptoms occur, including irritability, nervousness, headaches, and difficulty sleeping.

People usually begin to smoke as teenagers because of curiosity and peer pressure. If your friends or parents smoke, you are more likely to start smoking. The tobacco industry's promotion of its product with advertisements also influences teenagers.

Anyone who starts smoking is at risk for becoming addicted. The younger someone is when he or she starts smoking, the more likely it is that he or she will become addicted. Close to 90 percent of adult smokers took up the habit before age 19.

ADDITIONAL FACTS

1. *Cigarette smoking by adults decreased from about 42 percent of the population of the United States in 1965 to about 21 percent in 2006.*

2. *Currently, 45 million adults in the United States smoke cigarettes. About 24 percent of men and 18 percent of women are smokers.*

3. *Educational level is associated with smoking rates. The more educated a person is, the less likely the person is to smoke.*

◆◆◆

Landsteiner, Wiener, and Blood Typing

Not all blood is the same. This important milestone in the history of medicine was discovered in 1900 by the Austrian-born pathologist Karl Landsteiner (1868–1943), who identified the four different types of blood and made safe blood transfusions possible for the first time.

Early attempts at blood transfusions between animals and humans had been unsuccessful—doctors discovered that the human body rejects animal blood. But human-to-human transfusion often failed, too. While studying these transfusions, Landsteiner noticed that when he mixed the blood of certain people, the red cells clumped together, in what would be a dangerous clotting reaction in the body that could be fatal. But in some combinations, this negative reaction did not occur.

Landsteiner concluded that people had different types of blood, which determined if clumping would occur with a transfusion or if they would mix safely. The different categories, he hypothesized, were determined by whether a person's red blood cells contained a specific antigen.

He called two of the blood types A and B. Cells from these groups could not be mixed with each other, because clumping would result. Another group, which he called O, did not have any antigens and could safely be mixed with the other types. Another group, AB, carried both the A and B antigens.

Landsteiner moved to the United States and began working with the New York University physician Alexander Wiener (1907–1976), studying women whose blood seemed to be incompatible with that of their babies, a strange scenario first identified in 1939. Testing blood samples from both humans and animals, the scientists determined that the rhesus monkey—as well as six out of seven humans tested—had a previously unknown antigen, which they named the rhesus (Rh) factor. A small percentage of the population, they realized, was Rh-negative (now just referred to as negative), making their blood was incompatible with everyone else's.

Today, people with blood type O are known as universal donors because they can give blood to anyone of any blood type—however, they can receive only type O blood themselves. People with type AB can receive all types of blood. If a woman with Rh-negative blood carries a child with Rh-positive blood (inherited from an Rh-positive father), the woman needs medication injections so that her body does not build up antibodies that could harm the baby.

ADDITIONAL FACTS

1. *Blood group O is the most common blood type in the United States and throughout the world.*

2. *In 2008, four of Japan's top 10 best-selling books addressed the topic of blood type in relation to personality type. It is widely accepted in Japanese culture that the two factors are related.*

3. *During his studies on blood typing, Wiener worked with police to develop some of the first forensic blood tests and with lawyers to devise some of the first paternity tests.*

◆◆◆

Hives

At some point, about one in five people comes down with a case of raised, red, itchy welts that appear suddenly in one spot or across the body. The condition, called hives or urticaria, can last for a few days or a few weeks, and the bumps or welts can range in size from a pencil eraser to a dinner plate.

A variety of factors, such as allergies, stress, and reactions to foods or prescription or over-the-counter drugs, can trigger an outbreak. Extreme heat, perspiration, or exposure to the cold can also bring on hives. One of these stimuli can cause the body to release the chemical histamine, which sets off a series of inflammatory reactions. As a result, blood plasma leaks between small blood vessels in the skin, resulting in fluid-filled bumps. In one outbreak, hives can appear and disappear multiple times.

In the vast majority of cases, the welts go away on their own without any side effects. But in rare, severe cases, the swelling may lead to difficulty breathing or swallowing, requiring medical attention. Symptoms are usually treated with an over-the-counter or prescription antihistamine; cold compresses and wearing loose clothing also help. But the only way to eradicate the condition entirely is to avoid the trigger. That's why, for chronic cases, physicians often perform allergy tests, in which the skin is exposed to tiny amounts of potential causes. Once the offending substance is identified, patients know to steer clear of it.

ADDITIONAL FACTS

1. *The most common food triggers of hives include nuts, chocolate, shellfish, tomatoes, eggs, berries, milk, and food additives and preservatives.*

2. *A related condition is called angioedema, in which the swelling occurs beneath the skin instead of on its surface.*

◆◆◆

Embolism

The German physician Rudolf Ludwig Virchow (1821–1902) was a pioneer of public health, advocating modern sewage disposal and food safety inspections. But he began his brilliant career researching pathology. In 1847, he noticed a number of clots in the arteries of animals. Virchow theorized that the clots blocked bloodflow to the heart, resulting in heart attacks. Fragments from other, larger blood clots, such as those in leg or arm veins, could break off and travel to smaller, remote vessels, starving tissues of blood and oxygen. "That gives rise to the very frequent process on which I have bestowed the name of Embolia," he wrote.

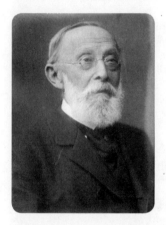

Today, experts know that this condition—called an embolism—can occur when clot fragments block blood vessels in the legs, feet, kidneys, intestines, or eyes. A clot close to the skin is generally harmless, but those in veins deep in the body, known as deep vein thrombosis, can be harmful. For instance, an embolism in an artery in the brain can cause a stroke, while one in the heart may lead to a heart attack. Another common form is a pulmonary embolism, in which a vein leading to a lung becomes clogged. Symptoms include shortness of breath, radiating chest pain, a bloody cough, and rapid heartbeat.

People with atherosclerosis (hardening of the arteries) and high blood pressure are at greater odds of experiencing an embolism. Having a sedentary lifestyle or a smoking habit or being overweight or obese increases the risk. Embolisms are treated in a variety of ways, depending on where they're located. Thrombolytic drugs can dissolve clots, while anticoagulants and antiplatelet medications can prevent new clots from forming. Other cases may require surgery, such as an artery bypass, clot removal, or angioplasty (opening the artery with a catheter).

ADDITIONAL FACTS

1. *Sitting for long periods of time can slow bloodflow, which may lead to the formation of clots in at-risk people.*

2. *Embolisms can also be caused by pieces of tissue, cholesterol crystals, clumps of bacteria, or amniotic fluid.*

✦✦✦

MAO Inhibitors

When people with depression do not respond to common antidepressants like Prozac or cannot tolerate their side effects, doctors may prescribe monoamine oxidase (MAO) inhibitors, a type of drug that targets chemical imbalances in the brain that may cause depression. Sold as a tablet or capsule under a variety of brand names, the drugs reduce the amount of monoamine oxidase, a chemical substance that breaks down neurotransmitters and causes imbalances in the brain. When these neurotransmitters are properly balanced, symptoms of depression often diminish.

Medications such as isocarboxazid (Marplan), phenelzine sulfate (Nardil), and tranylcypromine sulfate (Parnate) are examples of MAO inhibitors. MAO inhibitors are not recommended for children or teens and are usually not the first medicines prescribed for depression in adults because these drugs have serious side effects when combined with certain foods, beverages, or medications. Dangerously high blood pressure can occur, for example, if an MAO inhibitor is taken with fermented foods that have a high tyramine count—such as cheese, meat or sausage, fava beans, sauerkraut, or overripe fruit. Patients should also avoid alcoholic beverages, nonalcoholic beers or wines, and large amounts of caffeine while taking these drugs and for at least 2 weeks after stopping the medication.

Symptoms of unusually high blood pressure include chest pain, enlarged pupils, irregular heartbeat, severe headache, increased sweating, and a stiff or sore neck, and anyone experiencing them should be checked by a doctor immediately. Other side effects of MAO inhibitors can include dizziness, fainting, dry mouth, difficulty sleeping, blurred vision, loss of sexual desire, and appetite or weight changes—especially in older patients. Like all other antidepressants, MAO inhibitors have a black box warning on their labels regarding an increased risk of suicide, and patients should be monitored carefully for suicidal thoughts or behavior.

Research suggests that MAO inhibitors are as effective as other antidepressants in treating severe depression. In addition, they may be more effective than other antidepressants in treating those who have uncommon symptoms such as sleeping and eating too much or being overly sensitive to rejection.

ADDITIONAL FACTS

1. *Two MAO inhibitors, phenelzine and tranylcypromine, are often prescribed off-label to treat chronic headaches, panic disorder, and Parkinson's disease and for helping with smoking cessation.*

2. *Research on pregnant women has shown an increased risk of birth defects when MAO inhibitors are taken during the first 3 months of pregnancy.*

3. *A skin patch form of the drug selegiline (Emsam) was approved in 2006. Since the drug doesn't enter the gastrointestinal tract, this delivery method eliminates the dangers of dietary interactions.*

◆◆◆

Blindness

Anything that blocks the passage of light to the back of the eye or disrupts the transmission of optic nerve impulses to the brain will interfere with vision. A loss or lack of vision that can't be corrected with eyeglasses is known as blindness.

A person who is partially blind may see shapes and/or colors but can't focus properly or see details, while someone with total blindness is clinically referred to as having NLP, or "no light perception." The definition of *legally blind* in the United States and most of Europe is vision that's worse than 20/200 in the better eye; this means a legally blind person can't see with the same degree of clarity from 20 feet away what a normal person can see from 200 feet.

Worldwide, leading causes of blindness include cataracts, leprosy, trachoma, vitamin A deficiency, and infections such as onchocerciasis (or water blindness), a parasitic disease spread by flies. In developed countries where cataract surgery is common and quality of life is better, leading causes are diabetes, glaucoma, macular degeneration, and injuries usually involving detachment of the retina. Anyone experiencing sudden vision loss should be examined by a doctor immediately, because many forms of blindness must be treated quickly to ensure recovery.

The World Health Organization estimates that about 2.6 percent of the world's population is visually impaired or blind. Blind people can learn to function independently. They can read by touch with Braille, an international alphabet consisting of raised bumps. Some use white canes with red tips—the international symbol of blindness—or trained guide dogs to help them navigate safely around their neighborhoods.

In 2008, scientists attached a normal version of the gene RPE65 to a common cold virus (a safe and common delivery method in this type of research) and introduced it into the eyes of three young adults with a rare form of inherited blindness caused by an abnormal gene. The patients reported improved vision following the procedure, and researchers hope this type of gene therapy can be used in the future. Other ongoing studies include helping blind people "see" by way of sensors on their tongues that send pixilated images directly to the parts of the brain that are involved in vision.

ADDITIONAL FACTS

1. *Some blind people experience insomnia or have trouble sleeping at conventional times because they lack the daily rhythmic cues of light and darkness.*

2. *Training a guide dog for the blind may take up to 18 months. Guide miniature horses and helper monkeys are preferred by some because of their much longer life spans.*

3. *Strategies that allow blind people to handle normal daily activities include folding banknotes in different ways to indicate their denominations, labeling personal items and home appliances, and placing different types of food at specific positions on dinner plates.*

◆◆◆

Dihydrotestosterone Deficiency

In the early 1970s, the endocrinologist Julianne Imperato-McGinley made a long journey to a remote village in the mountains of the Dominican Republic, spurred by stories she'd heard about its children. When she arrived, she discovered that there was a group of children who, by all appearances, seemed to be girls at birth and had been raised as females. But during puberty, they began to transform into men: Their voices dropped, muscles developed, testes descended, and penises grew. In the village, these children were dubbed *guevedoces* (literally, "penis at 12") and *machihembras* (meaning "first woman, then man").

Back in the United States, Imperato-McGinley and other scientists continued to study this condition, which affected about 2 percent of the village children. After a few years, the researchers pinpointed the cause—a genetic mutation that resulted in low levels of the enzyme 5-alpha reductase (5AR). This enzyme is essential for the production of dihydrotestosterone (DHT), a powerful male sex hormone that causes male characteristics, including male pattern baldness and prostate growth. Production of DHT is stimulated at puberty by pituitary gland hormones, which is why the masculine features appear. After Imperato-McGinley's research was published, other reports surfaced of people with DHT deficiency around the world.

Imperato-McGinley's work also caught the eye of pharmaceutical researchers. If a DHT deficiency stymies prostate growth, they theorized, then it might just fend off enlargement of the prostate later in life. As a result, finasteride, a drug that inhibits 5AR, was released on the market in 1992. It's frequently prescribed for benign prostatic hyperplasia (enlargement of the prostate).

ADDITIONAL FACTS

1. *According to Imperato-McGinley's reports, 16 of the 19* guevedoces *adopted male roles later in life. The remaining 3 eventually lived as women. All of them were sterile, and not all had functioning penises.*

2. *Finasteride (brand name Propecia) is also prescribed to fend off male pattern baldness.*

◆◆◆

Tooth Cavities

Tooth cavities are caused by tooth decay, which is the second-most-common health disorder, after the common cold. Decay is a common cause of tooth loss in children and young adults, but it can affect anyone.

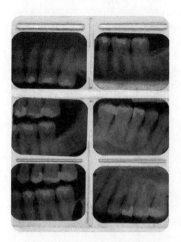

Tooth decay happens when plaque builds up on your teeth and is not thoroughly removed. Plaque formation begins when the normal bacteria in your mouth convert food into acids. Then the bacteria, acids, food debris, and saliva combine to form plaque, a substance that sticks to your teeth.

Plaque forms in particular on your back molars and just above the gum line. Certain acids in plaque dissolve the surface of your teeth, creating holes or cavities. Cavities usually do not hurt unless they grow very large, affect nerves, or cause a tooth to crack or break. When they progress this far, you may see holes in your teeth or have a toothache. An untreated cavity can lead to an abscess (a pocket of infected material within the tooth), destruction of the tooth's internal structures, and ultimately the loss of the tooth.

Most cavities are discovered during routine checkups. Dental x-rays show some cavities before they are visible to the eye. Sometimes the surface of a tooth that has a cavity is soft when probed with a sharp instrument.

Treatments for cavities include fillings, crowns, and root canals. The earlier the treatment is implemented, the less expensive and painful it is. To prevent cavities, you should have a professional cleaning every 6 months, brush twice a day with toothpaste that contains fluoride, and floss daily. As much as possible, avoid eating sugar, starches, and sticky foods, and refrain from frequent snacking.

ADDITIONAL FACTS

1. *Plaque starts to develop on your teeth within 20 minutes after eating.*

2. *Plaque that is not removed from your teeth hardens into tartar. Plaque and tartar irritate your gums and cause the gum diseases gingivitis and periodontitis.*

✦✦✦

Yellow Fever

US troops during the Spanish-American War had a lot more to worry about than just enemy soldiers and battlefield injuries. An even bigger threat at the time was yellow fever—a virus that caused flulike symptoms; jaundice (yellowing of the skin, from which the disease gets its name); and, often, internal bleeding, "black vomit," and death.

The epicenter of yellow fever infections was Cuba, where much of the fighting in the war happened. The disease had been recorded in the Caribbean for the first time in 1596 and was thought to have come over on slave ships from Africa. The disease was known to strike other parts of the continent—an epidemic hit Philadelphia in 1793, causing the government to flee as 10 percent of the city's population perished—but nowhere else was it as common as in Havana.

The United States temporarily took control of Cuba after winning the war, and in 1900 the US Army Medical Corps appointed the physicians Walter Reed (1851–1902) and James Carroll (1854–1907) to head a commission aimed at eradicating yellow fever. Mosquitoes had long been suspected as the agent of infection, and to test this hypothesis, Reed and Carroll divided soldiers into two groups—one of which lived among the clothing and bedding of yellow fever victims and one of which was kept in isolation but then bitten by mosquitoes. None of the first group fell ill, but 80 percent of the second did.

The next year, the government began a massive effort to eradicate mosquitoes, placing the campaign under the American military doctor William Gorgas (1854–1920). By eliminating any barrel, cistern, or tank where stagnant water could collect and using primitive pesticides—Gorgas poured kerosene into ponds to kill the insects—he managed to annihilate the mosquito population within 3 months, virtually eliminating yellow fever from Havana. Gorgas then targeted Panama, where the French had recently abandoned construction of the Panama Canal because of too many deaths from disease. Americans took over the operation in 1904, and within 2 years the Canal Zone was fever free. Similar programs were carried out, mostly with great success, in Brazil, Guatemala, Honduras, Mexico, Nicaragua, Peru, and El Salvador.

ADDITIONAL FACTS

1. *In 1925 in Africa, a new variety of yellow fever broke out, to which humans and monkeys are susceptible. Because there is no way to eliminate mosquitoes from the jungle, researchers developed a vaccine to fight the epidemic.*

2. *Reed remains the youngest student ever to graduate from the University of Virginia School of Medicine, where he completed a 2-year course and earned his degree at age 17. He obtained a second MD degree from New York University (NYU) Bellevue Hospital Medical College in 1870 at age 19.*

3. *Gorgas also graduated from the NYU Bellevue Hospital Medical College, in 1879. He went on to become surgeon general of the army and president of the American Medical Association.*

4. *Carroll allowed himself to be bitten by a mosquito that had bitten yellow fever victims, and 4 days later he came down with yellow fever. He survived but was left with heart disease, from which he died 17 years later.*

✦✦✦

Growth Plate

During childhood and adolescence, the bones grow at two specific points between the long shaft and the rounded ends. Each of these short stretches of fragile cartilage is called a growth plate, or an epiphyseal plate or physis.

The bone lengthens when the cartilage cells divide. After they stop reproducing, that area ossifies—or hardens—into bone, leaving behind a thin epiphyseal line. This typically occurs when people reach their adult height in their late teens or twenties. But even after that age, bones can still accumulate mass, or thickness. Much like skin cells, bone cells are constantly being made and broken down throughout life. The rate of turnover slows as you age; by age 30, most people reach their peak bone mass.

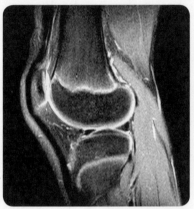

Because growth plates are among the weakest spots in the body—even more delicate than ligaments—they are vulnerable to injury. A tough tumble or fall can cause a growth plate fracture. Boys are twice as likely to suffer one, because they tend to develop more slowly than girls.

Most of the time, these injuries heal without any complications. However, in about one in six cases, they may lead to twisted or stunted bone growth. That's why many physicians may want to perform surgery or a series of follow-up x-rays on a fractured or broken bone in a child.

ADDITIONAL FACTS

1. *A bone growth disorder known as achondroplasia affects the epiphyseal plates and can lead to dwarfism.*

2. *Growth plate fractures account for 15 percent of all childhood fractures.*

◆◆◆

Lung Cancer

It's hard to believe that lung cancer was ever an obscure disease: About 150 years ago, it accounted for only 1 percent of cancers. But today, lung cancer is the leading cause of cancer death in the United States, claiming more lives than lymphatic, prostate, and breast cancers combined.

Why the drastic jump? The glamorous images of Hollywood stars smoking—and the growth in the popularity of cigarettes—in the early 1900s are culprits. (Studies show that cigarette smoke accounts for 82 percent of lung cancer deaths.) The increasing amount of air pollution, including exposure to asbestos, radon, and other chemicals, is another factor. That's because when you inhale these harmful particles, cancer-causing (carcinogenic) substances damage the cells that line the lungs' interior. These cells repair themselves, but chronic exposure can cause the cells to act abnormally and become cancerous.

There are two main types of lung cancer. Small cell lung cancer, which makes up 13 percent of cases, affects mainly heavy smokers and tends to spread rapidly. Non–small cell lung cancer is an umbrella term that accounts for the rest of lung cancers. In its earliest stages, the disease doesn't cause any symptoms. But as it progresses, it can cause a cough that doesn't go away, shortness of breath, chest pain, wheezing, and hoarseness. Sometimes sufferers cough up blood.

To diagnose lung cancer, a physician will perform an x-ray and a tissue biopsy. Treatments for the disease include chemotherapy, radiation therapy, targeted treatments, and surgery. The sooner the disease is detected, the better: Lung cancer patients have about a 50 percent chance of surviving longer than 5 years if it's caught—and treated—early on. If the cancer spreads, those odds drop to only 2 percent.

ADDITIONAL FACTS

1. *Lung cancer strikes more than 170,000 people a year and kills 157,000. Studies show that the rate of people dying of the disease is dropping in states with strong antitobacco programs.*

2. *The link between cigarettes and lung cancer was first written about by the German physician Fritz Lickint, who then went on an antismoking campaign in Germany. He was largely ignored.*

◆◆◆

Tylenol

A staple in any modern medicine cabinet, Tylenol is an over-the-counter pain reliever and fever reducer that works by cooling the body and changing the way the body senses pain. Tylenol's active ingredient and generic form, acetaminophen, was first used in medicine in 1894 and gained widespread use in the 1950s. It is a popular alternative to aspirin because it is gentler on the stomach.

Acetaminophen is part of a class of medications called analgesics (which relieve mild to moderate joint, muscle, or headache pain) and antipyretics (which reduce fever). Outside North America, it is sold as paracetamol; both generic names, as well as the brand name Tylenol, are derived from the chemical name of the compound, N-acetyl-para-aminophenol.

While acetaminophen is available without a prescription and is considered safe in small quantities, overdoses of this medication are responsible for more emergency room visits than any other drug on the market—up to 15,000 a year. Because so many medications contain acetaminophen, it's easy to take more than the recommended dosage without realizing it. Symptoms of an overdose may include nausea, vomiting, loss of appetite, sweating, extreme fatigue, unusual bleeding or bruising, pain in the upper right part of the abdomen, or yellowing of the skin or eyes. Even relatively small overdoses can severely damage the liver—especially if taken with alcohol.

More than 200 over-the-counter drugs contain acetaminophen, and it is often combined with other medications to treat symptoms other than general pain. Tylenol brand products, for example, include formulas specifically for cold and head congestion, sinus pain, menstrual cramps, arthritis, chest congestion, and cough and sore throat. Tylenol also markets nighttime products that contain antihistamines to induce drowsiness, extended-release formulas, liquid and chewable formulas, "meltaway" lozenges, and formulas for children and infants.

ADDITIONAL FACTS

1. *Combination acetaminophen products that contain nasal decongestants, antihistamines, cough suppressants, or expectorants should not be given to children younger than 2 years of age.*

2. *Chewable acetaminophen tablets may be sweetened with aspartame and should be avoided by people who have phenylketonuria.*

✦✦✦

Cerebral Aneurysm

A potentially fatal brain abnormality, cerebral aneurysms occur when arteries in the skull become swollen, thin-walled, and dangerously enlarged. These bloated vessels may then rupture or leak, spilling blood into the brain. About 27,000 cases of ruptured cerebral aneurysms are reported each year in the United States, usually in people between the ages of 30 and 60.

Cerebral aneurysms can be caused by infections, tumors, trauma to the head, or unhealthy arteries due to plaque buildup or high blood pressure. In some people, cerebral aneurysms form during fetal development and persist throughout life. They are most often found near the bottom of the skull. Aneurysms are common; millions of people have them, and most never burst.

However, when an aneurysm does burst, the bleeding into the brain may cause a stroke, nerve damage, or death. People who survive an aneurysm will have long-term health problems such as swelling in the brain or the blockage of important arteries. For people who experience a burst aneurysm, it may feel like "the worst headache of my life." High blood pressure, cigarette smoking, heavy alcohol use, and drug abuse (particularly the use of cocaine) increase a person's risk of the rupture of a cerebral aneurysm.

Even aneurysms that do not burst, though, may cause serious problems in some people. An enlarged vessel can bulge out against surrounding brain material, potentially causing eye pain, facial paralysis, and vision problems.

Aneurysms can be detected with a CT scan or MRI, and treatment options vary depending on their size and location. If the aneurysm is small and located in a low-risk area of the brain, doctors may simply leave it there.

ADDITIONAL FACTS

1. *A small number of patients will experience sentinel, or warning, headaches when an aneurysm leaks for days or weeks before rupturing.*

2. *Doctors use CT scans, MRIs or angiography (x-rays of blood vessels after injecting dye) to pinpoint the site of an aneurysm, usually after symptoms have already occurred.*

3. *A physician may perform surgery to repair damaged arteries, although it can be risky.*

4. *To treat the problem without surgery, a doctor may inject a substance via a thin tube threaded through the blood vessels to close off the aneurysm. It's estimated that 40 percent of patients whose aneurysms burst do not survive the first 24 hours, and up to another 25 percent die within 6 months. Those whose aneurysms are treated before they rupture generally have a better prognosis; they recover faster and require less rehabilitative therapy.*

◆ ◆ ◆

Adrenogenital Syndrome

Perched on top of each kidney is a triangle-shaped adrenal gland. In spite of its small, inch-long size, it plays a big role in the body, releasing male sex and steroid hormones, such as cortisol. But, for about 1 in 10,000 people, a recessive genetic disorder causes these glands to go out of whack. They slow their production of corticosteroids such as cortisol and pump an excess of androgen hormones, particularly androstenedione and other 17-ketosteroids, into the bloodstream. For men, this condition, called adrenogenital syndrome, isn't life altering; symptoms include an enlarged penis, small testes, acne, and short stature. But, for women, it can create an entire gender shift during the first decade of their lives or can lead to menstrual disorders and infertility when it appears after puberty in some women.

Because of the excess androgens, girls take on a male appearance at birth—even though they have the female chromosomes and a female reproductive system. Physically, the clitoris enlarges—in some cases, to the size of a penis—and the vaginal lips fuse to become an empty scrotum. In other words, these girls look like boys on the outside and are sometimes raised as male if the diagnosis is missed. Most parents are unaware of their child's condition until around puberty, when the testes don't descend. Some may choose to opt for cosmetic surgery altering the genitalia, and a physician typically prescribes hormones to correct the imbalance. Gender identity problems may require psychiatric treatment in such patients.

In adult women, adrenogenital syndrome can lead to other masculine attributes, such as a failure to menstruate and a deep voice. It can also trigger excessive hair growth: If you've ever seen a sideshow act with a bearded lady, chances are that you've just witnessed someone with adrenogenital syndrome.

ADDITIONAL FACTS

1. *Adrenogenital syndrome is most often caused by a genetic defect that lowers the levels of the enzyme 21-hydroxylase, which in turn slows corticosteroid production in the adrenal glands.*

2. *This condition is more common in Ashkenazi Jews, Italians, Latinos, and certain Eastern Europeans.*

3. *Amniocentesis, a procedure in which a sample of fetal cells is drawn from the fluid in the womb, can test whether a fetus has this syndrome.*

♦♦♦

Periodontal Disease

Periodontal disease is gum disease that threatens your oral health. Gum disease can range in severity from simple gum inflammation called gingivitis to conditions that damage the bone. Gum disease is extremely common, as about 80 percent of adults in the United States have some form of the disorder.

You probably have gingivitis if your gums are red and swollen and they bleed easily. Gingivitis usually gets better if you brush and floss every day and see your dentist regularly. If you do not treat gingivitis, you may develop periodontitis, in which the gums pull away from the teeth and form infected pockets. When periodontitis is left untreated, the underlying bones, gums, and connective tissues can be permanently damaged or destroyed, and eventually you may lose your teeth.

Gingivitis is caused by bacteria that occur normally in the mouth. Along with mucus and other particles, the bacteria form plaque, which sticks to your teeth. Plaque that is not removed by brushing and flossing hardens and becomes tartar, which is filled with bacteria. Normal brushing does not remove tartar; it can be removed only with a professional cleaning by a dentist or dental hygienist. In extreme situations, you may need medication, surgery, or bone and tissue grafts to treat gum disease or the damage it causes.

There are certain risk factors that increase the likelihood that you'll develop gum disease. These include smoking, hormonal changes in girls and women, some illnesses, stress, some medications, and genetic susceptibility. People who have rheumatoid arthritis may also be at increased risk of gum disease.

ADDITIONAL FACTS

1. *Gum disease may contribute to health problems in areas other than the mouth, including increasing the risk of heart attack or stroke.*

2. *Usually, people do not develop gum disease until they are in their thirties or forties. Men are more prone to gum disease than women are.*

3. *In pregnant women, gum disease has been associated with the risk of delivering preterm or low-birth-weight babies.*

◆◆◆

Laparoscopy

The practice of laparoscopy began with looking inside the body using a long, lighted tube and mirrors. In the 20th century, however, doctors saw its potential for more active treatments and use in surgical procedures as well.

In 1910, the Swedish physician Hans Christian Jacobaeus (1879–1937) performed what are considered to have been the first laparoscopic surgeries: He used a cystoscope—a narrow tube inserted into the urethra to examine the bladder—to determine the cause of abdominal complaints in patients with tuberculosis. The Johns Hopkins Hospital in Baltimore soon reported on a similar procedure of its own, called organoscopy. In New York City in the 1950s, Albert Decker (1895–1988)introduced the culdoscope for viewing the female pelvis through the vaginal canal.

Some of the first tools to be utilized laparoscopically were spring-loaded needles used for pneumoperitoneum (filling the abdominal cavity with air for easier visibility and maneuvering during surgery) and forceps used for electrocoagulation of bleeding areas. In 1961, the French gynecologist Raoul Palmer (1904–1985) performed the first laparoscopic retrieval of a woman's eggs for an attempt at in vitro fertilization. Around the same time, the German doctor Kurt Semm (1927–2003) performed the first appendectomy during a gynecologic procedure, without the need for a large incision in the abdomen. By 1970, gynecologists were routinely doing tubal ligation for sterilization by laparoscopy. In 1971, the New York gynecologist Bruce Young (1938–) introduced the umbilical incision for pelvic laparoscopy because a belly dancer requested that he leave no visible scar, and it was safer and easier to perform.

In the early 1970s, surgeons at Grant Hospital of Chicago standardized a technique for performing surgery through miniature incisions in the abdomen. This practice became widespread by the 1980s, especially after the introduction of video laparoscopy. The first laparoscopic cholecystectomy—removal of the gallbladder through four small abdominal incisions—was performed in 1987 in France. Today, gallbladder removal is the most common laparoscopic procedure performed, using scissors, graspers, and other tools only 5 to 10 millimeters in diameter. Because the gallbladder is like a small balloon, it can be sucked out of a 1-centimeter incision by first suctioning out the bile inside. Other procedures that can be done laparoscopically today include removal of the colon, kidney, and spleen; bariatric weight-loss surgery; and gynecologic and urologic surgery. Recovery time for these procedures is typically much less than for traditional surgery; sometimes patients can even leave the hospital the same day.

ADDITIONAL FACTS

1. *Laparoscopy is also known as minimally invasive surgery, keyhole surgery, or pinhole surgery.*

2. *Some laparoscopic surgery today is done robotically, which eliminates human error and allows doctors to operate from a remote location. The first transatlantic surgery ever performed, known as the Lindbergh operation, was a laparoscopic gallbladder removal in 2001.*

3. *The devices used as "ports" to introduce laparoscopic tools into the body cavity are called trocars.*

✦✦✦

Puberty

Except for infancy, puberty is the stage in life during which the body develops most rapidly. During this time, sex hormones start to change the body, turning girls into women and boys into men. In the United States, the average age at which puberty begins is 12 for girls and 14 for boys. This series of changes and events can stretch over 6 months or as long as 6 years, depending on the person, and it varies with ethnicity and geography as well.

First the adrenal glands begin to produce more hormones in boys and girls, stimulating some underarm and pubic hair to appear. Then a part of the brain called the hypothalamus kicks off a cascade of events that triggers puberty. The hypothalamus releases a hormone that instructs the pituitary gland (a pea-size gland at the bottom of the brain) to release two more hormones—luteinizing hormone and follicle-stimulating hormone—to initiate sexual development. In boys, these substances instruct the testes to start pumping testosterone and dihydrotestosterone, the male hormones, throughout the body. As a result, the testicles and penis grow, and hair starts to grow in the pubic area, in the armpits, and on the trunk, limbs, and face. Because of testosterone, the throat's larynx and vocal cords enlarge, resulting in a deeper voice.

In girls, the same hormones signal the ovaries to begin producing estrogen, causing the breasts to develop, fat to be deposited on the hips, and small amounts of male hormones to cause hair to grow in the armpits and pubic area. A few years after puberty commences, sufficient estrogen is being produced to stimulate the uterus, and a girl starts her first menstrual cycle. Subsequently, menstruation becomes regular as she ovulates (her ovaries release an egg) each month, and she's able to bear children. During puberty, the sex hormones in both boys and girls trigger rapid growth that generally brings them close to their adult height, which they reach after puberty. The growth stops when the sex hormones close the growth zones on long bones.

ADDITIONAL FACTS

1. *Testosterone causes the skin to generate more oil, which leads to adolescent acne.*

2. *Experiencing puberty a few years earlier or later than average is often hereditary.*

3. *The onset of puberty is earlier in parts of world with more sunlight exposure.*

◆◆◆

Pancreatic Cancer

Although your stomach may grumble when it's mealtime, the pancreas—a 6-inch-long organ that lies horizontally deep in the upper abdomen—also affects hunger. It secretes hormones that monitor and regulate blood sugar levels in the body, as well as enzymes that aid in digestion. Symptoms of pancreatic cancer include a loss of appetite and weight, as well as nausea, abdominal pain, and jaundice (a yellowing of the skin and eyes). The symptoms appear only late in the course of the disease.

One of the most lethal forms of cancer, pancreatic cancer strikes 38,000 people each year—and takes the lives of 34,000. Because the disease is difficult to detect and treat, the 5-year survival rate (the number of patients who are alive 5 years after diagnosis) is only about 5 percent.

Experts aren't exactly sure what causes pancreatic cancer, but they do know that people who have a family history of the disease, have a genetic syndrome that increases cancer risk (such as a BRCA mutation), or are African American are at a higher risk of developing it. Certain lifestyle factors, such as heavy drinking of alcohol, smoking, and being overweight, may also up the odds. Most people who get pancreatic cancer are older, in their seventies or eighties.

Unlike with breast cancer and mammograms, there are no standard screening tests for pancreatic cancer. To diagnose the disease, doctors examine the pancreas with an x-ray, MRI, CT scan, ultrasound, or biopsy. Pancreatic cancer is aggressive, which means that it quickly spreads to other parts of the body. That's why only a small number of cases have a good chance of being cured through the surgical removal of all or part of the pancreas. The majority of the time, chemotherapy or radiation therapy is employed to wipe out the cancerous cells. Currently, researchers are searching for ways to develop a vaccine for pancreatic cancer and drugs that would prevent cancerous cells from spreading to other parts of the body.

ADDITIONAL FACTS

1. *Pancreatic cancer is the fifth-leading cause of cancer deaths.*

2. *The actor Patrick Swayze (1952–), star of the movie* Dirty Dancing, *was diagnosed with pancreatic cancer in 2008.*

✦✦✦

Indomethacin

Indomethacin is a prescription drug that is used to fight fever, arthritis, gout, and other diseases. It belongs to a class of medications called nonsteroidal anti-inflammatory drugs, or NSAIDs. If used properly, indomethacin can reduce swelling and provide pain relief. But indomethacin must be taken carefully, because the drug can cause severe adverse reactions and even death in some people.

First approved in 1965, indomethacin is available in tablet, liquid, and suppository forms. The purpose of taking indomethacin is usually to alleviate pain; it generally does not cure the underlying disorder. It is often the first drug prescribed to treat attacks of gout, an extremely painful form of arthritis that has become increasingly common recently and usually strikes the big toe.

One disorder that indomethacin can cure is patent ductus arteriosus, a heart problem that often occurs in newborn infants. The condition arises when a newborn's circulatory system fails to adjust to being out of the womb, which may cause the infant's heart to work too hard. An injection of indomethacin given within a few days of birth will often take care of the problem.

Indomethacin shares many of the same possible negative side effects with other NSAIDs and may increase the risk of heart attack or stroke. It can also cause nausea, headache, and abdominal pain. In rare cases, fatal intestinal problems have resulted from taking the medication.

People taking indomethacin should not drink alcohol or take over-the-counter cold, allergy, or pain medications without talking to a doctor. These other drugs may contain similar ingredients (such as aspirin, ibuprofen, ketoprofen, or naproxen) and could lead to an accidental overdose.

ADDITIONAL FACTS

1. *Indomethacin is sometimes used off-label to slow preterm labor for up to 48 hours by slowing uterine contractions.*

2. *Like other NSAIDs, indomethacin often can relieve menstrual pain.*

3. *Indomethacin may worsen chronic health conditions such as epilepsy, Parkinson's disease, and psychotic disorders.*

❖❖❖

Brain Tumor

Any growth of abnormal cells in the tissue of the brain is known as a tumor. Such growths can be malignant (cancerous) or benign (noncancerous), but because of their proximity to important brain tissue and their enclosure within the skull, both types can be life threatening. Brain tumors are usually classified as low or high grade, depending on how fast they're growing.

About 52,000 new brain and nervous system tumors are diagnosed every year in the United States, and more than 13,000 people die of brain tumor complications annually. Research has shown that being male, Caucasian, or age 70 or older; being exposed to radiation or toxic chemicals at work; or having a family history of brain tumors increases a person's risk. Not everyone with these risk factors will get a brain tumor, however, and many people who do develop tumors do not have any of these risks.

Symptoms such as severe morning headaches; nausea or vomiting; changes in speech, vision, or hearing; balance and memory problems; and convulsions may occur when a tumor presses on a nerve or damages a certain area of the brain. The World Health Organization recognizes 126 different types of central nervous system tumors. The following are the most common.

Meningiomas account for 27 percent of tumors that start in the brain. They form in the meninges, the membrane lining the skull, and affect twice as many women as men. Because they rarely spread, they are often curable with surgery. Doctors may prescribe steroids to control swelling and inflammation or may follow a passive strategy known as watchful waiting to monitor the tumor's growth before considering surgery.

High-grade astrocytomas and glioblastomas originate in the astrocytes, the connective tissue cells of the brain. These tumors grow rapidly, invading nearby folds of the brain, and can be difficult to treat even with surgery, radiation, and chemotherapy. Astrocytomas and glioblastomas account for about 25 percent of all primary brain cancers.

Tumors that begin elsewhere and metastasize, or spread, to the brain are the most common brain tumors, especially since people are surviving primary cancers for longer periods of time.

ADDITIONAL FACTS

1. *Scientists are investigating whether cell phones may cause brain tumors, but no evidence has been found thus far.*

2. *After leukemia, brain tumors are the second-most-common type of cancer in children and young adults. Medulloblastoma, for example, is a rare type of tumor that afflicts mainly boys and young men.*

✦✦✦

Testicular Feminization

Testicular feminization, also known as androgen insensitivity syndrome, is seen when a person who is genetically male does not respond to the male sex hormone testosterone. As a result, female characteristics form to varying degrees. In complete testicular feminization, a person's outward appearance is all woman: He has a vagina and a female body, although the other internal reproductive organs—the uterus, ovaries, and fallopian tubes—are missing. The testes are internal and replace the ovaries. This occurs in about 1 in 20,000 births.

So, what causes this syndrome? Scientists have pinpointed genetic defects on the Y chromosome, which results in malfunctioning protein receptors in the cell. It's as if someone has changed the locks to keep out testosterone: When the male sex hormone attempts to bind to important tissues, it's blocked out and floats away.

Like the other ambiguous sex conditions, this syndrome is frequently detected during puberty. A person with testicular feminization may develop breasts but will fail to ovulate, menstruate, or grow underarm hair. Because these individuals have been raised as girls and identify as females, the majority choose to remain identified as women. Treatment options include surgery to remove any remaining testicular tissue and construct a more complete vagina, estrogen replacement therapy after puberty, and psychological counseling.

ADDITIONAL FACTS

1. *In 1953, the endocrinologist J. C. Morris suggested the term* testicular feminization *for the syndrome.*

2. *To diagnose testicular feminization, physicians often perform a pelvic exam and test hormone levels.*

✦✦✦

Alcohol

Alcohol is the intoxicating ingredient found in beer, wine, and liquor. It is made by fermenting of yeast, sugars, or starches. Occasional drinking of alcohol is extremely common in the United States.

For most people, moderate drinking is safe and may even have health benefits for the heart. Drinking in moderation is generally defined as no more than one drink a day for women and no more than two drinks a day for men. This definition refers to the amount consumed on a single day only and should not be used to average the number of drinks over a few days.

Alcohol is a central nervous system depressant. It is quickly absorbed from the stomach and small intestine into the bloodstream and broken down in the liver by enzymes. Since the liver can metabolize only a small amount of alcohol at a time, the excess alcohol circulates throughout the body. The more alcohol you drink, the more intoxicated you become.

There is no doubt that too much drinking is bad for you. Alcohol use slows reaction time and weakens your judgment and coordination, which is why you should never drink alcohol and drive. Binge drinking, or having five or more drinks at a time, increases your risk of accidents and assaults. Heavy drinking over years can lead to liver disease, heart disease, cancer, and pancreatitis. Drinking alcohol affects every organ in your body.

ADDITIONAL FACTS

1. *Some people should never drink, such as alcoholics, children, pregnant women, people taking certain medications, and people with certain medical conditions.*

2. *A standard drink in the United States is equal to 0.6 ounce (13.7 grams) of pure alcohol, 12 ounces of beer, 8 ounces of malt liquor, 5 ounces of wine, or 1.5 ounces of 80-proof distilled spirits or liquor, such as gin, rum, vodka, or whiskey.*

3. *The legal limit for blood alcohol content while operating a motor vehicle in the United States is 0.08 percent (80 milligrams per deciliter) for drivers who are at least 21 years of age. Drivers under 21 are not allowed to operate a motor vehicle with any amount of alcohol in their systems.*

◆◆◆

Joseph Goldberger and Pellagra

The link between poor nutrition, poverty, and a deadly disease called pellagra was first identified by the physician Joseph Goldberger in the early 21st century.

Goldberger (1874–1929) was born in Hungary and immigrated to New York City as a boy. After medical school at New York University, he enlisted in the United States Marine Hospital Service (later the US Public Health Service) and became well known for his skill at figuring out and fighting the causes of infectious diseases. He traveled the country battling yellow fever, typhoid fever, and Shamberg's disease, an itchy skin ailment caused by bed mites. In 1914, the United States surgeon general asked him to focus on pellagra, a skin disease that was reaching epidemic proportions throughout the country.

Pellagra, also known as *mal de la rosa*, was responsible for more than 100,000 deaths in the United States in the first 4 decades of the 20th century; the southern states were especially affected and had a much higher mortality rate. Doctors sometimes described pellagra as the disease of the four Ds, in reference to its four distinguishing symptoms: dermatitis, dementia, diarrhea, and death. When Goldberger began to study the disease, he was struck by the fact that in mental hospitals, orphanages, and other institutions, inmates became sick, but staff didn't. He decided, against popular opinion, that the disease could not be contagious, that something else had to be at play. When Goldberger requested that food shipments of fresh meat, milk, and vegetables be delivered to children in two Mississippi orphanages and to inmates at the Georgia State Asylum, pellagra at those institutions disappeared. He determined that some nutrient missing from a corn-based diet, popular in the poverty-stricken South, prevented the disease.

Goldberger spent the rest of his life searching for this "pellagra preventive factor," but never solved the mystery. He fell sick and died before realizing that the mystery nutrient was the B vitamin niacin, a discovery made in the next decade, largely thanks to Goldberger's work.

ADDITIONAL FACTS

1. *Frustrated and determined to convince his contemporaries that pellagra was not contagious, Goldberger and supporters held "filth parties" in which they shared bodily fluids with those of diseased people: They injected themselves with the blood of people with pellagra, swallowed capsules containing scabs of pellagra rashes, and rubbed affected people's mucus into their own throats and noses.*

2. *The pellagra epidemic was somewhat lessened by a plague of boll weevils that struck cotton fields in the South during the 1920s. The infestation forced many farmers to switch to other crops instead of relying totally on cotton, which in turn caused them to eat a healthier diet.*

3. *Pellagra has been suggested as a possible source of the myth of vampirism. Like vampires, people with pellagra are sensitive to sunlight, they often don't eat (because of diarrhea), and their tongues can swell and become red from malnutrition, evoking thoughts of blood.*

◆ ◆ ◆

Menarche

The term *menarche* contains the Latin word for "month" (*men*) and the Greek word for "beginning" (*arche*). Today it's a term used to describe the first menstrual cycle. The average age for menarche is from 11 to 14, although it can normally occur as early as 9 or as late as 15.

Menarche typically occurs a few years after the beginning of puberty, during which hormones prepare the body for reproduction. The pituitary gland starts to release two hormones—follicle-stimulating hormone and luteinizing hormone—which stimulate growth and the production of estrogen in the ovaries. Over 2 weeks, these levels climb until an egg is released from a follicle in one of the ovaries to travel down the neighboring fallopian tube. At this point, the hormone progesterone is added to the hormones made by the ovaries, causing the uterine lining to mature in preparation for a fertilized egg. But if the egg doesn't come into successful contact with sperm, the uterine lining is shed during menstruation.

The 28-day reproductive cycle takes a few tries before the body adjusts; most girls don't ovulate for the first year after menarche. During that time, the cycle is usually not regular; it can range anywhere from 21 to 40 days. Women have menstrual cycles once a month until menopause, which usually begins between ages 45 and 55.

In many societies and cultures around the globe, menarche has been heralded as a sacred rite of passage from girl to woman. The Kolosh Indians of Alaska, for instance, confined pubescent girls in a small hut for a year, while some Cambodian girls had to remain in bed under a mosquito curtain for 100 days. After these periods of confinement, the girls would emerge as marriageable women.

ADDITIONAL FACTS

1. *The earliest known menarche was supposedly at 8 months. The Peruvian girl, Lina Medina went on to give birth to a son when she was an estimated 6 to 8 years old.*

2. *Only the superficial part of the uterine lining is shed during menstruation. The basal layer remains and grows into a thick new lining in every normal cycle.*

◆◆◆

Skin Cancer

A glowing, tanned complexion seems healthy, but when achieved through unprotected exposure to the sun, it can be dangerous or even deadly. That's because changes in skin color, such as tans and sunburns, may indicate damage to skin cells caused by ultraviolet (UV) radiation. This can trigger mutations in skin cells and lead to cancer.

Skin cancer affects more than 1 million Americans every year; most—but not all—cases are considered to be sun related. There are three main forms of the disease. The most common kind, basal cell carcinoma, usually appears as a pearly, round, reddish bump or a scarlike lesion. Curable 99 percent of the time, this cancer has an extremely slow growth rate and usually does not spread to other parts of the body. If the bump is firm and red or if the lesion has a scaly, crusty surface, it's probably a squamous cell carcinoma. This cancer may grow and spread rapidly, but it's readily curable if diagnosed early. (Only 1 percent of squamous cell carcinomas are deadly.)

The most serious type of skin cancer is melanoma, which affects nearly 60,000 people each year. Compared with the other kinds, melanoma spreads more rapidly and is more resistant to treatments, such as chemotherapy. This cancer affects the melanocytes, pigment-producing cells in the skin, and appears as a flat, brown patch with uneven edges; a black or gray lump; or a raised brown patch with spots.

Because the majority of skin cancers are detected by patients themselves, experts recommend that all people know the ABCDEs of the disease. Look for moles that are asymmetrical (A) in shape, have blurry or jagged borders (B), become lighter or darker in color (C), are larger than ¼ inch in diameter (D), and/or are evolving, that is, changes (E), or raised above the skin's surface. A dermatologist can take a biopsy of the suspect mole to test for cancer. Most skin cancers are easily treated by removing the affected skin with surgery, such as cryosurgery (freezing off a small patch) or laser surgery. If the cancer has spread, radiation therapy or chemotherapy may be required.

ADDITIONAL FACTS

1. *Because the sun's rays are strongest from 10:00 a.m. to 4:00 p.m., the American Cancer Society recommends staying in the shade as much as possible during those hours.*

2. *Up to 80 percent of UV radiation passes through clouds, so sunscreen is needed even on gray, drizzly days.*

◆◆◆

Ayurvedic Therapy

One of the world's oldest medical systems is Ayurveda, which means "the science of life" in Sanskrit. Ayurvedic medicine originated in India several thousand years ago and uses materials and techniques such as herbs, oils, and massages to cleanse and balance the body, mind, and spirit.

Two Sanskrit books written more than 2,000 years ago are considered to be the main texts on Ayurvedic medicine. They describe eight branches of medicine: internal medicine; surgery; treatment of head and neck diseases; psychiatry; toxicology; sexual vitality; gynecology, obstetrics, and pediatrics; and care of the elderly and rejuvenation.

Ayurveda remains highly popular in South Asia and especially in India, where almost 80 percent of the population still relies to some degree on the ancient practices. Most major cities in India have an Ayurvedic college and hospital. In the United States, a 2002 survey found that about 750,000 Americans (about 0.4 percent of the population) had used Ayurvedic medicine at some point.

Ayurveda has several key foundations that pertain to health and disease, including the notion of interconnectedness, the importance of personal constitution, and the three life forces that act upon all people.

Interconnectedness means that all beings in the universe are, in a sense, part of a single whole, and that keeping in harmony with this web of existence is crucial for health. A person's constitution, or *prakriti,* also plays a critical role in overall health. Finally, the three life forces, or *doshas,* are believed to control basic bodily functions like breathing, digestion, and the beating of the heart.

Ayurvedic medications are not regulated by the Food and Drug Administration. Some can be toxic if taken in large quantities or in combination with other drugs, and several studies have found that many over-the-counter Ayurvedic remedies (all manufactured in Southeast Asia) contain lead, mercury, or arsenic.

ADDITIONAL FACTS

1. *Research is currently being done on several Ayurvedic treatments, including using turmeric for cardiovascular conditions, the herb gotu kola to treat Alzheimer's disease, and botanicals such as ginger, turmeric, and boswellia to treat inflammatory disorders such as arthritis and asthma.*

2. *A 2008 report by researchers at Boston University found that 21 percent of Ayurvedic treatments purchased on the Internet contained impurities.*

3. *Students who receive their Ayurvedic training in India can earn either a bachelor's or a doctoral degree there. The United States has no national standard for training or certification of Ayurvedic practitioners, although a few states have approved Ayurvedic schools as educational institutions.*

✦✦✦

Arteriovenous Malformations

Arteriovenous malformations (AVMs) are short circuits in the circulatory system believed to arise during fetal development or shortly after birth. Most of the suspected 300,000 people with AVMs exhibit minor—if any—symptoms, but about 12 percent of cases can result in headaches, seizure, stroke, or even death. The malformations can form anywhere in the body, but are especially dangerous when they occur in the brain.

Normally, oxygen-carrying blood flows into the brain and other organs through arteries and tiny vessels called capillaries, nourishing the surrounding tissue before traveling back to the heart through the veins. AVMs are areas that lack the tiny capillaries, where blood flows straight from the artery (heading away from the heart) into the vein (heading back toward the heart). The location of this connection between the artery and vein is called a fistula, or shunt. The nearby area of tissue, which misses out on blood and nutrients, is called the nidus of the AVM.

Though headaches and seizures are the most common signs of AVMs, these malformations can cause a wide range of other symptoms—including muscle weakness, loss of coordination, memory deficits, hallucinations, and mental impairment—depending on their locations in the body.

Each year, about 4 percent of people with AVMs experience hemorrhaging, or internal bleeding, when increased blood pressure and flow cause fistula vessels to rupture. Most episodes are not severe enough to produce significant damage, but some may cause a stroke or altered bloodflow, sparking progressive neurological problems.

Some of the symptoms of AVM can be eased by medications, but surgery is the only true way to treat them. However, surgery of the central nervous system carries its own risks. Whenever an AVM is detected, the patient should be monitored carefully for signs that may indicate an increased risk of hemorrhage.

ADDITIONAL FACTS

1. *Three surgical options exist for the treatment of AVMs: Conventional surgery is best for relatively small AVMs in superficial portions of the brain or spinal cord. For anything larger or in a riskier area, embolization (introducing a glue, coil, or tiny balloon into the bloodstream through a tiny catheter to form a clot and divert bloodflow) or radiosurgery (aiming high-dose beams of radiation at the AVM to alter the blood vessel walls) is usually performed in lieu of or in addition to conventional surgery.*

2. *An AVM can be detected by a CT scan or an MRI. But because so few people experience symptoms, most AVMs are discovered accidentally during examination for another condition or during autopsy after death.*

3. *There are some genetic conditions known to cause AVMs, such as Osler-Weber-Rendu disease and polycystic kidney disease.*

◆◆◆

Rokitansky Syndrome

Throughout his lifetime, Baron Karl von Rokitansky (1804–1878), an Austrian pathologist, performed more than 30,000 autopsies in his research. During one of them, he came across something startling—a woman born without a fully formed uterus, cervix, and vagina. This birth defect later become known as Rokitansky or Mayer-Rokitansky-Kuester-Hauser (MRKH) syndrome, named in part after three other scientists who also studied the condition. Although fewer than 20,000 cases of MRKH have been diagnosed worldwide, experts believe many others go unreported; some estimate that as many as 1 in 5,000 women are affected.

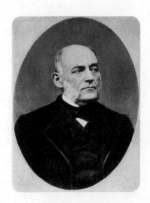

Although the exact cause of the syndrome isn't clear, it's known that the reproductive system fails to completely develop when the fetus is about 3 months old. The ovaries and fallopian tubes form, but the uterus, cervix, and upper portion of the vagina either are missing or don't fully take shape (called agenesis); in some cases, there may be kidney abnormalities. Many women with MRKH have a very shallow vagina, known as a vaginal dimple. While most vaginas are about 5½ inches deep, a vaginal dimple measures less than 2 inches. As a result, sexual intercourse can be difficult or impossible.

Despite these missing reproductive organs, a woman with MRKH, by all physical appearances, leads a normal existence. She possesses a complete set of 46 female (XX) chromosomes, experiences the same physical and hormonal changes other young women go through during puberty, and undergoes ovulation every month. The main difference is that, without a functioning uterus, she is unable to menstruate or become pregnant. If an MRKH couple wishes to have a child, the pair may opt for in vitro fertilization and a surrogate mother. Although many women with this syndrome choose not to seek treatment, others undergo procedures to create a vagina through dilation (a gradual stretching) or surgery.

ADDITIONAL FACTS

1. *Some researchers believe that MRKH may stem from a defective gene, possibly on chromosome 22.*

2. *MRKH is one of a group of birth defects of the vagina or uterus known as müllerian anomalies. They affect up to 10 percent of women.*

3. *What we now call MRKH syndrome is described in medical literature as far back as Hippocrates'* Nature of Women.

◆◆◆

Food Poisoning

Food poisoning is caused by food contamination, usually by bacteria, parasites, or viruses. Symptoms can vary from mild to serious and include upset stomach, abdominal cramps, nausea and vomiting, diarrhea, fever, and dehydration. Symptoms usually last a few hours to a few days. Most of the time, increasing your fluid intake is the only treatment needed, but occasionally hospitalization and intravenous fluid replacement become necessary.

Food poisoning occurs for a number of reasons. Some foods already have bacteria on them when you buy them. Meat may be tainted during slaughter. Fruits and vegetables may come in contact with fecal material or other causes of disease when the produce is growing or being processed. However, food can also become contaminated if you leave it out for 2 hours or more at room temperature. Sometimes food contamination occurs during preparation of food. Additionally, dangerous chemicals can cause food poisoning if they come in contact with food during its harvesting or processing.

To prevent food poisoning, food should be kept refrigerated or should be thoroughly cooked. When the temperature of food is between 40° and 140°F, bacteria multiply the most rapidly. The best way to destroy bacteria in contaminated food is with thorough cooking. Meat should be cooked to an internal temperature of 165°F, and poultry should reach an internal temperature of 180°F. Additionally, your refrigerator should be set to 40°F or lower, and your freezer should be kept at 0°F.

Young children, people with compromised immune systems, pregnant women and their fetuses, and older adults are at the greatest risk from bacterial infections. Certain microorganisms rarely can cause the spontaneous abortion of a fetus or the death of an adult. Children are at particular risk from the bacteria *Escherichia coli* O157:H7, which can lead to kidney failure and death.

ADDITIONAL FACTS

1. *Seventy-six million people in the United States get sick from contaminated food annually. The majority of these infections are not reported. However, 5,000 people die of food poisoning each year.*

2. *It's estimated that 1 in 10,000 eggs is contaminated with the bacterium* Salmonella. *Produce such as spinach, lettuce, tomatoes, sprouts, and melons can be contaminated with* Salmonella, Shigella, *or* E. coli *O157:H7.*

❖❖❖

Influenza Epidemic of 1918

Getting the flu today is certainly no fun—but for most of us, it's not a matter of life or death. The influenza epidemic that swept the world in 1918, however, was another story. In as little as 6 months, the flu killed more than 25 million people; that's more than three times the number of people killed in World War I, and makes it's the deadliest epidemic in history.

In the spring of 1918, reports of influenza surfaced quietly, with few deaths and quick recoveries. In the fall it returned—and this time, turned quickly to pneumonia, for which there was no effective treatment at the time. The plague spread rapidly across the globe on ships transporting people and goods on the heels of the recently ended Great War. Especially hard hit were the cities of Freetown, Sierra Leone; Brest, a French naval port; and Boston. In Boston, 10 percent of the population contracted the flu, and 60 percent of sufferers died. The illness decimated US troops at home and abroad; by October, 34,000 soldiers had died in battle, compared with 24,000 from the flu.

Throughout the United States, public gatherings were banned. Schools, churches, cinemas, and businesses were closed, and people wore face masks outside their homes. Because many medical personnel had gone abroad for the war, doctors and nurses often traveled long distances to see patients and either became ill en route or found themselves unprepared and unable to help upon reaching their destinations.

Overall, the United States lost more than 500,000; England and Wales, 200,000; and Samoa, a quarter of its population. Thankfully, the flu vanished abruptly in 1919. although less-severe outbreaks have occurred several times since. Scientists first thought that bacteria had caused the 1918 epidemic. In 1933, however, researchers correctly identified the influenza A virus as the culprit; they discovered influenzas B and C over the next 2 decades and devised vaccines to protect against them. Because flu viruses mutate so quickly, it's recommended today that people get a new flu vaccination every year.

ADDITIONAL FACTS

1. *The particular flu strain that caused the epidemic was often referred to as Spanish flu—although it originated in the United States.*

2. *Aside from getting a flu vaccination, one of the best ways to fight the spread of flu is to wash your hands frequently and cover your mouth when you cough or sneeze.*

3. *Influenza returned in a pandemic form in 1957 and again in 1968, each time killing tens of thousands of Americans.*

✦✦✦

Acne

Every year, Americans spend more than $100 million on over-the-counter products to treat acne. That's because this skin ailment is a frustrating and unsightly condition that affects about 85 percent of teenagers and young adults, along with 12 percent of women and 3 percent of men until about age 44.

Acne occurs when hair follicles, the openings in which hairs grow, become clogged with oil, dead skin cells, and bacteria. As a result, a lubricating substance called sebum that's normally secreted from these openings blocks them, creating bumps called whiteheads. (If the plug is close to the skin's surface, it can darken into a blackhead.) Bacteria that reside on the surface of the skin can multiply and infect the area, resulting in inflammation. That's what causes a red and swollen pimple.

The severity of acne depends on how deeply a follicle becomes clogged. Papules and pustules are red bumps with white pus just beneath the skin's surface, while nodules are the more painful lumps resulting from buildup deep in the follicle. Cysts are boil-like bumps beneath the skin's surface; these blemishes can lead to scarring.

Acne is often brought on by the increased levels of hormones, such as testosterone, that are generated during puberty. These hormones cause the skin to release excess sebum. Exposure to oily substances, such as cosmetics or heavy lotions, may also increase risk. For mild cases, over-the-counter topical treatments that kill bacteria and dry up oil are effective. More serious cases may be treated with antibiotics (to kill bacteria) and, for women, oral contraceptives (to regulate hormones). Newer therapies include isotretinoin, laser treatments, and ultraviolet light therapy.

ADDITIONAL FACTS

1. *Acne often runs in families; if your parents had acne, it's likely that you'll have it as well.*

2. *Contrary to popular belief, what you eat doesn't increase the likelihood of developing pimples.*

3. *Washing your face too frequently with harsh cleansers may actually set the stage for acne.*

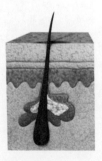 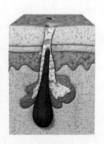 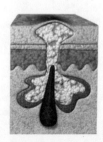

✦✦✦

Lactose Intolerance

For nearly 50 million Americans, a glass of milk or slice of cheese can bring on a stomachache, bloating, and diarrhea. These people are lactose intolerant, or unable to digest lactose, a sugar found in dairy foods. Why? The cells that line their small intestines don't produce sufficient amounts of an enzyme called lactase, which breaks down milk sugar into simpler forms that can be absorbed by the body.

As a result, milk products can trigger uncomfortable symptoms, which also include gas, cramps, and nausea. These problems usually start a half hour to 2 hours after eating milk products and can range from mild to severe. Most people who have this condition were born with it; certain ethnic and racial populations are at greater risk. In fact, as many as 75 percent of Jewish, Native American, and Mexican American adults, along with 90 percent of Asian American adults, are lactose intolerant to some degree.

Other people can develop the problem as they age, because the body gradually produces less lactase as you consume fewer dairy products after childhood. An intestinal problem, such as Crohn's disease or gastroenteritis, may also cause a temporary bout of lactose intolerance, since inflammation may prompt the small intestine to cease lactase production.

Although there are supplements that contain the lactase enzyme, they offer only temporary relief. Fortunately, people who are lactose intolerant can now buy a variety of lactose-free dairy products in the dairy aisles of most grocery stores. Because milk products are a primary source of calcium, experts recommend taking a calcium supplement.

ADDITIONAL FACTS

1. *Babies born prematurely are more likely to be lactose intolerant.*

2. *To diagnose lactose intolerance, a physician may perform a hydrogen breath test, a lactose tolerance test, and a stool acidity test.*

◆◆◆

Steroids

Drugs referred to as steroids can be classified into three categories: corticosteroids, female hormones, and male hormones. Corticosteroids are widely prescribed by doctors and sold over the counter to help control inflammation in the body, and the female hormones estrogen and progesterone are used for hormone replacement and birth control medications.

In contrast, male hormones of the anabolic type are often manufactured illegally and used to produce and maintain muscle in athletes. Anabolic steroids are synthetic hormones that mimic the chemical structure of testosterone—a natural hormone responsible for masculine characteristics such as increased muscle mass, facial hair growth, and a deep voice. Like testosterone, androgenic anabolic steroids stimulate muscle growth and help prevent muscle breakdown.

These medications were developed in the late 1930s to treat hypogonadism, a condition in which a boy's testes do not produce enough testosterone for normal growth and sexual development. Steroids are still used today to treat delayed puberty, some types of impotence, and complications of HIV infection or other diseases. But shortly after the discovery of steroids, scientists ascertained that these substances could also cause muscle tissue to grow. Soon, bodybuilders and weight lifters began abusing the drugs.

In the United States, it is illegal to take anabolic steroids without a prescription. Drugs such as androstenedione, or andro, however, are still commonly used by athletes, from football players to cyclists. Androstenedione can be taken orally, injected into the muscle, or rubbed onto the skin in the form of gels or creams. It is often used in an on-and-off pattern called cycling or in slowly escalating doses in a process called pyramiding.

Overuse of steroids, however, can lead to unwanted side effects. Steroids can prompt testosterone to build to dangerous levels in the body, causing impotence, reduced testicle size, acne, baldness, and breast growth in men. Women who use steroids may have their menstrual cycles disrupted, develop excessive facial and body hair and a deeper voice, and experience long-term fertility problems.

Steroids can also stunt growth in teenagers by causing bones to mature too fast and stop growing at an early age. Use of steroids has been linked to liver tumors, abnormal enlargement of the heart muscle, blood abnormalities that contribute to heart disease, and violent, aggressive behavior known as 'roid rage.

ADDITIONAL FACTS

1. *Some research has shown that 5 percent of teenage boys and 2.5 percent of teen girls have used some form of anabolic steroids.*

2. *The process of combining several different types of steroids is known as stacking. By doing this, users believe that the different steroids will interact to produce an effect on muscle size that is greater than the effects of using each drug individually.*

◆ ◆ ◆

Meningioma

Meninges are layers of protective membranes surrounding the brain and spinal cord, and tumors that form in these areas are called meningiomas. They are the most common type of tumor that originates in the brain. Most meningiomas (90 percent) are noncancerous, but they can still be life threatening or cause complications such as vision loss or paralysis by pressing on important parts of the brain or spinal cord.

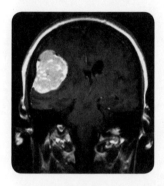

For a tumor of this type to occur, something—genes, environmental exposure, or a combination of the two—needs to alter the cells in the meninges so that they begin to multiply rapidly. It is common in children who received radiation therapy for leukemia. The condition is also more common in women, which has led scientists to think that female hormones may play a role.

Most people develop a meningioma after age 40, although it's possible at any age. It is usually a very slow-growing tumor and often doesn't cause symptoms or require immediate treatment. Doctors can detect a meningioma through a CT scan or MRI of the brain, often after the tumor grows large enough for a patient to experience symptoms, such as seizures, persistent headaches, hearing loss, or muscle weakness. Surgery may be performed, although it's not always possible to remove the entire tumor if it is in a sensitive area, such as near the eyes. If the meningioma can't be completely removed, the doctor may opt to administer radiation in an attempt to destroy the rest of the tumor and reduce the risk of recurrence.

ADDITIONAL FACTS

1. *Studies have linked meningiomas to exposure to weed killers and pesticides used in farming. Women appear to be at particularly increased risk if they have spent many years around these chemicals.*

2. *If a patient chooses not to undergo treatment for a benign meningioma, he or she usually will undergo a brain scan every few months to monitor its growth.*

3. *Infection and inflammation of the meninges, caused by either a virus or bacteria, is called meningitis. It can cause brain damage, hearing loss, or learning disability, and in rare cases, it can be fatal.*

✦✦✦

Hermaphroditism

In ancient Greek and Roman mythology, a handsome god named Hermaphroditus was walking by a lake when a water nymph spotted him and immediately fell head over heels in love. He rebuffed her advances, so when he went for a swim, the lovelorn nymph embraced him tightly and prayed that they might never be separated. The gods granted her wish, and their bodies fused into one person with both female and male attributes. Today, a person with physical aspects of both sexes is called a hermaphrodite, in reference to this tale. Many advocates, however, argue that this term is stigmatizing and prefer the use of the word *intersex* instead.

There are varying degrees of the condition. True hermaphrodites have both ovarian and testicular tissues, while pseudohermaphrodites have the internal reproductive organs of one sex but the outward appearance of the other. (Examples include those with adrenogenital syndrome and testicular feminization.) Most cases of full hermaphroditism can be attributed to a genetic defect. One of the most common is an additional sex chromosome, so that there are 47 chromosomes instead of the normal 46. As a result, these individuals have an XXY set rather than an XX or XY. Rarely, a person may have the internal organs of both sexes, or an ovotestis.

Beginning in the 1960s, babies with this hermaphroditism were assigned to one sex, usually dictated by the more prominent genitalia. They then underwent surgery to remove the inconsistent genitals. However, in the 1990s, a group of psychologists and other experts started a movement against this procedure. They explained that intersex isn't a medical emergency and that a child who undergoes such surgery may grow up with a sense of loss and misplacement. Ultimately, they argued, the child should make that decision later on in life.

ADDITIONAL FACTS

1. *Intersex conditions occur in about 1 in 1,500 to 2,000 births.*

2. *According to 16th-century literature, a hermaphrodite living as a woman was put to death for impregnating her master's daughter.*

✦✦✦

Mercury Contamination

Mercury is an extremely toxic element found in nature and as a pollutant in the environment. It is particularly dangerous because mercury contamination can exist without our realizing that it's there. For example, fish or shellfish can be contaminated with the most toxic form of mercury, called methylmercury, and you cannot taste or smell it.

Almost all fish and shellfish contain traces of mercury. Fish become contaminated because industrial waste has been dumped into streams or the ocean or released into the air and fallen into streams and oceans. Fish absorb the mercury as they feed in the water.

Fortunately, the risk of mercury poisoning from eating fish and shellfish is generally not a health concern. Fish and shellfish are important components of a healthy diet, because they contain high-quality protein, are low in saturated fat, and are good sources of omega-3 fatty acids. However, it is particularly dangerous for a developing fetus to be exposed to methylmercury. Fetuses are 5 to 10 times more sensitive to the substance than adults are. Methylmercury can affect the immune system, alter genetic and enzyme systems, and damage the nervous system, including coordination and the senses of touch, taste, and sight.

Pregnant women, women who may become pregnant, nursing women, and young children should avoid types of fish that tend to have higher levels of mercury, such as king mackerel, shark, swordfish, and tilefish. People in these high-risk categories should also have no more than 12 ounces a week of other kinds of fish and shellfish. Young children should consume even less than 12 ounces of fish and shellfish per week.

ADDITIONAL FACTS

1. *Another form of mercury, called elemental mercury, can be released from a broken thermometer. Though it is less toxic than methylmercury, elemental mercury causes tremors, gingivitis, and excitability when it is inhaled over a long period. If elemental mercury is ingested, it usually passes though the digestive system without causing harm.*

2. *The larger and older a fish is, the higher the level of methylmercury it contains. This is because larger fish have had more time to accumulate the substance from contaminated water.*

◆◆◆

Banting, Best, and Insulin

Diabetes had baffled physicians for centuries when, late in the 19th century, a series of connections was made between this mysterious "sugar disease" and the pancreas, paving the way for the lifesaving insulin treatments we take for granted today.

Since then, insulin has saved millions of lives. In the United States alone, about 23.6 million people have diabetes, many of whom depend on daily insulin injections for survival.

Diabetes comes in two forms, type 1 and type 2, and robs the body of its ability to metabolize sugar. The disease has a genetic basis, but is most commonly seen with an unhealthy lifestyle, especially obesity, when it is referred to as type 2 diabetes. Type 1 diabetes usually begins in childhood or adolescence, as opposed to type 2 which usually appears in late adulthood. Symptoms of type 1 include excessive urination, weight loss, and thirst leading to drinking large amounts of water. If untreated, it can quickly lead to vomiting, coma, and death. Type 2 diabetes is most often asymptomatic, but may be associated with increased frequency of skin infections, urinary tract infections, and poor healing.

The modern understanding of diabetes began to emerge in 1869, when Paul Langerhans (1847–1888), a German biologist, first identified a part of the pancreas now called the islets of Langerhans. After his death, studies in 1889 showed that removing these islets caused laboratory animals to develop diabetes. Scientists deduced that something in the pancreas must be responsible for metabolizing sugar, and thus preventing diabetes in a healthy person. This substance was called insulin, after the part of the body where it is produced.

Replacing insulin, researchers theorized, might offer a treatment for diabetes. Efforts to isolate the substance for medical use were unsuccessful, however, until 1921, when Canadian surgeon Frederick Banting (1891–1941) and his assistant Charles Best (1899–1978) were able to inject insulin into a diabetic dog at their lab in Toronto. Subsequent insulin injections on a human subject were also a success, saving the life of a young Toronto boy who was on the verge of death.

In recognition of his accomplishment, Banting won the Nobel Prize in Physiology or Medicine in 1923 at the improbably young age of 24. He shared the honor with John Macleod (1876–1935), in whose lab Banting had performed most of his research. Banting gave half of the prize money to Best.

ADDITIONAL FACTS

1. Diabetes *is Greek for "siphon." Ancient Greek physicians made reference to this disease, which caused sugar-laden urine, frequent urination, persistent thirst, and eventually rapid weight loss and death. Doctors used to diagnose diabetes by tasting a patient's urine.*

2. *Many unsuccessful treatments for diabetes were proposed before the discovery of insulin. One treatment involved feeding patients pieces of pancreas, hoping it would help the diseased organ.*

◆ ◆ ◆

Growth Spurt

For the first 2 decades of life, children and young adults grow steadily. But no one grows at a perfect pace; there are weeks or months of slower growth interspersed with mini growth spurts.

The period of fastest growth is during the first year of life. Infants can sprout 10 inches in length—nearly tripling their birth weight. During these growth spurts, babies may eat, sleep, and fuss more than usual. After the first year, babies develop at a slower rate; by age 2, children tend to grow 2 to 3 inches a year until adolescence.

That's when they hit their second-most-prominent growth spurt. Between the ages of 8 and 15, children reach puberty. At that time, the pituitary, a pea-size gland near the base of the brain, releases chemicals that step up the production of sex hormones, which results in maturational body changes. The pituitary gland also pumps out growth hormone, which stimulates cells to reproduce. A child becomes taller when bone cells divide and grow, widening and lengthening the bone. Because girls tend to undergo puberty a few years before boys, they hit their growth spurts at an earlier age. Although growth tends to cease after puberty (around age 16 or 17), young adults can continue to grow well into their twenties.

ADDITIONAL FACTS

1. *The tallest man to live, Robert Wadlow (1918–1940), grew to be 8 feet 11 inches. By the age of 8, he was already 6 feet tall.*

2. *Children tend to grow faster in the spring.*

✦✦✦

Celiac Disease

Although awareness of celiac disease, a digestive condition that interferes with the absorption of nutrients from food, has grown over the past decade, the ailment can be traced back to the 1st century. The Greek physician Aretaeus of Cappadocia (2nd century) wrote, "If [foods] pass through undigested and crude, and nothing ascends into the body, we call such persons coeliacs." Aretaeus's description went largely ignored until 1888, when the renowned English physician Samuel Gee (1839–1911) wrote about the condition.

Today, scientists know that celiac disease is a genetic autoimmune disorder that affects the digestive process. When someone with the condition consumes gluten, a protein found in wheat, rye, and barley, the immune system begins attacking the small intestine and the small protrusions, called villi, that line the interior are lost. Since these villi absorb nutrients from food and transfer them to the bloodstream, celiac disease can cause malnourishment. As a result, people with celiac disease often experience related conditions, such as osteoporosis, anemia, and fatigue. About one in four sufferers also has dermatitis herpetiformis, an itchy, blistering skin rash that occurs on the elbows, knees, and buttocks.

Although experts estimate that some 3 million people suffer from celiac disease, only 3 percent of them have ever been diagnosed. That's because symptoms of the condition are often confused with those of other illnesses, such as irritable bowel syndrome and chronic fatigue syndrome. Physicians first run blood tests to check for higher-than-normal levels of certain antibodies, a sign of an autoimmune disorder. If these screenings suggest celiac disease, a tissue sample of the small intestine is taken to check for damaged villi.

Unfortunately, there's no cure for the condition. The only treatment is following a gluten-free diet, which means avoiding grains, pasta, cereals, and most processed foods. Because many food manufacturers are producing gluten-free foods made with potato, rice, soy, and buckwheat flour, among others, those with celiac disease can follow a balanced diet.

ADDITIONAL FACTS

1. The word celiac is derived from the Greek koelia, meaning "abdomen."

2. Celiac disease runs in families: Research suggests that 4 to 12 percent of first-degree relatives of a person with the disease also have it.

✦✦✦

Green Tea

For as long as 5,000 years, people have consumed tea leaves steeped in boiling water. But tea—and green tea, especially—is much more than just a beverage: Studies suggest that it may aid in weight loss, reduce cholesterol levels, and even help treat or prevent cancer. Once available only as a drink, green tea is now available as an extract in capsule form and is an ingredient in weight-loss and energy supplements, and even topical beauty treatments.

Green tea is made from the same plant, *Camellia sinensis,* as white, black, and oolong teas. The difference is in the processing: Green and white teas are made from unfermented leaves and contain the highest concentrations of polyphenols, a type of antioxidant. (Herbal and rooibos teas aren't really teas at all, but are made from different mixtures of plants.) One of the most powerful antioxidants in green tea is called epigallocatechin gallate, or EGCG. Tea also contains caffeine (although white and green teas have two to three times less than black, and all teas have significantly less caffeine than an equal serving of coffee), which contributes to its ability to improve alertness.

Traditionally valued in China and India for its properties as a stimulant and diuretic, modern medicine has shown that green tea can also boost mental processing. Research also suggests that it can slow the growth of some cancers and benign skin tumors; increase metabolism and help burn fat; and reduce inflammation associated with arthritis, Crohn's disease, and ulcerative colitis.

Most research has studied the impact of 1 to 10 cups of green tea a day, and the beverage is safe for most adults when used in these quantities. However, people taking blood-thinning medications may find that the vitamin K in green tea makes their treatments less effective. For those taking concentrated doses of green tea in capsule form, a few cases of liver problems have also been reported.

ADDITIONAL FACTS

1. *It is suspected (but not proven) that green tea and EGCG may help protect against sun damage, so they are now popular ingredients in sunscreens and other skin-care products.*

2. *Early research using a green tea combination product was thought to have shown some success in helping women conceive, although more research on green tea alone needs to be done.*

3. *When sold as a beverage, green tea is often classified by the region in which it was grown. The most expensive varieties from southwest China can cost up to $150 a pound.*

✦✦✦

Anosmia (Kallmann Syndrome)

Loss of the ability to smell is called anosmia, a sensation that almost everyone experiences when suffering from a cold, allergies, or a sinus infection. But occasionally, anosmia can be a long-term or permanent disorder in which a person either is born without or loses the sense of smell as a result of head trauma, medication side effects, a brain tumor, or enlarged structures in the nasal cavities. People with no sense of smell react to the world in a different way: They have a limited sense of food flavor, can't detect smoke or other dangerous odors, and can't appreciate the aromas that other people take for granted.

One cause of anosmia is Kallmann syndrome, a rare inherited disorder that affects mostly men. People with Kallmann syndrome are born with little or no sense of smell, fail to go through puberty, and are often sterile and have small genitalia. This stems from a deficiency of gonadotropin-releasing hormone (GnRH) being produced in the hypothalamus; GnRH is a chemical that plays a role in sexual maturity and helps regulate the olfactory bulbs, which give us our sense of smell. The condition can also be associated with color blindness and other vision problems, although scientists are not sure why.

Kallmann syndrome can be treated, in part, by restoring the deficient hormones through infusion pumps or injections. This can induce fertility, but only temporarily. The disorder can also have a psychologically isolating effect on its victims.

In people who don't have Kallmann syndrome, some loss of the sense of smell occurs normally with aging. Some people may be born anosmic for one particular odor, such as fish or sweat, a condition called specific anosmia. Loss of smell may also be caused by Alzheimer's disease, endocrine system disorders, lead poisoning, nutritional disorders, radiation therapy, or medications such as amphetamines, estrogen, or nasal decongestants.

ADDITIONAL FACTS

1. *People with anosmia can't perform certain basic tasks, like smelling milk to tell if it has gone bad, and must take special precautions against such dangers.*

2. *Doctors can diagnose anosmia by using scratch-and-sniff odor tests or by testing with familiar odors such as coffee, lemon, grape, vanilla, and cinnamon.*

3. *Many people who are born with anosmia report having lied as children and pretended that they could smell things that other people could—mimicking others' facial expressions, for example—so that they'd appear normal.*

✦✦✦

Sex Change Surgery (John Money)

Male. Female. John Money (1921–2006), a New Zealand–born psychologist, devoted much of his career to researching everything about the sexes and the various states in between. During his career as the director of Johns Hopkins University's Psychohormonal Research Unit in Baltimore, Money coined the terms *gender identity* (a person's self-classification as male, female, or in-between) and *gender role* (a person's behavior that defines how they are identified as male, female, or in-between).

Money is perhaps best known—and most criticized—for his work advocating sex change operations for children with ambiguous genitalia (most often caused by genetic conditions, such as hermaphroditism) before the age of 3. This played out devastatingly in 1967, when a young Canadian couple asked him for help. One of their twin boys (born in 1965) had suffered a botched circumcision, and Money told them that with hormones and a sex change surgery, the boy could be raised as a girl. It was the first sex reassignment for a developmentally normal (nonhermaphrodite) infant, and the child was raised as Brenda. But even so, Brenda always identified with males—tearing off dresses, playing sports, walking with a swagger.

When Brenda's parents finally explained his history to him when he was 14, he immediately decided that he wanted to be reassigned as a male, David Reimer. He stopped estrogen therapy, underwent surgery to construct a penis, and went on to marry a woman. But after a number of marital and professional failures, along with his brother's suicide, David himself committed suicide in 2004. A few years before Reimer's death, a paper and subsequent book drew attention to his case—and critics argued that Money had played the role of a scientist who strong-armed the results that he wanted to see. Colleagues said that the psychologist was devastated by the backlash and became withdrawn in his later years.

ADDITIONAL FACTS

1. *David Reimer's (1965–2004) story became known as the John/Joan case and was documented in the book* As Nature Made Him: The Boy Who Was Raised a Girl.

2. *In his free time, Money collected anthropological art he gathered from traveling around the world. He later donated it to a gallery in Gore, New Zealand.*

❖❖❖

Vitamins

Vitamins are substances found in food that are essential to children's normal growth and development and to all people's lifelong health. There are 13 vitamins that your body needs. They are vitamins A, C, D, E, and K, and the vitamins known as the B complex: biotin, folate, niacin, pantothenic acid, riboflavin, thiamin, vitamin B_6, and vitamin B_{12}.

Each vitamin has specific jobs. Without enough of certain vitamins, you could develop a deficiency disease. For example, if you don't take in enough vitamin D, you could develop rickets. Vitamin A prevents night blindness. Elderly people with low levels of vitamin B_{12} may be at greater risk of brain atrophy, or shrinkage of the brain.

You can usually obtain all the vitamins you need by eating a balanced diet that includes a variety of foods. However, you may need to take a multivitamin for optimal health. Unfortunately, you cannot skip nutritious foods and rely on vitamin supplements, because it's impossible to get all the nutrition the body needs through supplements alone.

There are three main benefits to focusing on whole foods rather than dietary supplements. Food supplies you with optimal nutrition because whole foods provide a complex combination of nutrients, which supplements don't offer. Many whole foods also contain dietary fiber, which can help prevent constipation, heart disease, and type 2 diabetes. And the right foods contain protective substances that are not available in supplements; for instance, phytochemicals, found in fruits and vegetables, protect you against cancer, and antioxidants combat cell and tissue damage.

It may be beneficial for you to take multivitamins if you eat fewer than 1,600 calories a day; if you are a woman who is pregnant, trying to get pregnant, or breastfeeding; or if you have a medical condition that affects how your body absorbs nutrients, such as chronic diarrhea, food allergies, or food intolerance. People who eat a vegetarian diet may need to take a vitamin B_{12} supplement. For most people, a balanced diet based on the USDA MyPyramid provides all the vitamins the body needs.

ADDITIONAL FACTS

1. *Vitamins D and K are the only vitamins your body can make. Otherwise, you can get vitamins only from the food or supplements you consume.*

2. *Unfortunately, with vitamins as with many other things, more is not always better: Too much of some vitamins can make you sick.*

◆◆◆

Artificial Joints

As the body ages, our joints suffer and arthritis can develop. Protective cartilage wears away and bones rub together, causing pain and loss of motion—most commonly in the knees and hips.

Doctors theorized for decades that the most effective way to reduce this pain and discomfort might be to simply replace the damaged joint. But finding a safe and effective replacement turned into a major medical challenge.

Early (and unsuccessful) attempts to replace or smooth the surfaces of joints included the use of muscles, fat, pig bladder, gold, magnesium, and zinc. None had the combination of safety and strength needed to replicate a human joint.

One of the doctors working to devise an artificial joint was Boston surgeon Marius Smith-Petersen (1886–1953), whose first design was a molded glass replacement, The glass joint failed to work, but Smith-Petersen continued his research on mold arthroplasty, as he called it, and eventually found better success with plastic and stainless steel.

Efforts to design a working joint replacement received a boost in 1936, when the metallic alloy Vitallium was invented. Part cobalt, part chromium, the alloy was strong enough to walk on and safe enough to insert into the body. The first reported hip replacement with Vitallium took place in 1940 at Johns Hopkins Hospital in Baltimore. New York City doctor Edward Haboush (1904–1973) solved a related problem by devising a way to adhere the artificial joint to the existing human bone. And the English surgeon Sir John Charnley (1911–1982) addressed the issue of pain and function by replacing the hip socket (instead of just the ball) with a Teflon implant in 1958. When Teflon didn't work, he tried polyethylene, which worked wonderfully. He borrowed a polyethylene adhesive, known as bone cement, from dentists and used it to secure the artificial joint firmly to the bone—resulting in a "total hip replacement."

At the same time, treatments for knee arthritis were being developed, including a hinged prosthesis and a metal spacer to prevent rubbing between the bones. In New York City in 1972, John Insall (1930–2000) developed the prototype for today's knee prostheses, with components for all three surfaces of the knee—the femur, tibia, and patella, or kneecap.

ADDITIONAL FACTS

1. *Today, more than 100,000 hip replacements and 150,000 knee replacements are performed annually in the United States, using arthroplasty techniques and metal and plastic parts.*

2. *In 1960, the Burmese surgeon San Baw (1922–1984) performed the first hip replacement with an ivory prosthesis; over the next 20 years he used more than 300 of these replacements, citing an 88 percent success rate for patients being able to walk, squat, ride a bicycle, and play football a few weeks after surgery.*

3. *Physicians got the idea of using stainless steel for prostheses from the shipping industry, which first used this steel to resist corrosion in ships at sea.*

✦✦✦

Growth Hormone

A pea-shaped gland located at the base of the brain, the pituitary gland has a crucial job in the body: It secretes growth hormone, which stimulates cells in the body to grow and reproduce.

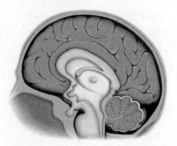

When growth hormone attaches to certain cells, they respond by growing and dividing. Growth hormone encourages the synthesis of proteins and breaks down stored fat for use as energy. That's why it's important that the body has the right balance of hormones. Too much growth hormone can lead to gigantism, in which a person continues to grow to 8 feet or more in height. Too little growth hormone may lead to dwarfism, a condition characterized by short stature, with a height of under 4 feet 10 inches.

Children, in particular, have larger amounts of growth hormone. But beginning at age 40, the pituitary gland starts reducing the amount that it produces. Some people believe that this dip may lead to the frailty associated with aging, such as weaker bones. Yet studies show that healthy adults who take growth hormone raise their risk of a host of health problems, such as diabetes and heart disease. Synthetic growth hormone, however, is often useful for treating children of extremely short stature.

ADDITIONAL FACTS

1. *Growth hormone was first discovered in 1956 and, 2 years later, was derived from human cadavers to treat dwarfism. In 1985, a synthetic form of this hormone was approved for use.*

2. *Some bodybuilders and athletes abuse synthetic human growth hormone in order to build more muscle mass.*

◆◆◆

Osteoporosis

Imagine if a simple act, such as bending over or even coughing, could break one of your bones. This scenario is a reality for the 10 million Americans with osteoporosis. The progressive condition causes bones to become fragile and brittle, so that even a small amount of stress is dangerous. In fact, nearly half of all women and one in four men will experience an osteoporosis-related bone fracture sometime during their lives.

Under a microscope, bone looks like the inside of a honeycomb. Collagen fibers are interlaced with hard calcium-phosphate complexes and living bone cells. The measure of bone's thickness and density is called bone mass. With osteoporosis, the bone mass declines, and the matrix is dotted with gaps and holes, like a poorly knitted sweater.

Osteoporosis takes years to develop, affecting mainly people ages 50 and above. The stage is set as early as childhood: For the first few decades of life, bone grows much faster than it is broken down. By age 18, up to 90 percent of bone mass has formed, and it reaches its peak by age 30. After that point, you start to lose bone mass more quickly than you can replace it. Because women's bodies have lower levels of the bone-protecting hormone estrogen as they enter menopause, they're at greater risk for osteoporosis.

Certain lifestyle moves, such as bulking up on bone-building vitamin D and calcium, can help safeguard your skeleton as you age. Weight-bearing exercise, such as running and strength training, can also stimulate bone formation; your skeleton adapts to gravity and the shock of impact by building more bone cells. Doctors screen for osteoporosis by using an x-ray or ultrasound to gauge bone density in the spine, hip, and wrist—the three areas most likely to be affected by osteoporosis. To prevent harmful fractures, doctors prescribe bone-protecting drugs, such as selective estrogen receptor therapy and bisphosphonates.

ADDITIONAL FACTS

1. *About 5 to 7 years after reaching menopause, most women have lost about 20 percent of their bone mass.*

2. *People who smoke or have smoked, have thin frames, or have suffered an eating disorder are more likely to develop osteoporosis.*

3. *People of Caucasian and Asian descent or with family histories of the disease are also at greater risk for osteoporosis.*

❖❖❖

Black Cohosh

Black cohosh, also known as both *Actaea racemosa* and *Cimicifuga racemosa,* is a member of the buttercup family that is used to alleviate the symptoms of menopause, such as hot flashes. Preparations of black cohosh are made from its roots and underground stems, called rhizomes.

Black cohosh was widely used by Native Americans, and it became a popular cure-all in 19th-century America—especially among a group of alternative practitioners who called the herb macrotys. This group often prescribed black cohosh for conditions of women's reproductive organs, including menstrual problems, inflammation of the uterus or ovaries, infertility, and labor pains or complications.

Scientists aren't sure how black cohosh might work. It's possible that its active compounds, such as fukinolic acid, work like the female hormone estrogen—although studies in this area have been contradictory. Women who have reached menopause generally have lower levels of estrogen in their bodies, and this can contribute to symptoms such as hot flashes, mood swings, weight gain, and vaginal dryness. Most reports on the benefits of black cohosh emphasize relief from hot flashes and mood swings.

In 2001, the American College of Obstetrics and Gynecology issued a statement that black cohosh, when taken for 6 months or less, may be helpful for women with menopause symptoms. Although preliminary research is encouraging, few studies have been placebo controlled and dosage has been inconsistent, so no official recommendation has been made by any government health organization.

Black cohosh appears to be safe when taken as directed, although it can cause headaches, stomach discomfort, and a feeling of heaviness in the legs. (A very small percentage of people have reported liver damage, as well.) The herb usually is not used for long periods of time, however, and studies have followed women for only 6 months or less. Women who are pregnant or who have breast cancer or liver disorders should not take black cohosh without talking to a doctor.

ADDITIONAL FACTS

1. *Other common names for black cohosh include black snakeroot, bugbane, bugwort, rattleroot, rattle-top, and rattleweed. Insects tend to avoid it, which accounts for some of these names.*

2. *One widely used commercial brand of black cohosh is a tablet called Remifemin. Other preparations, such as solutions that mix black cohosh extract with alcohol, have been less well studied.*

3. *Black cohosh should not be confused with blue cohosh* (Caulophyllum thalictroides), *a nicotine-like herb also used to treat menstrual and gynecological problems that also has not been thoroughly tested for effectiveness and safety.*

✦✦✦

Asperger's Syndrome

In 1944, the Austrian pediatrician Hans Asperger (1906–1980) described a puzzling tendency he noted among certain children in his practice. These children displayed impressive vocabularies and formal patterns of speech—but encountered difficulties in carrying out basic social interactions. "Little professors," Asperger called them.

Asperger's syndrome (AS), as this pattern of behavior is now known, is a common form of autism, a spectrum of disorders that typically involve language and social deficiencies coupled with obsessive interests and, sometimes, high intelligence.

For instance, children with AS often have a singular interest in a particular topic, to the point where they converse about nothing else—memorizing catalog after catalog of camera model numbers, for example, while caring little about photography.

Autism disorders are believed to form early in fetal development, and symptoms are usually present by age 5 or 6. Unlike children with other forms of autism, those with AS retain their early language skills. AS is distinguished by inappropriate behavior in social settings, unusual speech patterns, and difficulty understanding body language.

Children with AS may also exhibit clumsy or repetitive motor movements such as hand flapping or twirling and may find it difficult to perform physical tasks that others take for granted, such as riding a bicycle. With effective treatment, however, they can learn to cope in the workplace as adults—though personal interactions often remain difficult.

Individuals with AS may also suffer from anxiety and depression, and treatment often involves medication for those conditions. Therapy also seeks to address obsessive tendencies and communication problems, and it often includes training on social interaction. Most professionals agree that intervention should start as early as possible.

Prevalence estimates for AS vary widely, partly because it can be hard to distinguish between AS and high-functioning autism. One school of thought—led by the University of Cambridge professor Simon Baron-Cohen—argues that these two conditions should not be thought of as disabilities, but rather as interesting and unique ways of thinking.

ADDITIONAL FACTS

1. *Individuals with AS often have excellent auditory and visual perception and may notice tiny changes in patterns and arrangements. However, they may have deficits in tasks involving spatial perception or visual memory. They may also be unusually sensitive—or insensitive—to touch, texture, taste, smell, and other stimuli.*

2. *AS, as well as milder forms of awkward behavior and communication problems, appears to run in families. Scientists believe that a number of inherited genes combine to help determine the severity and symptoms of AS.*

Syphilis

The disease syphilis has been called a laundry list of names throughout history. It's been known as the great pox and the French disease after an epidemic among French soldiers. But modern science settled on *syphilis* in honor of a shepherd in ancient Greek mythology who was cursed by the gods to suffer from a horrible disease. Physicians have dubbed it "the great imitator" because its signs and symptoms mimic those of many other diseases.

So what, exactly, is this condition of many monikers? An infection caused by the bacterium *Treponema pallidum,* syphilis is transmitted by direct contact with a sore. These sores primarily occur on the penis, vagina, anus, or rectum; they can also appear on the lips or in the mouth. Pregnant women can pass on the disease to their babies. (Contrary to popular belief, syphilis cannot be transferred through toilet seats, hot tubs, or baths.) Every year, about 36,000 Americans contract syphilis.

Because symptoms can lie dormant, many people can carry the disease for years before they realize they have it. On average, however, it takes about a month for the first sign to appear. In this primary stage, a sore (called a chancre) or multiple sores develop. They often heal on their own, but, if left untreated, the disease will progress after the sore is gone. The next stage leads to a rash on the hands and feet, fatigue, chills, and sore throat. People who aren't treated will damage their internal organs, such as the heart, brain, liver, bones, and joints. Luckily, the disease is easy to diagnose with a simple blood test. A course of antibiotics, typically penicillin, will usually wipe out the bacteria.

ADDITIONAL FACTS

1. *The Italian physician and writer Girolamo Fracastoro (c. 1478–1553) gave the disease the name syphilis in 1530.*

2. *People with syphilis are up to five times more likely to contract HIV, because the virus is more easily transmitted through the sores.*

3. *An untreated case of syphilis can lead to aneurysms that compress vocal cords, causing the sufferer to speak in a husky voice. This became known as a "prostitute's whisper" in the 14th century.*

❖❖❖

Antioxidants

Antioxidants are substances that bolster your immune system by protecting you from the harmful effects of oxygen released by chemical reactions in your body. The name *antioxidants* stems from their ability to help prevent and possibly even repair the damage caused by the process of oxidation.

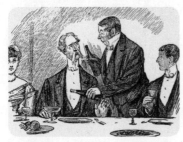

Oxidative damage occurs either when your body breaks down food, creating oxygen, or when you're exposed to environmental toxins, such as tobacco smoke and radiation. This damage causes your cells to stop functioning properly. Over time, the harm to the cells becomes irreversible and leads to illnesses such as diabetes, cancer, and heart disease.

You can prevent oxidative damage by making sure your diet includes antioxidant substances, such as beta-carotene, lutein, lycopene, selenium, and vitamins A, C, and E. These compounds are found in many of the foods that you probably already eat, such as fruits and vegetables; nuts; grains; some meats, poultry, and fish; and even red wine. Foods containing antioxidants should be eaten at every meal for the maximum benefit. Since the process of digestion causes the oxidative process, the best way to combat the damage is to have antioxidants—either from food or from supplements taken daily—already in your bloodstream when you're eating.

ADDITIONAL FACTS

1. *The antioxidants in a daily glass of red wine may help prevent the development of certain cancers. The same benefit has not been shown from having a daily glass of white wine, beer, or liquor.*

2. *The brain is vulnerable to oxidative damage. As a result, antioxidants are commonly used in medications to treat brain injuries and are being investigated as medications for Alzheimer's disease and Parkinson's disease.*

3. *The antioxidant process is similar to stopping a cut apple from browning after it's been exposed to the air. If you dip a cut apple in orange juice, which contains the antioxidant vitamin C, it will stop the oxidation process and the apple's flesh will stay white.*

4. *As many as 30 percent of Americans take antioxidant supplements.*

◆◆◆

Alexander Fleming and Penicillin

The discovery of the world's first and best-known "miracle drug" happened quite by accident, thanks to the messy laboratory and quick thinking of Alexander Fleming.

A military physician during World War I, Fleming (1881–1955) witnessed firsthand the terrifying toll bacterial infections took on British troops. He began looking for an effective treatment after the war ended in 1918. In his experiments at St. Mary's Hospital in London, Fleming first discovered a naturally occurring chemical called lysozyme. The enzyme is produced in the body and is present in some fluids, including teardrops. However, Fleming determined that while the substance kills bacteria, it is too weak to treat serious infections. He continued his investigations.

Then in 1928 he stumbled upon an interesting discovery while cleaning up his lab. He saw that mold was growing in a petri dish where he had been cultivating staph bacteria, and the mold actually seemed to have killed the bacteria around it. He examined the mold and found that it was from the *Penicillium* genus. He presented his findings the next year, but they received little interest and his work was largely forgotten for several years.

In 1935, however, cancer researchers at Oxford University happened across Fleming's old articles about lysozyme and *Penicillium*. They began experimenting with penicillin, injecting it into live mice with bacterial infections. When those results were promising, they tried the injections on human subjects. A policeman who was near death after a scratch had become infected showed great improvement when he was treated with penicillin. But supply was short, and when the researchers ran out in a few days, the policeman got sick again and died. They quickly realized the need for mass production.

By this time, England had entered World War II, and resources for drug production were tight. The researchers turned to the United States, where they received funding from the Rockefeller Foundation and located a production facility in Peoria, Illinois. When the United States joined the war as well in 1941, the government pressed private chemical companies to begin producing the drug, which was still extremely scarce in the early stages of the conflict. These efforts had a major impact; by the end of the war, the US was producing 650 billion units of penicillin every month.

ADDITIONAL FACTS

1. *Fleming shared the Nobel Prize in Physiology or Medicine with the Oxford researchers Sir Howard Walter Florey (1898–1968) and Ernst Boris Chain (1906–1979) in 1945.*

2. *Technically, penicillin was discovered before Fleming's findings in his laboratory. The scientists John Tyndall (1820–1893) and Ernest Duchesne (1874–1912) documented the penicillin phenomenon in 1875 and 1897, respectively.*

3. *In 2000, doctors in Costa Rica published the manuscripts of the scientist Clodomiro Picado Twight (1887–1944), who reported on the antibacterial actions of penicillin fungus between 1915 and 1927.*

◆◆◆

Thyroid

The thyroid, a 2-inch-long, butterfly-shaped organ that sits at the front of the throat, plays one of the most important roles in the body.

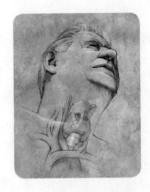

The control center of the endocrine system, the thyroid pumps out hormones that help determine how smoothly and quickly the body runs when converting calories to energy, contracting the heart muscle, or recalling a memory, among other things. In other words, the thyroid affects every cell. When the organ generates too few or too many hormones, it can affect all the systems in the body; these problems are called thyroid disorders.

Because there are no telltale symptoms of a thyroid disorder, the vast majority—up to 13 million cases—go undiagnosed. Thyroid disease most frequently presents symptoms at puberty, more in adolescent girls than in boys. Symptoms of hypothyroidism, or an underactive thyroid, include fatigue, weight gain, muscle and joint pain, forgetfulness, and mood swings. This condition is detected with a blood test that measures the amount of thyroid-stimulating hormone in the body. If the results reveal hypothyroidism, a doctor will usually prescribe a thyroid hormone replacement pill.

An overactive thyroid, or hyperthyroidism, leads to anxiety, sudden weight loss, a racing heartbeat, and insomnia. An antithyroid medication that slows the gland's production of hormones can treat the condition. More serious cases may require a radioactive iodine treatment that destroys the thyroid without harming other parts of the body. People who undergo this procedure must take thyroid hormone replacement pills for the rest of their lives. Not infrequently, symptoms that begin in adolescence will subside spontaneously or after a year of drug therapy.

ADDITIONAL FACTS

1. *About 5 percent of Americans have hypothyroidism, while 1 percent have hyperthyroidism. Women are much more likely to experience either condition than men are.*

2. *Adults need about 150 milligrams of iodine a day for thyroid hormone production. The mineral is found in fish, seaweed, and iodized salt.*

3. *Because thyroid disorders are so prevalent in women, some doctors recommend that women have their thyroids checked every 3 years beginning at age 35.*

◆◆◆

Diverticulitis

A healthy colon is a 5-foot tube of smooth muscle tissue. But some people's colons develop small bulges caused by weak spots in the muscle. More than half of all people over age 60 have this harmless condition, which is called diverticulosis. But when these marble-size pouches of intestinal lining become inflamed and infected, it becomes diverticulitis.

Up to one in four people with diverticulosis develops diverticulitis. The most common sign is severe pain on the lower left side of the abdomen; others include fever, nausea, cramping, and a change in bowel habits. A physician diagnoses the condition with a physical exam, blood tests, and CT scans of the abdomen. In the majority of cases, a course of antibiotics is prescribed to combat the infection. If not treated promptly, the infection can lead to an abscess, or a collection of pus, in the colon wall. When this abscess bursts or pus leaks out, peritonitis occurs. This severe condition causes serious illness and can be fatal without proper medical treatment.

Another complication of diverticulitis is a fistula. When damaged tissues come into contact and fuse, creating an abnormal communication, a fistula is formed. Fistulas—along with recurring cases of diverticulitis—are treated with the surgical removal of the troublesome section of the colon.

The best way to ward off these diverticular diseases is to consume a high-fiber diet. Experts believe that constipation causes people to strain during bowel movements, exerting pressure on the colon and weakening the lining. Although adults need 25 grams of fiber a day from foods such as fruits, vegetables, and whole grains, most consume less than half that amount. Drinking plenty of fluids and eating salads and whole grain cereals also help maintain regular bowel function and keep the colon healthy.

ADDITIONAL FACTS

1. *Diverticular diseases are rare in Asia and Africa, where most people eat high-fiber diets.*

2. *Diverticulosis affects both sexes equally, but diverticulitis is more common in women.*

✦✦✦

Midwife

Since America's colonization, midwives have been caring for pregnant women and attending births in the United States. Today, certified nurse-midwives can run their own practices, perform clinical exams, and even prescribe medicine—not just during pregnancy, but at all stages of a woman's life. However, most states require that a midwife practice have a physician backup or supervisor.

The profession of nurse-midwifery was established in the 1920s, in response to the alarming rate of infant and maternal mortality in the United States. A group of obstetricians, nurses, and mothers formed the Maternity Center Association (MCA) in New York City to address the problem. The MCA looked at foreign countries with outstanding maternal and child health records, and saw that the most prominent figure in the birth cycle was the nurse-midwife.

The first nurse-midwives in America came from England. They joined the Frontier Nursing Service, which was established in Kentucky to send nurses on horseback to isolated areas in the Appalachian Mountains. The first nurse-midwifery school was established a few years later. Today there are more than 7,000 certified nurse-midwives, and members of the profession attend about 8 percent of US births each year. They no longer care only for isolated or poor women and children; plenty of affluent customers today appreciate the personalized, holistic health care that nurse-midwives provide.

Certified nurse-midwives are registered nurses who have completed graduate-level training in midwifery and passed a national certification exam. They can practice in homes, birth centers, clinics, and hospitals and can prescribe medication, and their services are often reimbursed by insurance. Many patients visit their midwives for annual checkups and for guidance on women's health issues such as birth control, breast cancer, and menopause.

Most states license nurse-midwives, but only for care of healthy patients, not for treatment of disease or complications of delivery.

Other types of non-nurse-midwives, including certified midwives and direct-entry midwives, have different rights to practice depending on state laws. Another type of midwife figure is the doula—a woman whose role is to provide physical and emotional support to women and their partners during labor and birth, but not to diagnose medical conditions or give medical advice. A doula is not usually licensed or certified to have had specific training.

ADDITIONAL FACTS

1. *Practitioners of midwifery are known as midwives, whether they are women or men. The word comes from the roots mid, meaning "with," and wif, meaning "woman."*

2. *In many areas of the world, traditional midwives, renamed traditional birth attendants by the World Health Organization and other groups, are the only available providers for childbearing women. They are usually local women with some experience but little or no specific training, much as midwives were in America before licensing was required.*

◆◆◆

Brain Atrophy

The loss of tissue and neurons in the brain as a result of disease, injury, or old age is called cerebral or brain atrophy. Brain atrophy can be generalized, meaning that tissue is shrinking all over, or it can be focal, affecting only a limited area and impairing only the functions that that part of the brain controls.

Atrophy of the brain is not a medical diagnosis, but rather an anatomical description of what a doctor might see in an MRI or CAT scan. Accelerated brain atrophy is commonly associated with Alzheimer's disease and other forms of dementia in the elderly. But all people show some degree of atrophy as they age, as the brain naturally shrinks in size and volume. Age-related atrophy takes place mainly in the frontal lobes, which are responsible for "executive functions" such as planning, controlling, and inhibiting thought and behavior. Atrophy in other areas of the brain can affect coordination, language skills, and intelligence. Decreased bloodflow to the brain is thought to cause most cases of atrophy.

Other diseases that can lead to earlier- or greater-than-normal cerebral atrophy include cerebral palsy, encephalitis, Huntington's disease, multiple sclerosis, stroke, traumatic brain injury, and infectious diseases such as AIDS. Many of these conditions are associated with memory impairment, seizures, and communication problems.

Mental and social forms of stimulation—such as doing puzzles, reading, and interacting with friends—are important parts of preventing brain atrophy. Regular physical activity and good nutrition also appear to help reduce or reverse the rate of brain atrophy in older adults with dementia. Research suggests that people with low levels of vitamin B_{12}, which is found in meat, dairy, and eggs, may have more brain shrinkage than those with normal levels of the vitamin.

ADDITIONAL FACTS

1. *Research shows that brain atrophy can affect elderly people's judgment and their ability to inhibit unwanted thoughts, sparking depression, gambling problems, socially inappropriate behavior, and unintentional prejudice and racism.*

2. *Brain atrophy often involves aphasias, sensory disorders that take two forms. Receptive aphasia makes it difficult to "receive," or understand the meaning, of words spoken by others. Expressive aphasia makes it difficult to express oneself in words, leading to symptoms like strange word choices, inability to think of a word or to name common objects, and incomplete phrases or sentences.*

◆◆◆

Chlamydia

Chlamydia is one of the most overlooked sexually transmitted infections (STIs), yet it's also one of the most prevalent. Although as many as 10 million Americans are exposed to it every year, it's thought that only 20 percent are ever diagnosed and properly treated. That's because chlamydia's trademark symptoms are easily confused with those of other conditions. Most often, the disease causes discharge from the penis or vagina, along with slight pelvic pain.

One reason that chlamydia is often overlooked is because scientists and doctors knew less about the bacterium that causes it, *Chlamydia trachomatis,* than about other strains. Because the bacterium is not easily grown in a laboratory setting, it wasn't identified until 1965. What's more, until the past few decades, diagnosis of the disease required a complicated laboratory test that took as long as a week to complete and was offered at only a few locations.

Today, doctors can screen for chlamydia with a simple culture or smear and treat it with a weeklong course of tetracycline or erythromycin antibiotics. Unfortunately, sometimes physicians mistake the symptoms for those of another STI, gonorrhea, and prescribe an incorrect medication. In women, this allows the bacteria to travel up to the uterus and fallopian tubes. The resulting infection, called pelvic inflammatory disease, may leave the female reproductive tract scarred, affecting a woman's ability to have children. However, untreated gonorrhea may do exactly the same thing, and a patient who has one of these diseases is at greater risk of contracting the other.

ADDITIONAL FACTS

1. *Some 10 percent of college students have an episode of chlamydia infection.*

2. *A chlamydia infection raises a woman's risk of ectopic pregnancies, and if she's pregnant when infected, it increases the chance of premature birth and postpartum infection.*

3. *After exposure through sex, it takes 1 to 4 weeks for symptoms to appear.*

◆◆◆

Vitamin C

Vitamin C, which is also called ascorbic acid, is a vitamin that your body requires for good health. Your body uses it to form collagen in bones, cartilage, muscle, and blood vessels and to help with the absorption of iron. Vitamin C can be found in fruits and vegetables, especially citrus fruits, such as lemons, limes, and oranges. Currently the recommended daily intake of vitamin C is 90 milligrams for men ages 18 and older and 75 milligrams for women 18 and older. Pregnant and breastfeeding women need larger quantities and should check with their doctors. Children require different amounts of vitamin C based on their ages.

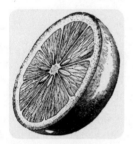

Vitamin C deficiency can lead to scurvy, which is a serious disease that can even lead to sudden death. This is rare and happens only in cases of severe deficiency. Scurvy may occur in people who are malnourished or in infants whose only source of nourishment is breast milk. Patients with scurvy are treated with vitamin C, and their symptoms usually improve within 24 to 48 hours.

There are many proposed uses for vitamin C. In particular, researchers continue to investigate the use of this vitamin to prevent or treat colds and respiratory infections, although for the most part they've been unable to show that it causes any significant reduction in the risk of developing a cold. However, the vitamin may shorten the duration of colds in the general population. In people living in very cold temperatures or those who exercise at extreme levels, vitamin C may lead to as much as a 50 percent drop in the risk of developing a cold. Vitamin C has not been shown to be beneficial in the prevention of cataracts, heart disease, or cancer, although research is constantly being done to evaluate its effects.

ADDITIONAL FACTS

1. *Your body cannot store vitamin C, so it is extremely rare to develop vitamin C toxicity.*

2. *Consuming more than 2,000 milligrams of vitamin C a day may lead to upset stomach and diarrhea.*

3. *Scurvy was widespread in the British navy until limes were added to the sailors' diets. This is believed to be the reason British sailors were called limeys.*

✦✦✦

Cardiac Catheterization

In the early 1900s, scientists were steadily searching for new ways to see into and manipulate the beating human heart. It was clear that more and more people were dying of cardiovascular disease, clogged arteries, and heart attacks, but it wasn't until cardiac catheterization was put into use that doctors could see what was really going on inside a living person's circulatory system.

One of the inventors of the technique was Werner Forssmann (1904–1979), who was a medical student in Germany when he decided to test the idea on the most readily available guinea pig: himself. In 1929, Forssmann took an x-ray of himself after slipping a long, thin, tube into his arm and sliding it up his vein. It turned out that he had pushed the catheter all the way into the right atrium of his heart. This opened the door to a whole new set of possibilities: Two years later, Forssmann performed the experiment again, this time injecting a liquid known to show on x-ray film—essentially performing the first angiocardiogram.

Building on these experiments, André Frédéric Cournand (1895–1988) and Dickinson Richards (1895–1973) continued studying cardiac catheterization on laboratory animals at Bellevue Hospital in New York City. They demonstrated that the procedure was safe—again, by testing it on Cournand himself—and used it in a clinical setting for the first time in 1941.

Cardiac catheterization allowed for a new way to study the heart and lungs by permitting doctors to draw blood directly from the heart. By attaching tiny devices to the catheter's tip, doctors could also take blood pressure readings and measure oxygen and carbon dioxide levels as blood flowed through the body. For their discovery, Forssmann, Cournand, and Richards shared the 1956 Nobel Prize in Physiology or Medicine.

ADDITIONAL FACTS

1. *Today, cardiac catheters are inserted into veins or arteries in either the arm, neck, or leg.*

2. *A catheter with a balloon at the tip may be used for cardiac angioplasty, or percutaneous coronary intervention, a technique used to compress plaque and enlarge a narrowed blood vessel.*

3. *A cardiac catheterization can last from 1 to several hours. Although patients are usually given a sedative beforehand to help them relax, they generally must remain awake during the procedure.*

◆◆◆

Adenoids

Adenoids are clumps of spongy tissue that lie on each side of the throat, between the nose and the roof of the mouth. Although they're usually grouped together with the tonsils, adenoids aren't visible when you open your mouth.

Like the tonsils, these masses of lymphatic tissue help protect the body by acting as filters. Each adenoid is covered with a thin layer of mucus and cilia, hairlike projections that propel the mucus down the throat. This mucus and the adenoids themselves trap harmful bacteria and viruses each time you breathe or swallow. What's more, these glands also produce antibodies to help fight off infections.

Experts believe that adenoids play an important role during early childhood. In fact, adenoids usually start to shrink at age 5, so by the time someone reaches his or her teenage years, the tissues have practically disappeared altogether. It's during those early years that adenoids can become infected and enlarged or swollen. This occurrence usually goes hand in hand with tonsillitis; symptoms include a sore throat, swollen glands, a stuffy nose, and an ear infection.

If the infection is caused by bacteria, your doctor may prescribe a course of antibiotics. But if the medication doesn't clear up the symptoms or if a child suffers from recurring infections, the doctor may recommend surgical removal of the adenoids, called an adenoidectomy. It usually takes children about a week to recover from this procedure, which is often accompanied by the removal of the tonsils.

ADDITIONAL FACTS

1. *Because enlarged adenoids cause a stuffy nose, forcing the person to breathe through his or her open mouth, one symptom is a vacant facial expression.*

2. *An adenoidectomy done at the same time as a tonsillectomy is commonly called a T and A.*

◆◆◆

Cystitis

On the Greek island of Kos is the teaching hospital founded by the ancient Greek physician Hippocrates (460–377 BC), also known as the founder of modern medicine. The structure was built onto a hillside, and each section corresponded to the appropriate section of the human body: The building on the hilltop was home to the study of mental illness, while the departments devoted to the bowels and bladder were at the base of the hill. It was in this lower section of the hospital that cystitis—infection of the bladder—was first studied.

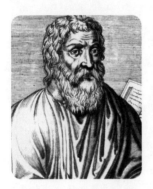

Cystitis is triggered by a bacterial infection of the urinary bladder. Bacteria, most commonly *Escherichia coli,* make their way up through the urethra and multiply in the urinary tract. The resulting infection leads to a frequent, urgent need to urinate and a burning or painful sensation when urinating. Other symptoms include cloudy or bloody urine, a low fever, and pelvic pain. These days, cystitis is diagnosed with a urine analysis, in which a sample is screened for bacteria, blood, or pus and a culture is done to identify the offending organism. The most common treatment is antibiotics to kill the bacteria; symptoms usually clear up within a few days. Sometimes the cause is a sexually transmitted organism.

The bladder can also become inflamed without a bacterial infection. Chemical irritants, such as products in bubble baths and spermicidal jellies, as well as trauma from sexual intercourse, can cause irritation. About 1 million people suffer from interstitial cystitis, chronic bladder inflammation that has been linked to an autoimmune disorder. Although there's no cure for interstitial cystitis, doctors can prescribe treatments to ease the condition, such as nerve stimulation or medications to relieve pelvic pain and urinary frequency.

ADDITIONAL FACTS

1. *Because they have shorter urethras, women are more likely to develop cystitis.*

2. *Pregnant women are particularly at risk, because pregnancy can interfere with the complete emptying of the bladder.*

3. *Compounds in cranberries have been shown to protect against cystitis by blocking bacteria from adhering to the urinary tract walls.*

◆◆◆

Rolfing

"This is the gospel of Rolfing: When the body gets working appropriately, the force of gravity can flow through. Then, spontaneously, the body heals itself."
—Ida P. Rolf

Rolfing structural integration is a method of soft tissue manipulation, similar to a deep massage, that aims to improve posture, relieve stress, and ease chronic pain. Founder Ida P. Rolf (1896–1979), a pioneer in the field of medicine in the 1920s, was intrigued by alternative healing practices such as homeopathy, chiropractic, and yoga. She felt that the body functions best when its bones are properly aligned and that structural imbalances negatively affect the body's muscles, tendons, and ligaments. This belief led her to establish a method she called structural integration: slow-moving pressure applied with the knuckles, thumbs, fingers, elbows, and knees to the muscles and the soft tissues around them.

Rolf movement is taught as a sequence of sessions—known as the 10 Series—devoted to specific structural and movement themes. The first session typically focuses on using breathing patterns to release pent-up "holdings" in the ribs, lungs, and diaphragm. Subsequent sessions address movement patterns in the feet, ankles, knees, hips, arms, neck, and head.

Proponents of Rolfing claim that it can improve athletic coordination, prevent repetitive stress injuries, and be used as a prophylactic measure in children with potential structural problems. They stress that Rolfing is not just a deep tissue massage, and the Rolfers must be highly skilled. Practitioners first detect problem areas, then "discriminate" by focusing on the muscles that have been pulled out of place by stress or injury. Finally, they "integrate the body, relating its segments in an improved relationship, bringing physical balance in the gravitational field," according to the Rolf Institute of Structural Integration—something that a simple massage cannot do.

Some clinical studies have shown that Rolfing may be effective at reducing anxiety, improving movement in cerebral palsy patients, boosting well-being in patients with chronic fatigue syndrome, and treating lower-back disorders, although more research is needed in these areas. Patients with osteoporosis, skin damage, or bleeding disorders and those who are taking blood-thinning medications should avoid Rolfing.

ADDITIONAL FACTS

1. *It's estimated that more than 1 million people have received Rolfing work. The term is now a registered service mark in 27 countries.*

2. *According to the Rolf Institute of Structural Integration, more than 1,550 specialists worldwide offer Rolfing services.*

3. *Rolf held a doctorate in biochemistry from Columbia University.*

◆◆◆

Parkinson's Disease

In his 2000 autobiography *Lucky Man,* the actor Michael J. Fox (1961–) describes his battle with Parkinson's disease (PD) as a "Jekyll-and-Hyde melodrama" that cycles between times when his medication is working and times when it's not, when he is possessed by the symptoms of his condition: rigidity, shuffling, loss of balance, and difficulty communicating, among others.

In a healthy brain, the chemical dopamine regulates movement by sending the proper signals to your brain. So, when the cells responsible for dopamine production break down, the body has trouble moving the way it's supposed to. Symptoms of PD usually begin at about age 50 and slowly worsen over many years.

The four main symptoms of the disease are trembling arms and legs (tremor), stiff muscles, slow movement (bradykinesia), and problems with balance. Tremor often begins first, in just one arm or leg. But in time, PD affects muscles throughout the body and can lead to problems such as constipation or difficulty swallowing. Some patients also show signs of dementia.

Aging and exposure to environmental toxins (such as herbicides and pesticides) seem to be risk factors for PD, and having one or more close relatives with the disease increases a person's chances as well. But scientists have not been able to find any direct causes.

PD can't be detected in the blood, and diagnosis is often based on a doctor's physical exam. A medication called levodopa seems to relieve symptoms, so a doctor may prescribe it to see how a patient reacts in order to decide on a diagnosis.

Levodopa (also called L-dopa) and another drug, carbidopa, are often combined to help produce dopamine in the brain. Other types of medications, including dopamine agonists, may also be prescribed. PD drugs can have unpleasant side effects, however, including hallucinations, confusion, and even compulsive gambling. The medicines' effectiveness can also peter out after a few years, so doctors often try to keep patients with mild symptoms off medication for as long as possible.

ADDITIONAL FACTS

1. *For patients who have unstable reactions to levodopa, a surgical treatment called deep brain stimulation may be used. Tiny electrical wires are placed in the brain and send signals to the areas that control movement.*

2. *Depression is common in people with PD and sometimes develops even before motor symptoms.*

3. *Unconscious movements such as blinking, smiling, and swinging the arms while walking may be diminished or lost in people with PD. Some people with PD develop a staring expression or no longer seem animated when they speak.*

◆◆◆

Gonorrhea

There are a handful of misconceptions about why gonorrhea is also known as the clap. Applause and hand-smacking references aside, the truth is that the slang term is derived from the 16th-century French word *clapoir,* referring to a sexual sore. Probably it was the chancre of syphilis, another disease often present with gonorrhea. In gonorrhea, the most common signs, including a burning sensation when urinating, blood in the urine, and vaginal discharge, are less noticeable and usually briefly present. This sexually transmitted infection (STI) affects roughly 1 million Americans every year, the majority of them under the age of 30. Symptoms appear 1 to 14 days after exposure.

The infection is caused by a strain of bacterium called *Neisseria gonorrhoeae*, which thrives in the mucous membranes found in the genital tract and urethra and causes inflammation. Up to half of all gonorrhea cases go undetected, because symptoms can be mild and usually clear up on their own within a short time—a week to a few months. But it's important that sexually active adults get screened for STIs. In many women, gonorrhea can spread throughout the reproductive tract, affecting the fallopian tubes and ovaries. This condition, called pelvic inflammatory disease, may lead to pain and sterility.

Gonorrhea is diagnosed through a test of the urine or vaginal discharge. In the majority of cases, one course of penicillin or tetracycline is enough to wipe out the bacteria. However, because of the microbes' growing resistance to antibiotics, a larger dose or stronger medication, such as cefoxitin, is sometimes required.

ADDITIONAL FACTS

1. *The bacterium that causes gonorrhea was discovered by the German physician Albert Neisser (1855–1916) in 1879. He went on to identify the bacterium responsible for leprosy.*

2. *In rare cases, gonorrhea contracted through sexual contact can lead to eye infections.*

3. *Resistant strains of gonorrhea appeared in servicemen returning from duty in the Vietnam War.*

✦✦✦

Vitamin E

Vitamin E is a nutrient essential to the human body. It helps your body form red blood cells and use vitamin K. Vitamin E is also an antioxidant that protects your body from damage caused by free radicals, which are unstable substances that can harm cells, tissues, and organs. Free radicals are also believed to affect certain age-related conditions.

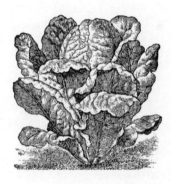

Vitamin E is found in many foods, including asparagus, corn, margarine, nuts, olives, seeds, spinach and other green leafy vegetables, vegetable oils, and wheat germ. If you are on a low-fat diet, you need to make careful food choices to ensure that your vitamin E intake is adequate. However, too much vitamin E can be harmful. Amounts in excess of 400 IU per day may lead to bleeding problems, since vitamin E can act as an anticoagulant (blood thinner). The amount of vitamin E found in most multivitamins is generally not harmful.

Vitamin E deficiency is rare. It is likely to occur in people who cannot absorb dietary fat, those with certain kinds of rare genetic abnormalities, and very low-birth-weight infants. Sometimes people with zinc deficiency also have decreased levels of vitamin E. Insufficient levels of this vitamin can lead to neurological problems associated with nerve degeneration, which causes tingling and burning sensations in the hands and feet.

ADDITIONAL FACTS

1. *It's recommended that individuals ages 14 and older take 15 milligrams of vitamin E a day. Children need different amounts of vitamin E based on their ages. Breastfeeding women may require more vitamin E and should check with their doctors.*

2. *Vitamin E supplements are usually sold as alpha-tocopheryl acetate, a form of alpha-tocopherol that has antioxidant properties.*

3. *Vitamin E exists in eight different forms. The most active form in humans is alpha-tocopherol.*

◆◆◆

Flexible Endoscopy

The ability to see inside the body—whether to perform surgery, make a diagnosis, or chart the process of growth and repair—is invaluable to almost all fields of medicine. To do this, doctors today use a technique called flexible endoscopy.

As far back as the Roman Empire, doctors sought ways to peer into the living body; the remains of primitive efforts by ancient doctors to build such a device have been found at archaeological digs in Italy. In Germany in 1805, Philip Bozzini (1773–1809) developed a tubular probe prototype—lit at one end by a candle—which he called a *Lichtleiter* (light-guided instrument). The term *endoscope* was first used in 1853, when the French physician Antoine Jean Desormeaux (1815–1894) used a similar device. In 1868, the German doctor Adolf Kussmaul (1822–1902) was the first to use one of the devices to see inside a human stomach by enlisting a sword swallower to ingest an 18-inch metal tube with mirrors attached throughout and light directed in from the top. Such rigid tubes caused injury and irritation, so a flexible version was developed in 1932.

The next step—the invention of an endoscopic camera—required extremely small lenses, tiny sources of bright light, and suitable film. The first prototype, unveiled in 1950 by the Olympus Corporation in Tokyo, required manual activation of the flashbulbs and winding of the film. Development progressed quickly, and the "gastrocamera" became widely used as a diagnostic tool for early stage stomach cancer. The development of glass fiber in the 1960s allowed the creation of new endoscopes that were thinner and more flexible. This made possible the first gastrocamera with an "eye," meaning that doctors could actually watch while taking photos.

Physicians now use endoscopes to examine the bladder, esophagus, large intestine, and other parts of the body—often pairing the scopes with tiny surgical tools for minimally invasive, or laparoscopic, surgery. Some endoscopes today take live video footage, while others can perform ultrasound imaging of surrounding tissue.

ADDITIONAL FACTS

1. *A high-definition television version of the endoscopic camera was released in 2002, radically improving the quality of images and the accuracy of diagnoses.*

2. *Scientists hope to soon develop a capsule endoscope that can be swallowed by the patient and will relay pictures wirelessly as it moves through the body.*

3. *When endoscopy is used on certain body parts, it may have specific names:* arthroscopy *for use in the joints,* bronchoscopy *for the lungs,* colonoscopy *or* sigmoidoscopy *for the large intestine,* cystoscopy *or* urethroscopy *for the urinary system, and* upper gastrointestinal endoscopy *for the esophagus and stomach.*

◆◆◆

Bone Age

Most parents can imagine how a child will look as an adult, based on what traits run in their families. But there's a true crystal ball when it comes to height: a bone age test. This simple screening, which reveals the maturity of a child's skeletal system, can predict when a child will enter puberty, how tall the child will be as an adult, and how long it will take to reach that height. Doctors use bone ages to check for growth disorders and other problems that may interfere with development.

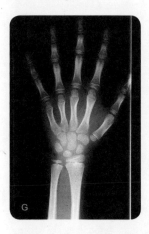

To assess bone age, doctors compare a single x-ray of a child's left wrist and hand with a standard measure of bone development. The x-ray reveals softer, less mineral-packed areas called epiphyses, or growth plates. These areas are where bone cells reproduce and calcify, forming new bone. As a child ages, this zone becomes thinner; if the plate width, or bone age, is different from that of other children of the same age, that may suggest a growth problem.

A delayed bone age may indicate a genetic growth disorder, such as Turner's syndrome, or a condition that affects growth hormones, such as hypothyroidism. Doctors also use bone age to treat orthopedic problems by measuring a child's projected growth. On the other hand, an accelerated bone age may suggest precocious puberty, in which a child undergoes puberty at an early age, or it may indicate an overactive adrenal gland.

ADDITIONAL FACTS

1. Bone age is also known as skeletal age.

2. Having a bone age that differs from one's chronological age doesn't necessarily mean that there is a growth problem. Children develop at different rates.

◆ ◆ ◆

Heartburn (GERD)

If you frequently experience heartburn—a burning sensation in your chest after a meal—chances are you're one of the estimated 25 million Americans who suffer from gastroesophageal reflux disease (GERD). Also dubbed acid reflux, this condition causes the acidic digestive juices in the stomach to back up into the esophagus, the tube that connects your mouth to your stomach.

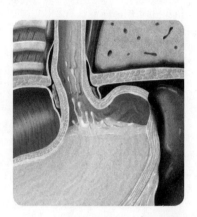

Usually, after you swallow, a valve called the lower esophageal sphincter (LES)—a band of muscle at the bottom of the esophagus—clamps shut. But when the LES loosens or opens sporadically, stomach fluids can flow back up. Pressure on the stomach, the result of pregnancy or obesity, can cause this to occur; diabetes and asthma are also culprits. Over the long term, constant exposure to this acidic backwash can irritate the lining of the esophagus and may lead to inflammation, ulcers, and, in rare cases, cancer.

To prevent heartburn, experts recommend cutting back on foods that can trigger it, such as caffeine, chocolate, fatty foods, citrus fruits, tomatoes, peppermint, spices, and garlic. Gravity can also work to your advantage; staying upright or taking a walk after eating can help. Since smoking revs up the production of stomach acid, kicking that habit can also improve symptoms.

Over-the-counter antacids that neutralize the juices can be effective. A physician can also prescribe acid-suppressing medications. Because these drugs work so well, surgical procedures to tighten the esophagus are rare and usually a last resort.

ADDITIONAL FACTS

1. *One in 10 adults suffers a bout of heartburn at least once a week.*

2. *Experts say avoiding eating before going to bed and elevating the head of the bed 6 to 9 inches can also help alleviate GERD.*

3. *It's called heartburn because the burning sensation is in the area of the chest thought by early medical practitioners to be the site of the heart.*

◆◆◆

Physical Therapy

People with orthopedic conditions such as joint pain or sports injuries often attend physical therapy sessions to practice techniques for reducing pain, restoring movement and function, and preventing disability. In many cases, physical therapy can even take the place of surgery.

Physical therapy is known in some countries as physiotherapy. Its roots can be traced back to the ancient Greeks, who wrote that the capacity to move is a vital element of health and well-being. More than 173,000 physical therapists are employed in the United States, according to federal statistics.

In order to practice, physical therapists must receive a master's or doctoral degree from an accredited physical therapy program and pass national and state exams to receive a state license. Some specialize in particular types of physical therapy, focusing on children, for instance, or athletes. Physical therapy can be helpful for people with bone injuries; neurological disorders like Parkinson's disease; heart problems; repetitive stress disorders such as carpal tunnel syndrome (a wrist injury) or shin splints (a running injury), or connective tissue injury for those who have had a stroke, traumatic brain damage.

As part of a treatment plan, physical therapists often prescribe a regimen of therapeutic exercise to strengthen injured areas. Physical therapists may push a joint to its extreme range of motion to stretch it and extend movement, or they may massage a muscle to promote proper function. They teach patients stretches and exercises they can do at home, as well as self-care techniques for sore muscles and injury. For example, to treat a foot or ankle injury before the injured person can get to a doctor, physical therapists advise a process of rest, icing the injury, applying a compression bandage, and elevating the injured area so that it is positioned higher than the heart—a simple and effective procedure known by the acronym RICE. In some cases, physical therapists may apply hot packs or use ultrasound equipment to treat some types of injuries.

ADDITIONAL FACTS

1. *In 2006, the American Physical Therapy Association announced a new workplace disorder named BlackBerry thumb, which involved chronic finger pain due to typing on tiny electronic comunication devices.*

2. *Physical therapists often have certified, registered, or licensed assistants (PTAs), who complete a 2-year associate's degree program.*

3. *The World Confederation for Physical Therapy, which was founded in 1951, has designated September 8 as World Physical Therapy Day.*

❖❖❖

Alzheimer's Disease

A crippling and irreversible form of dementia that affects nearly half the over-85 population, Alzheimer's disease (AD) is one of the most common old-age afflictions. AD, which causes memory loss, personality changes, and problems communicating, usually begins after age 60. But despite its prevalence, AD should not be considered a normal part of aging, as growing evidence suggests that safeguards can be taken to reduce an individual's susceptibility to it.

Physical evidence of AD was first observed in 1906 by the German doctor Alois Alzheimer (1864–1915). While performing an autopsy on a mentally ill woman, Alzheimer found mysterious abnormalities in her brain tissue. These clumps of tangled nerves are now considered the only definitive physical marker of AD. Because they are visible only after death, doctors must diagnose "possible" or "probable" AD while a patient is still alive. Other conditions overlap with AD, making the clinical diagnosis difficult.

Even so, specialists in AD can correctly identify it up to 90 percent of the time by performing tests of memory, problem solving, and attention. Other changes in the brain that suggest AD—including cell death and lower-than-normal levels of certain chemicals that carry messages back and forth—may also be visible in brain scans.

AD begins in the brain's memory and language centers, and early symptoms may be confused with normal age-related forgetfulness. But gradually, symptoms become worse and people with AD lose their ability to communicate, grow moody and anxious, and may forget the names and faces of family members. Because people with AD may also wander away from home or forget how to handle basic tasks, they eventually need constant care.

The exact cause of AD is unknown, but age and family history increase a person's risk. Scientists have identified a gene that triggers production of a specific form of apolipoprotein E (ApoE), which helps carry cholesterol in the blood. Everyone has ApoE, but about 15 percent have the form that raises AD risk.

High blood pressure, high cholesterol, and low levels of the vitamin folic acid appear to increase the risk of AD, while growing evidence suggests that exercise, social interaction, and mental activities (such as doing crossword puzzles or playing cards) may protect against the disease. There is no treatment, but medication may temporarily help keep symptoms from worsening, especially when the illness is diagnosed early.

ADDITIONAL FACTS

1. *AD patients generally live from 8 to 10 years after they are diagnosed, though some may live with AD for as long as 20 years.*

2. *Scientists think that as many as 4.5 million Americans have AD. Notable people who have developed it include the former US president Ronald Reagan (1911–2004), the actress Rita Hayworth (1918–1987), and the actor Charlton Heston (1924–2008).*

✦✦✦

Herpes

Affecting more than 45 million Americans, herpes is one of the most common sexually transmitted infections. Caused by the herpes simplex virus 1 (HSV-1) or 2 (HSV-2), the virus is one of the few that can be transferred through skin-to-skin contact. Unfortunately, there's no cure for herpes; while it can be effectively treated with medication, the virus remains in your body throughout your lifetime.

Once a person is exposed to herpes, the virus takes as long as 3 weeks to spread throughout the body. As it circulates through the body, it may affect the nervous system and cause flulike symptoms or aches and pains. But the telltale sign is a painful lesion around the mouth (with HSV-1) or on the genitals (with HSV-2), which may take up to a year to appear. The lesion usually begins as one or more blisterlike pimples that burst, leaving behind an open sore. Depending on the person, outbreaks can occur infrequently (or even never) or as often as weekly. Emotional or physical stress, which weakens the immune system, or fever may trigger an attack. An antiviral medication, such as valacyclovir (Valtrex) or famciclovir (Famvir), can help reduce the number and severity of these outbreaks.

The largest impact on herpes sufferers is the psychological toll it can take. But in pregnant women, a herpes attack can have serious consequences for the fetus. If there are active lesions at the time of delivery, the baby may be infected and may suffer a generalized infection causing multiple organ damage, including brain damage, if it comes into contact with a large quantity of the virus. As a result, mothers usually undergo a Caesarean section if they are having their first vaginal infection or have visible signs of an active genital infection.

ADDITIONAL FACTS

1. *The herpes viruses are usually dormant in the local nerve cells until something stimulates them to grow and produce sores on the skin or in the mucous membranes, such as the mouth.*

2. *Because of oral sex, there are plenty of cases of HSV-2 on the mouth and HSV-1 on the genitals.*

3. *A person's first outbreak is generally the most serious.*

4. *The cold sores and fever blisters that are commonly seen are outbreaks of herpes.*

◆◆◆

Vitamin D

Vitamin D is a nutrient that is essential to good health. This vitamin helps your body absorb calcium, which is necessary for forming and maintaining strong bones and teeth. Vitamin D may also help protect your body from osteoporosis, cancer, high blood pressure, and several autoimmune diseases.

There are two forms of vitamin D that are important to the human body: calciferol, or vitamin D_2, and cholecalciferol, or vitamin D_3. You can get vitamin D_2 by eating foods that naturally contain it, such as fish, eggs, and cod liver. You can obtain both vitamin D_2 and vitamin D_3 from food supplements or foods that are fortified, such as milk. Your body can make vitamin D_3 when your skin is exposed to ultraviolet B rays from sunlight. As little as 10 minutes of sun exposure a day should prevent you from being vitamin D deficient.

Populations at risk of vitamin D deficiency include the elderly, the obese, exclusively breastfed infants, individuals getting limited sun exposure, and people who have fat malabsorption syndrome or inflammatory bowel disease. Without enough vitamin D, your body cannot absorb calcium and must take calcium from its stores in your skeleton. In children, vitamin D deficiency can lead to rickets, which results in skeletal deformities. Lack of the vitamin in adults can lead to osteomalacia, which causes muscular and bone weakness.

Populations at particular risk for vitamin D toxicity from an excess of the vitamin include those with histoplasmosis, hyperparathyroidism, kidney disease, sarcoidosis, or tuberculosis. However, anyone can develop vitamin D toxicity by regularly taking the vitamin in excess. Too much D leads to bone loss and hypercalcemia, which can have life-threatening complications. To treat the condition, a doctor will stop the patient's intake of vitamin D and calcium and monitor his or her progress.

ADDITIONAL FACTS

1. *It is believed that all individuals from 50 to 70 years old need 10 micrograms daily, and those who are over 70 need 15 to 20 micrograms a day. (One microgram equals 40 IUs.)*

2. *Pregnant and breastfeeding women should check with their physicians about vitamin D supplementation.*

✦✦✦

Jonas Salk, Albert Sabin, and the Polio Vaccine

When outbreaks of poliomyelitis plagued the United States and Europe in the late 1800s and early 1900s, the public rallied to help find a cure and poured money into research. What they got were two vaccines from the researchers Jonas Salk and Albert Sabin that largely eradicated the disease over the next 50 years.

At the turn of the 20th century, polio struck as many as 50,000 people—mainly children—in a single year. The virus paralyzed breathing muscles and could be fatal, and it left most victims permanently crippled. A vaccine was tested in 1935, but it killed six of the children in the study; it wasn't until 1950 that the medical community felt ready to give vaccination another try.

Jonas Salk (1914–1995), a researcher at the University of Pittsburgh, proposed an injectable vaccine made from a killed virus, and a double-blind trial of nearly 2 million children was arranged. In 1955, the inactivated polio vaccine was declared safe, and Salk was hailed as a national hero. The vaccine was speedily licensed and mass produced, and more than 450 million shots were given over the next 4 years. As a result, the incidence of paralytic polio in the United States fell from 18 cases per 100,000 to fewer than 2 per 100,000.

Another vaccine containing live, weakened virus was approved in 1961 after extensive testing on children in the Soviet Union, the Netherlands, Mexico, and other countries. The new formula, developed by the University of Cincinnati researcher Albert Sabin (1906–1993), had a very small risk of actually causing polio, but it also promised extended immunity and could be taken orally, in liquid drops or sugar cubes that dissolved on the tongue. The oral polio vaccine largely replaced Salk's version as the predominant vaccine used in the United States and most other countries. By the 1970s, the annual incidence of polio in the United States had declined a thousandfold from prevaccine levels, to an average of 12 cases a year.

ADDITIONAL FACTS

1. *Both types of polio vaccines generally require three doses, with a fourth "booster" given when a child reaches school age.*

2. *The World Health Organization in 1988 called for the global eradication of polio by the year 2000. Complete elimination by the target date didn't happen, but the number of new cases each year had been reduced to approximately 1,000 to 2,000 (down from more than 250,000).*

3. *In November 2005, four Amish children in Minnesota were diagnosed with polio. None of them had been vaccinated.*

✦✦✦

Cryptorchidism

As a baby boy grows within his mother's womb, his testicles typically develop inside his abdomen. Shortly before birth, they drop into the scrotum, a bag of skin behind the penis. But for up to 5 percent of boys, one or both of their testicles does not descend properly. This condition, called cryptorchidism, is most common among babies born prematurely.

Physicians check for cryptorchidism shortly after delivery. About 70 percent of the time, the testicle can be found, and it will usually descend on its own. But in the remaining cases, the testicle may still be located in the abdomen or may not have fully developed.

If the testicle hasn't dropped by 6 months of age, a pediatrician may recommend a minimally invasive surgery. During this procedure, called an orchiopexy, a small incision is made in the groin and the testicle is repositioned in the scrotum. It usually takes about a week for the boy to recover. If left untreated, cryptorchidism may increase the risk of hernias, trauma, fertility problems, and even testicular cancer.

In some boys, the testicles may appear to have left the scrotum from time to time, but that doesn't automatically indicate cryptorchidism. It may be a sign of retractile testes, in which the testicles are usually in the scrotum but, on occasion, pull back up into the groin. A physician can distinguish this condition from cryptorchidism. Retractile testes is a normal variant and does not need to be treated.

ADDITIONAL FACTS

1. *The term* cryptorchidism *is derived from the Greek words* crypto, *which means "hidden," and* orchid, *meaning "testes."*

2. *The condition affects up to 30 percent of boys born prematurely.*

◆ ◆ ◆

Kidney Stones

Every year, more than 3 million unlucky people head to the doctor to be diagnosed with a kidney stone when a pebblelike formation travels down the urinary tract. Since the beginning of civilization, humans have been plagued by this painful condition. In fact, scientists have discovered evidence of kidney stones in a 7,000-year-old Egyptian mummy.

Today, 10 percent of men and 5 percent of women will experience a kidney stone (also known as renal lithiasis) by the age of 70. Like the filter in an aquarium, the kidneys filter out waste from the blood. As a result, small, hard deposits of minerals and acid salts eventually accumulate on the surfaces of the kidneys. These substances typically dissolve in urine, but when the urine is concentrated—due to dehydration or some other reason—they may stick together to form a hard mass.

Ranging in size from a grain of sand to a golf ball, kidney stones don't have any symptoms when they remain in the kidney. But when they travel through the urinary tract, severe pain and nausea occur. In the majority of cases, kidney stones will pass on their own after a few days or even weeks. But about 15 percent of cases require treatment, such as extracorporeal shock wave lithotripsy, in which shock waves are used to break the stone into smaller pieces. Doctors can also remove the stone in a minimally invasive procedure or insert a small stent to keep the passage open.

Experts aren't exactly sure what causes kidney stones to form, but they know that a family history of the disease increases a person's chances of suffering from it. Gout, high levels of uric acid or calcium, oxalosis (an excess of a substance called oxalate in the body), high blood pressure, and obesity also raise the odds. Dehydration and a diet that's high in protein and sodium are risk factors as well.

ADDITIONAL FACTS

1. *Global warming has another unexpected side effect: Scientists say that the increasing temperatures will result in a jump in the number of people with kidney stones. That's because the heat will lead to dehydration, a risk factor for the condition.*

2. *Some people are susceptible to kidney stones that are made up mainly of calcium that binds to a chemical called oxalate. In these instances, doctors may recommend cutting back on foods high in oxalate, which include spinach, chocolate, and black tea.*

❖❖❖

Vegetarianism

Analyses of global food trends have found that the Western diet, popular in the United States, focuses heavily on meat—too heavily, as far as many nutritionists and health experts are concerned. However, many people in the United States and all over the world make the choice to be vegetarians: people who follow a diet of mainly plant-based foods and don't eat meat, fish, or poultry.

Vegeterians are divided into several categories. Ovo-vegetarians eat dairy and eggs, while lacto-vegetarians include dairy products—but not eggs in their diet. Vegans eat no animal products at all and consume only foods from plant sources. Many people consider themselves semivegetarians or "flexitarians," meaning that they eat fish or poultry or may occasionally eat red meat.

Throughout history, a number of religions—including Brahmanism, Buddhism, and the Seventh-Day Adventist Church—have advocated vegetarianism, mainly to prevent the killing or cruel treatment of animals. Vegetarianism has been shown to reduce carbon emissions and be better for the environment, and it is also more economical, as meat is more expensive than plant-based foods in most places.

Vegetarian diets tend to be higher in fiber and lower in fat, an inherently healthier diet. But when a vegetarian diet isn't planned carefully, it may leave people deficient in protein, vitamin B_{12}, vitamin D, calcium, iron, and zinc, which come mainly from animals. Therefore, it's important to incorporate other sources of these nutrients into the diet. Eggs, milk, nuts, legumes, tofu and other soy-based products, and vitamin supplements are popular choices.

Health benefits linked to vegetarianism include reduced risks of heart disease, osteoporosis, and cancer, as well as a longer life expectancy. German research published in 2005 found that for every 100 deaths in the general population, there were just 59 deaths in a study group consisting of nearly 2,000 vegetarians and flexitarians. However, giving up animal products entirely does not seem to be the healthiest approach: For every 100 deaths among vegans, there were just 66 among vegetarians and 60 among occasional meat eaters.

ADDITIONAL FACTS

1. *Vegetarians can be at increased risk for gum disease from a lack of vitamin D and calcium. The Academy of General Dentistry suggests that vegetarians discuss food substitutions and vitamin supplementation with their dentist or a nutritionist.*

2. *According to the* Oxford English Dictionary, *the word* vegetarian *debuted in 1839 and was popularized in 1847 after the founding of a group called the Vegetarian Society.*

3. *In their writings, the early philosophers Plutarch (c. AD 46–c. 119), Ovid (43 BC–c. AD 17), and Seneca (c. 4 BC–AD 65) expressed their opposition to eating meat (or "dead carcass," as Plutarch put it). Other famous vegetarians include Plato (c. 428–c. 348 BC), Pythagoras (c. 580–c. 500 BC), and Socrates (c. 470–399 BC).*

◆◆◆

Dementia

As people get older, their memories may not be as sharp as when they were younger. They may forget minor details or have trouble concentrating, but these symptoms shouldn't be serious enough to affect their daily activities. When forgetfulness becomes a dangerous or life-altering problem or the person is disoriented with regard to time, place, or other people, the condition may be diagnosed as dementia.

Alzheimer's disease is the most common cause of dementia, but there are many other causes. Age is the biggest risk factor; by age 85, about 35 percent of people have some form of dementia. Symptoms usually result from damage or changes to the brain, including strokes, tumors, or head injuries. Disorders such as Creutzfeldt-Jakob, Huntington's, and Parkinson's diseases may also be to blame. In some cases, symptoms like those of dementia stem from treatable conditions, such as depression, underactive thyroid, vitamin B_{12} deficiency, or a buildup of fluid in the brain, called hydrocephalus. Memory loss and confusion may also result from medication use or interactions between medications or supplements.

Sometimes dementia develops suddenly and quickly; other times it progresses slowly, over many years or even decades. Memory loss is usually the first sign. As the condition progresses, people may forget the names of relatives, get lost in places they know well, or forget how to perform simple actions such as combing their hair or brushing their teeth. If dementia gets bad enough and can't be treated, patients may require constant care.

To diagnose dementia, a doctor will ask a patient questions, perform simple memory tests, and talk to family members. Blood tests may check for treatable causes, and brain scans can show whether brain tissue is shrinking—a probable sign of dementia. Medication can be prescribed to slow the condition's progression, and studies show that keeping the brain busy with activities like playing cards or doing crossword puzzles can help stave off dementia as well. Family members can make life easier for a person with dementia by posting reminder notes around the house and keeping important phone numbers next to the telephone.

ADDITIONAL FACTS

1. *Research shows that physical activity—such as daily walks or other moderate exercise—can help slow the progression of dementia in patients in the early stages. Scientists believe that people who are physically healthy get more blood and nutrients to their brains, keeping brain tissue healthy longer.*

2. *More than 70 percent of Americans with dementia are cared for at home by family caregivers. In one study, more than a third of caregivers reported six or more symptoms of depression.*

3. *It is believed that high cholesterol levels may also increase the risk for developing dementia.*

♦♦♦

Human Papillomavirus

More than half of young, sexually active adults have human papillomavirus (HPV) at some point in their lives. That's because there are more than 70 strains of this virus, many of which can be spread through skin-to-skin contact. In the overwhelming majority of cases, the virus will vacate the body in 3 to 5 years without leaving a trace. But there are also a handful of types, usually spread through sexual contact, that can lead to more serious problems.

The first group of strains are considered low risk, because while they lead to unsightly genital and venereal warts, they're harmless. To remove the warts, doctors can cut, freeze, or laser them off. The more threatening version of HPV is a handful of high-risk types that trigger cellular changes in the cervix. This may lead to cervical cancer if left untreated. If caught early enough, though, the infections are usually cured. Even when they progress to cervical cancer, they're rarely fatal, since surgery has a high rate of success, except in the most advanced cases.

One major development in the fight against high-risk HPV and cervical cancer is a vaccine called Gardasil, which is administered as a course of three injections. Approved by the Food and Drug Administration in 1996 for women ages 9 to 26, this vaccine protects against two types of HPV that cause 70 percent of cervical cancer cases and two more that result in about another 20 percent, potentially preventing 90 percent of genital wart cases that might lead to cancer. Scientists arbitrarily set 26 as the cutoff age, because women older than 26 have generally already been exposed to those HPV strains.

ADDITIONAL FACTS

1. *High- and low-risk strains of HPV can be spread through vaginal, oral, or anal sex.*

2. *Using a condom can reduce the risk of contracting HPV.*

3. *HPV is a virus that can lead to cancer in the vagina, external genitalia, or penis, as well as the usual site, the cervix.*

✦✦✦

Calcium

Calcium is a mineral that is more plentiful in the human body than any other mineral. Most of your body's calcium is stored in your bones and teeth to make them strong. Your body also uses calcium to help your muscles, blood vessels, and nervous system work and to aid the functioning of hormones and enzymes.

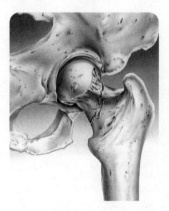

Since your body cannot make calcium and uses it for so many functions, it's important to get enough calcium in your diet. Milk, cheese, yogurt, and leafy green vegetables are all excellent sources of this mineral. If you don't consume enough calcium, you should take a supplement or eat calcium-fortified foods (such as orange juice, bread, and cereals).

The amount of calcium you need depends on your age. It's generally recommended that adults take in 1,000 to 1,200 milligrams of calcium daily, optimally through diet. Children and teenagers need more calcium than young adults. If you are calcium deficient, your body will have to break down bone to get the mineral, making your bones weaker and more likely to fracture over time.

As you get older, small amounts of bone are removed and new bone is formed through a normal process called remodeling. However, after age 35, more bone is lost than is replaced. Women who have reached menopause lose even more bone more rapidly. As a result, older women need more calcium to prevent osteoporosis, a condition of decreased bone mass. Osteoporosis affects both men and women and is the reason older people are more susceptible to breaking bones.

ADDITIONAL FACTS

1. *Calcium supplements frequently contain vitamin D, which our bodies need to absorb calcium. However, the two nutrients do not need to be taken together to be effective.*

2. *Generally, it's recommended that adults who are seldom exposed to sunlight take 33 micrograms of vitamin D daily. Though most people have adequate sun exposure and do not need vitamin D supplements (because sunlight helps the body manufacture this vitamin), it's believed that all adults over the age of 50 should take a vitamin D supplement.*

3. *Calcium supplements can be made from any of several different calcium compounds, including calcium carbonate, calcium citrate, and calcium phosphate. The important aspect of these compounds for nutritional value is the amount of elemental calcium, which is the actual amount of calcium in the supplement.*

◆◆◆

Howard Rusk and Rehabilitative Medicine

In the early 20th century, people with disabilities were generally cared for only by surgeons—who tried to "fix" them with operations but didn't give much thought to their lives afterward. It wasn't until after World War II that a former military doctor named Howard Rusk (1901–1989) convinced the nation that disabled people could be taught to improve their conditions and contribute meaningfully to society.

Rusk is known today as the father of comprehensive rehabilitative medicine. His ideas were largely shaped by two major events that occurred during his early medical career: the polio epidemic in the United States and World War II, both of which left behind large numbers of young, seriously handicapped people. An internist from St. Louis, Rusk enlisted in the army and was put in charge of medical services at the Jefferson barracks in Missouri. He quickly realized that his injured or disabled patients seemed to improve faster if they were challenged physically and intellectually, so he began designing activities to keep them busy and get them back on their feet. Increasingly, he became interested in soldiers who had become permanently disabled.

Soon Rusk was put in charge of rehabilitation programs at all air force hospitals. In 1943, he opened a special convalescent center in Pawling, New York, dedicated to the rehabilitation of servicemen, including concepts of physical, psychological, and vocational services. The program was so successful that it quickly ran out of space and was transferred to Long Island—and within 3 years, Rusk had introduced similar programs at 12 more air force medical centers. In the next few years, President Harry S. Truman (1884–1972) made rehabilitation standard policy throughout all armed services branches.

After the war, Rusk joined the faculty of New York University School of Medicine and founded what is now a world-renowned rehabilitation facility. He was concerned with "what happens to severely disabled people after the stitches are out and the fever is down," he said in a 1982 interview. His practice of treating the whole person and not just the injury or disability earned him the nickname "Dr. Live-Again."

ADDITIONAL FACTS

1. *Rusk's many celebrity patients included Joseph P. Kennedy (1888–1969), the U.S. Ambassador to Great Britain and father of President John F. Kennedy (1917–1963), Supreme Court Justice William O. Douglas (1898–1980), and the baseball player Roy Campanella (1921–1993), who were treated at the Rusk Institute of the New York University Medical Center, the first institute for rehabilitation medicine in the world.*

2. *From 1946 to 1969, Rusk was a columnist and part-time associate editor for the* New York Times *and wrote weekly about public health and disability issues.*

3. *Howard Rusk Jr. succeeded his father in 1982 as president and chief executive officer of the World Rehabilitation Fund. The fund has helped train more than 6,000 doctors and specialists in more than 150 countries and helped provide more than 4 million people with artificial limbs and braces.*

◆◆◆

Down Syndrome

The British physician John Langdon Down (1828–1896) was a man far ahead of his time. Not only did he argue for the higher education of women, but he was also passionate about the humane treatment of the mentally handicapped. In fact, Down went on to become the medical superintendent of a mental institution in Surrey. While there, he described the physical features of a "mongoloid" disorder, which included mental retardation, flattened facial features, upward-slanting eyes, a small head, and unusually shaped ears. This condition went on to be named, in his honor, Down syndrome.

Even though Down first identified the condition in 1866, the genetic cause was not discovered until nearly a century later. In 1951, a French geneticist named Jérôme-Jean-Louis-Marie Lejeune (1926–1994) found that people with the disorder had an extra copy of chromosome 21.

Today, researchers know there are three ways for a child to wind up with that extra chromosome. In about 90 percent of Down syndrome cases, the sperm or egg cell experiences abnormal division, resulting in three copies of chromosome 21—called trisomy 21—in every cell in the body. With mosaic Down syndrome, the cells experience abnormal division after fertilization; these children have some cells with the extra chromosome 21, but not all. The last, and most uncommon, form occurs when part of chromosome 21 becomes attached to another chromosome. This form is called translocation Down syndrome.

Children with Down syndrome suffer from mental retardation, as well as a heightened risk of heart defects, leukemia, weakened immune systems, and dementia. Modern science and earlier intervention have increased the average life span of people with Down syndrome dramatically. In the early 20th century, most babies with the condition didn't live past age 10. Today, however, people with Down syndrome frequently live to age 50 and beyond.

ADDITIONAL FACTS

1. *Mothers who give birth at an older age are more likely to have children with Down syndrome. By age 45, the risk increases to 1 in 30.*

2. *Blood tests and ultrasounds can calculate the risk that a baby in the womb has Down syndrome.*

3. *Modern prenatal diagnostic testing with chorionic villus sampling (taking a tiny piece of placenta) or amniocentesis (using a needle to remove a teaspoon of fluid from around the baby in the uterus) can accurately detect Down syndrome.*

✦✦✦

Ulcer Disease

Even though other scientists called him crazy, the Australian researcher Barry J. Marshall (1951–) was convinced that the bacterium *Heliocobacter pylori* led to peptic ulcer disease. At the time, experts believed that the condition, which causes open sores to develop in the stomach, small intestine, or esophageal lining, was caused only by excess stomach acid. To prove his hypothesis, Marshall drank a solution of the bacteria, much to his assistant's horror. Sure enough, he began to show symptoms of ulcers—vomiting, fatigue, and weight loss—after a week, and tests revealed ulcers. Marshall recovered completely and went on to win a Nobel Prize in 1995 for his discovery.

Today, researchers estimate that roughly 85 percent of ulcer disease cases are caused by *H. pylori*, a spiral-shaped bacteria that infects about half of the US population. For most people, it doesn't cause any problems. But in some, it can damage the mucous lining in the digestive system, producing inflammation and, eventually, an ulcer or lesion. Because there's no mucus to protect the stomach lining from hydrochloric acid, eating a meal can lead to intense gastrointestinal pain that can last anywhere from a few minutes to many hours. The bouts of pain often flare up at night and every few days or weeks.

Besides *H. pylori*, there are a few other reasons people can develop ulcers. Regularly using painkillers called nonsteroidal anti-inflammatory drugs (NSAIDs), such as aspirin and ibuprofen, can irritate and inflame the lining of the stomach and small intestine. Since smoking and alcohol consumption increase the amount of stomach acid produced, these habits can also lead to ulcer disease. But, contrary to popular belief, stress and spicy foods aren't culprits—although they can aggravate symptoms and delay healing.

Ulcer disease is diagnosed with an x-ray or an endoscopy, in which a tiny camera is inserted through the throat to examine the stomach lining. Blood and stool tests can determine whether *H. pylori* is the culprit; worldwide, the pesky bacterium accounts for about 85 percent of cases. Antibiotics can remedy the situation. Other medications, including acid-blocking drugs, over-the-counter antacids, and cytoprotective agents (such as Pepto-Bismol), can help relieve symptoms.

ADDITIONAL FACTS

1. *To protect the stomach lining, it's best to take aspirin and other NSAIDs with food.*

2. *Stomach cancer and other conditions that increase the production of stomach acid, such as Zollinger-Ellison syndrome, are rare causes of peptic ulcers.*

✦✦✦

DHA and Omega-3 Fatty Acids

The term *healthy fat* may sound too good to be true, but that's exactly what docosahexaenoic acid (DHA) and other omega-3 fatty acids are. They are monounsaturated, which means they are liquid at room temperature—think oil instead of butter. (The other healthy fats are polyunsaturated fats, such as olive oil.)

DHA is a long-chain omega-3 that is naturally present in fatty fish such as mackerel, salmon, sardines, trout, and tuna. In the human body, DHA is found primarily in the brain and eyes, and it is important for development of these organs. Adults with the highest levels of DHA are up to 47 percent less likely to develop dementia than those with lower levels of the substance, according to studies, and the fatty acids also help the development of visual and cognitive abilities in infants.

Another type of long-chain omega-3, eicosapentaenoic acid (EPA), also has numerous health benefits. Together, DHA and EPA have been shown to lower the LDL ("bad") cholesterol level, heart rate, and blood pressure and boost HDL ("good") cholesterol. Studies show that about 500 milligrams a day of DHA and EPA—the amount you'd get from eating about 8 ounces of fatty fish a week—is enough to produce benefits in an adult.

The American Heart Association recommends that all adults eat fish at least twice a week. And for fetal and infant brain and tissue development, the European Commission advises that all pregnant and breastfeeding women consume an average of at least 200 milligrams of DHA a day. (Guidelines and expert recommendations in the United States have flip-flopped in recent years because of concerns over mercury poisoning during pregnancy. According to the Food and Drug Administration, pregnant women should not eat king mackerel, shark, swordfish, or tilefish and should limit albacore tuna to 6 ounces per week.) For those who choose not to eat fish, both fish oil and algal oil supplements are good sources of DHA. Certain foods and beverages are also now available in omega-3-fortified versions.

ADDITIONAL FACTS

1. *A shorter-chain omega-3 called alpha-linolenic acid (ALA) is found in plant foods such as flaxseeds, walnuts, and canola oil. The human body can convert ALA into DHA in very small amounts, but it's important to consume both kinds directly.*

2. *A 2008 study found that farmed tilapia, a popular fish in the United States, has low levels of omega-3s and high levels of unhealthy omega-6 fatty acids because of the inexpensive, unhealthy food the fish have been fed.*

3. *Breast milk contains DHA and is the preferred source for infant nutrition. Babies who are not breastfed should receive a formula containing DHA and arachidonic acid, another healthy fat.*

❖❖❖

Huntington's Disease

In 1872, the American doctor George Huntington documented a genetic disorder that caused patients to have incessant jerky, involuntary movements. It came to be known as Huntington's chorea—a Greek word meaning "dance"—or Huntington's disease (HD). The disorder appears to cause a dramatic accumulation of cholesterol in the brain, disrupting the network of brain cells that controls motor and cognitive skills.

Symptoms of HD usually develop in middle age and include uncontrolled movements, clumsiness, mood swings and irritability, and trouble remembering new things. Concentration becomes increasingly difficult, and people with HD may have trouble feeding themselves or swallowing.

The rate of progression varies, although those who develop symptoms at a younger age often have more aggressive cases. Young people who develop HD may experience seizures or muscle rigidity and tremors that mimic Parkinson's disease. Most people live about 10 to 30 years after signs of HD first appear, and they usually die as a result of a complication such as an infection or a fall.

HD is an autosomal dominant disorder, meaning that a single copy of the defective gene, from either parent, will produce the disease. In other words, a parent who is a carrier of the HD gene has a 50 percent chance of passing it on to his or her offspring.

Doctors use a genetic blood test, along with brain scans and family history, to diagnose HD. Anyone who has a parent with HD can choose to take this test, even if they have no symptoms, to determine whether they carry the defective gene—although some people in this situation decide they would rather not know. In 1 to 3 percent of HD cases, however, no family history can be found.

There is no cure for HD, but tranquilizers and antipsychotic drugs can help prevent sudden movements and violent outbursts. Antidepressants and lithium may also be prescribed to control obsessive-compulsive rituals and extreme mood swings. Regular exercise keeps muscles stronger and more flexible, and proper nutrition is important: People with HD may burn as many as 5,000 calories a day and may need extra vitamins and supplements.

ADDITIONAL FACTS

1. *The number of Americans who have Huntington's disease is estimated at 30,000.*

2. *Although the drug is not specifically approved for this use, some doctors administer botulinum toxin injections in certain areas, such as the jaw, to relieve involuntary muscle clenching.*

3. *Couples at risk of passing the HD gene on to their children may consider in vitro fertilization with preimplantation screening, in which embryos are checked for the gene mutation before they're implanted in the woman's uterus.*

❖❖❖

Cervical Cancer

Where the uterus tapers into the vagina, there is a 1½- to 2-inch stretch called the cervix. This area is highly vulnerable to changes caused by human papillomavirus (HPV), which can lead to cervical cancer. Every year, more than 11,000 women in the United States develop this devastating disease—and some 3,000 die of it.

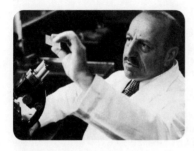

The number one weapon in the fight against cervical cancer is the Pap test. Invented by the physician George Papanicolaou (1883–1962) in 1942, the test involves scraping cells off the cervix with a small brush or spatula. The sample is then studied by a pathologist, who looks for any abnormal cells that may be precancerous. If such cells are spotted, a gynecologist can perform a biopsy to check for cancer and remove the area before it has a chance to develop into a tumor. Because it takes several years for cells to turn cancerous, most cases of HPV are diagnosed and caught before they take a troublesome turn. In fact, since the advent of the Pap test, cervical cancer has fallen from being the most prevalent type of gynecological cancer to the third most common (behind ovarian and uterine cancers).

Pap tests, however, are only about 80 percent accurate, which is why doctors order repeat screenings for at-risk patients. Current techniques can search for HPV in Pap tests by identifying the presence of the HPV type's DNA with very high accuracy. Symptoms of cervical cancer include bloody vaginal discharge with an unpleasant odor, vaginal bleeding, and pelvic pain. Treatments include chemotherapy, radiation, and surgery, among others.

ADDITIONAL FACTS

1. *Smoking, having multiple sex partners, using birth control for many years, having one's first intercourse at an early age, and having given birth to more than five children all are associated with an elevated risk of cervical cancer.*

2. *The time it takes for mildly abnormal cells detected with a Pap test to develop into invasive cancer is usually 10 years or more.*

◆◆◆

Vitamin B$_{12}$

Vitamin B$_{12}$ is a nutrient that your body requires for optimal health. It's needed to make red blood cells, to help your nervous system work properly, and to synthesize DNA, which is the genetic material in all your cells. Vitamin B$_{12}$ is found in meat and dairy products.

A deficiency of this vitamin is extremely rare, since the body can store several years' worth. People who are at risk for vitamin B$_{12}$ deficiency include the elderly, vegetarians who do not eat meat or dairy products, and people who have trouble absorbing vitamin B$_{12}$ from their stomachs or small intestines. Those who have trouble absorbing vitamin B$_{12}$ include people with a disease called pernicious anemia, people who use medicine for heartburn and ulcers over the long term, and people who have had surgery on their stomachs or intestines.

If your vitamin B$_{12}$ level is slightly low, you probably will not have any symptoms. But if your level of the vitamin becomes significantly low, you may develop anemia, dementia, depression, or problems with your nervous system. People who have a low level of vitamin B$_{12}$ and a high level of homocysteine, an amino acid in the blood, may have a greater risk of heart disease and stroke.

If your doctor diagnoses you with low vitamin B$_{12}$, you will need to take special B$_{12}$ pills, because over-the-counter multivitamins do not contain enough of this vitamin for people who are deficient in it. There is also a vitamin B$_{12}$ shot, which is usually given every 1 or 2 days for 2 weeks, then once a month thereafter.

ADDITIONAL FACTS

1. *Elderly people with low levels of vitamin B$_{12}$ may have an increased risk of brain atrophy, or shrinkage, which is associated with Alzheimer's disease and decreased cognitive function.*

2. *To take in a day's supply of vitamin B$_{12}$, you could eat one chicken breast, one hard-boiled egg, and 1 cup of plain low-fat yogurt, or have 1 cup of milk and 1 cup of bran cereal.*

3. *Some people with vitamin B$_{12}$ deficiency experience burning sensations in their hands and feet as the first symptoms. This is called peripheral neuropathy and may have other causes as well.*

◆◆◆

Sulfa Drugs and World War II

Throughout most of history, military forces during times of war have traditionally lost more men to sickness, disease, and infection than to battlefield action. So during World War II, the treatment of wounds and the containment of disease were top priorities of the US Army and Navy. Even though penicillin had been developed by this time, the miracle drug had not gone into widespread production. Instead, physicians relied on the only antibiotics available: the recently discovered sulfa drugs.

When the United State entered the war in 1941, sulfanilamide was the drug of choice for meningitis within the US Army. Sulfa drugs were also used to treat diarrhea and dysentery; fever; and wounds, burns, and related infections.

By 1943, however, the US Navy was fighting a losing battle against crowding, poor living conditions, and a rapid spread of *Streptococcus* bacteria that caused scarlet fever and strep throat. The navy cleaned and disinfected barracks, isolated people who were thought to be carriers, and moved training camps away from areas of high incidence.

When these methods failed to reduce the virus's spread, the navy decided on a mass chemoprophylaxis (the act of administering medication in hopes of preventing disease spread) with sulfa drugs. Recruits at five naval training centers received small daily doses of sulfadiazine, while others at the same centers were observed as control subjects. In as little as 1 week, the illness rate in the medicated groups had dropped dramatically—to just 15 percent of the control group's rate at one center. Within 3 months, the navy opened up the treatment to all recruits at the test centers and expanded the program to three additional facilities.

The program was a striking success, saving the navy an estimated 1 million man days and between $50 million and $100 million in 1944 dollars. In less than a year, however, bacteria had become resistant to the drugs, and in the last months of the war, the navy abandoned its daily medication program. Safer antibiotics, including penicillin, became available soon after, and the use of sulfa drugs declined after the war.

ADDITIONAL FACTS

1. *On December 5, 1941, the New York City surgeon John Moorhead gave a lecture in Honolulu advising the treatment of wartime wounds with sulfa drugs. Two days later, Pearl Harbor was attacked, and Moorhead and members of his audience put these guidelines into practice caring for the injured.*

2. *Sulfa drugs helped bring the US military death rate from meningitis down to a mere 4 percent in World War II, compared with 31 percent in World War I.*

3. *Between December 1943 and June 1944, about 1 million men participated in the sulfa drug chemoprophylaxis program, 600,000 as recipients and 400,000 as controls.*

✦✦✦

Turner Syndrome

Most people receive one sex chromosome, an X or Y, from each parent. Two X chromosomes signifies a female. But in about 1 in 2,000 to 2,500 births, a baby girl has a missing or partially missing X chromosome. This condition is known as Turner syndrome.

Turner syndrome is typically diagnosed at an early age. Because of the missing genes, many girls affected by the disorder have physical abnormalities. They are usually short in stature (on average, their height doesn't exceed 4 feet 8 inches) and may also have drooping or lazy eyes, low-set ears, a receding lower jaw, a webbed neck, a broad chest, and flat feet. At birth, a girl with Turner syndrome also tends to have swollen hands and feet. If a physician suspects the disorder, he or she will conduct a karyotype—a snapshot of a person's complete chromosomal lineup—to screen for the condition.

Besides the visible symptoms, females with Turner syndrome are affected in other ways, as well. Many are born without fully functioning ovaries. Without these female reproductive organs, their bodies produce insufficient amounts of estrogen. As a result, most girls with Turner syndrome fail to undergo many of the changes associated with puberty, such as developing breasts or menstruating. What's more, they're also at greater risk for heart defects, kidney problems, hypothyroidism, and scoliosis.

Once a girl is diagnosed with Turner syndrome, she typically requires frequent monitoring by a physician. Growth hormones and estrogen therapy can help her develop properly. Because hearing loss is common among these children, a hearing aid may also be necessary.

ADDITIONAL FACTS

1. *Turner syndrome is named after the American endocrinologist Henry Turner (1892–1970). He first noted the symptoms of the condition in 1938.*

2. *Only girls can have Turner syndrome.*

♦♦♦

Colitis

Ulcerative colitis is a chronic disease that causes the linings of the colon and rectum to become inflamed and pocked with painful sores, or ulcers. Affecting some half-million Americans, the condition causes flare-ups of bloody diarrhea, fever, and abdominal pain that can last a few days or weeks. Colitis and Crohn's disease (a similar condition that can affect any area of the gastrointestinal tract, including the small intestine) are the two main types of inflammatory bowel disease.

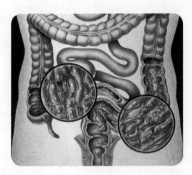

Although experts aren't exactly sure what causes colitis, one theory is that it's an autoimmune disease. This means that a person's own immune system mistakes foods and healthy bacteria for harmful foreign invaders. As a result, white blood cells attack the large intestine, leading to inflammation and ulcers. Colitis may also have a hereditary link; research shows that 20 percent of those with the ailment have a close relative with either colitis or Crohn's disease.

Most sufferers develop colitis between the ages of 15 and 30, although a small percentage have their first attack in their fifties or sixties. The severity of the disease varies widely: Some people may experience only mild symptoms in flare-ups that occur every several months or even years, while others may suffer long-term severe effects, such as weight loss, anemia, and associated arthritis, as well as eye or skin inflammation, with more frequent and acute attacks. Children can experience stunted growth as a result of the condition.

Fortunately, treatment with drugs is often successful. Antibiotics and steroids may help, as can a handful of medications that short-circuit or control inflammation. In more severe cases, surgical removal of part of the colon may be required.

ADDITIONAL FACTS

1. *Ulcerative colitis is more common among Caucasian people and those of Jewish descent.*

2. *Having the condition raises the risk of colon cancer.*

◆◆◆

Pritikin Program

The Pritikin Program for diet and exercise was created by Nathan Pritikin (1915–1985), a diet guru who gained popularity in the 1970s. Pritikin often referred to his program as "mankind's original meal plan" and emphasized the importance of fruits, vegetables, whole grains, and seafood.

During World War II, Pritikin—an inventor at the time—saw documents showing that European deaths from heart disease and diabetes had dropped dramatically during the war. Intrigued, he began following the work of a cardiologist who was studying the benefits of a low-cholesterol, low-fat diet (which mimicked the wartime food rations on which many Europeans survived) on seriously ill heart attack patients. Things got personal when Pritikin himself visited this cardiologist. Pritikin's cholesterol level was more than 300 milligrams per deciliter, and a stress electrocardiogram showed that his arteries were closing up quickly. He was diagnosed with coronary heart disease at age 41.

At the time, the standard prescription for heart disease patients was to stop exercising or doing anything strenuous. But Pritikin was determined to get healthy. He became a vegetarian and also started running 3 to 4 miles a day. Within 4 years, his cholesterol was down to 120 and signs of his heart disease had disappeared. Over the next 25 years, Pritikin participated in more than 100 published studies detailing the benefits of his diet and exercise program. He wrote several books, and in 1975 opened the Pritikin Longevity Center—a health resort that focuses on nutrition, exercise, and lifestyle-change education.

The Pritikin eating plan recommends at least five servings of unrefined, complex carbohydrates a day, at least five vegetable and four fruit servings, two calcium-rich foods, and no more than one serving of animal protein—preferably fish, shellfish, or lean poultry. When the plan is followed strictly, fat accounts for just 10 percent of the diet. The program also includes a daily exercise regimen that combines cardiovascular conditioning (such as brisk walking), strength training, and stretching.

ADDITIONAL FACTS

1. *To date, nine books have been published on the Pritikin Program, including three by Nathan's son Robert Pritikin. In* The Pritikin Principle, *Robert tweaks his father's message and focuses on calorie density—the number of calories per pound in a specific food.*

2. *In 1977, the television program* 60 Minutes *followed three men with severe heart disease as they attended 1-month programs at the Pritikin Longevity Center. All three men improved dramatically, regained much of their energy, experienced less chest pain, and were able to stop taking most of their medications.*

3. *When Nathan Pritikin died in 1985 from complications related to leukemia, the results of his autopsy were published in the* New England Journal of Medicine. *They showed that his arteries were free of any sign of heart disease—a remarkable phenomenon for a man 69 years old, the pathologist wrote.*

◆◆◆

Muscular Dystrophy

There are more than 30 types of muscular dystrophy (MD), a group of diseases in which a defective gene causes weakness and degeneration of skeletal muscles. MD can strike at any age, can progress slowly or quickly, and can vary in severity from mildly disabling to fatal.

The most common form of muscular dystrophy, Duchenne MD, is caused by a deficiency of dystrophin, a protein that helps maintain muscle. This version strikes mainly boys between the ages of 3 and 5 and progresses rapidly. Most victims can't walk by age 12 and later need a respirator to breathe. Early warning signs in children include frequent falls, large calf muscles, difficulty running and jumping, and a tendency to walk on the toes or balls of the feet. A less severe form of MD is called Becker MD. Both disorders are passed from mother to son by way of a defective gene on the X chromosome, which a boy inherits from his mother. Girls get another X from their fathers, which protects them from the disease.

Other forms include facioscapulohumeral MD, which begins in the teenage years and causes weakness of the face, arm, and leg muscles; and myotonic MD, the disorder's most common adult form, characterized by cataracts, heart problems, prolonged muscle spasms, and gaunt facial features.

Symptoms of MD include muscle weakness, an apparent lack of coordination, and progressive crippling as muscles around the joints become stiff and lose mobility. In the late stages of MD, fat and connective tissues completely replace muscle fibers.

MD can be diagnosed with a blood test for creatine kinase, an enzyme released by damaged muscles. Electrical impulse tests, ultrasound, and muscle biopsy may also be used to test for damage and confirm the diagnosis.

There is no way to stop or reverse MD, but physical therapy and orthopedic appliances can make living with MD less debilitating. Doctors can perform corrective surgery to relieve joint pain, and they may prescribe drugs such as corticosteroids, anticonvulsants, immunosuppressants, and antibiotics to delay cell damage and fight infection. Braces can provide support for weakened muscles, although canes, walkers, or wheelchairs may be necessary in advanced cases.

ADDITIONAL FACTS

1. *Because respiratory infections may become a problem in later stages of MD, patients should be vaccinated against pneumonia and get a flu shot every year.*

2. *The Duchenne and Becker forms of MD rarely occur in women—but women who have one X chromosome with the defective gene for these disorders are carriers and sometimes develop heart muscle problems and mild muscle weakness.*

3. *The first Muscular Dystrophy Association Labor Day Telethon—now an annual event hosted by Jerry Lewis (1926–) and benefiting "Jerry's Kids"—was broadcast in 1966. It was the first televised fundraising event of its kind to raise more than $1 million.*

❖ ❖ ❖

Birth Control

Throughout time, people have used a wide assortment of concoctions and devices to fend off pregnancy. Ancient Egyptian women applied a mixture of crocodile dung, honey, and sodium carbonate to their vaginas, while the infamous Italian lover Casanova (1725–1798) used condoms made of linen and sheep intestines. Even as late as the 1960s, the disinfectant Lysol was popular among women as a spermicide. Fortunately, science has made major progress when it comes to birth control.

Today, there are a number of different forms of contraception, although no form is 100 percent foolproof. They fall into several groups: The first, called barrier methods, block sperm from entering the uterus. Condoms, cervical caps, sponges, and diaphragms all fall into this category. These contraceptives are affordable, attainable, and convenient, but they also have a higher failure rate: In 11 percent of couples using the male condom, for instance, the woman becomes pregnant.

The second common birth control form is hormonal; these medications release the female sex hormones estrogen and progestin in the woman's body to prevent the ovaries from releasing an egg. The first birth control pill was developed by the medical researchers Gregory Pincus (1903–1967) and John Rock (1890–1984) in 1957. Ten years later, some 12.5 million women worldwide were taking the once-a-day pill.

Other methods of hormonal contraception include the birth control patch (applied weekly), the vaginal contraceptive ring (inserted monthly), and hormonal shots and implants (administered every month to 5 years). Hormonal forms are effective—the Pill, when used correctly, is 99 percent successful—but they do not protect against sexually transmitted diseases, as condoms do. Intrauterine devices (IUDs) are another very effective contraceptive strategy; once inserted, they remain 95 to 97 percent effective for up to 10 years. Lastly, some people may opt for sterilization—a permanent surgical procedure. Women can have their fallopian tubes "tied," while men can have a vasectomy, in which the vas deferens tubes are cut.

ADDITIONAL FACTS

1. *Margaret Sanger (1883–1966), a birth control activist in the 1950s, was inspired to advocate for birth control by her mother, who died at age 50 after bearing 11 children.*

2. *In 1873, the US government passed a law, written by the antiobscenity crusader Anthony Comstock (1844–1915), that made all forms of contraception illegal. The law was struck down in 1965.*

3. *By federal law, sterilization procedures require a counseling session, followed by a 30-day wait and a second written consent.*

✦✦✦

Vitamin A

Vitamin A is an essential nutrient for good health. Your body needs this vitamin to develop and maintain healthy teeth, skin, skeletal and soft tissues, and mucous membranes. Vitamin A creates the pigments in the retina of the eye and is needed for good vision. It may also be critical to breastfeeding and reproduction. It's recommended that males ages 14 and older take in 900 micrograms of vitamin A daily and that females ages 14 and older get 700 micrograms a day.

You can obtain vitamin A by eating meat, kidneys, liver, codfish, halibut, fish oil, eggs, cheese, cream, whole milk, and some fortified foods. However, most of these foods are high in saturated fat and cholesterol. Your body can also produce vitamin A when you eat carotenoids, which are dark-colored dyes found in plant foods. One of the most common carotenoids is beta-carotene, which is found in apricots, broccoli, cantaloupe, carrots, pink grapefruit, pumpkin, spinach, sweet potatoes, winter squash, and most dark green, leafy vegetables. These sources of beta-carotene do not have fat or cholesterol and are healthier options for ensuring that you take in adequate amounts of vitamin A.

The best way to get your daily requirement of vitamin A is to eat a balanced diet. If you are vitamin A deficient, you're more susceptible to infectious diseases and vision problems. But if you consume too much vitamin A, you can also become sick.

Vitamin A poisoning occurs when an adult takes several hundred thousand international units of the vitamin. Large doses of vitamin A taken during pregnancy can cause birth defects, and babies and children can become sick after taking smaller doses of vitamin A or products that contain it, such as retinol. Eating too many foods that contain beta-carotene, such as carrots, can temporarily turn your skin yellow or orange.

ADDITIONAL FACTS

1. *Women who are pregnant or breastfeeding should check with their doctors about taking vitamin A.*

2. *Children need different daily amounts of vitamin A based on their ages.*

3. *Retinoids are derivatives of vitamin A and are used to treat skin disorders such as acne.*

◆◆◆

Organ Transplants

The first organs to be successfully transplanted were kidneys, in the early 1950s. Since then, doctors have learned to safely transplant hearts, lungs, and other organs, improving, extending, and saving countless lives.

Early efforts to transplant human organs ended in failure because the body rejected the new, transplanted tissue. Only when scientists realized that identical twins could receive transplants without risk of rejection was the first successful transplant performed. In 1954, the surgeon Joseph Murray (1919–) carried out the first successful kidney transplant on a pair of 23-year-old identical twins at Brigham and Women's Hospital in Boston. Whether a transplant is likely to succeed depends on the similarity of donor and recipient, which is measurable by their sharing of immune markers called human leukocyte antigens (HLAs). A perfect match is six out of six of the major HLA markers, as are found in identical twins.

But few people have identical twins. After Murray proved the feasibility of transplants, scientists spent the next several decades searching for a way to make the surgery possible for nontwins—and even for people who weren't related at all. To prevent the body from rejecting the new organ, researchers developed a powerful drug in the 1960s called cyclosporine, which suppressed the immune system. At first, immune-suppressing drugs were extremely dangerous, and many patients died shortly after surgery. By the 1980s, however, medications had improved and survival rates increased. Doctors have now successfully transplanted most body parts, including hands and, in 2005, a face for a French woman who had been mauled by dogs. Face transplants remain a controversial procedure because of the ethical and identity issues involved.

For conditions such as cirrhosis (a disease of the liver) and kidney failure, patients can receive organs from a living donor, often a friend or relative. Heart and lung transplants are usually considered only as last resorts and must come from recently deceased victims whose organs have been kept alive on artificial life support. (It is possible to transplant a lung from a living donor, but it's very risky and very rare.) Today, the demand for organs has far surpassed the supply of donated organs available. In the United States, patients must go on a waiting list as part of the Organ Procurement and Transplantation Network, a division of the US Department of Health and Human Services.

ADDITIONAL FACTS

1. *Since 1982, more than 400,000 people in the United States have received new kidneys, hearts, livers, lungs, pancreases, or intestines.*

2. *Doctors at Massachusetts General Hospital in Boston are currently studying ways to use pig organs for human transplants.*

3. *A kidney transplant in 1950 allowed a woman to live for 5 more years, even though her body rejected the organ after only a few months. The 1954 operation is considered the first successful transplant, however, because that kidney functioned properly for at least a year.*

✦✦✦

Klinefelter's Syndrome

Klinefelter's syndrome is one of the most common sex chromosome disorders among males, affecting up to 1 in 500 births. A completely random occurrence, the condition arises when a boy inherits an extra X chromosome from one of his parents. Instead of the typical XY, boys with Klinefelter's syndrome have an XXY set.

The condition was first identified in 1942 by the physician Henry Klinefelter of Massachusetts General Hospital in Boston. He published a report on nine men with enlarged breasts, small testes, sparse facial and body hair, and an inability to produce sperm. These symptoms are the result of the low testosterone levels that are associated with Klinefelter's syndrome.

Most cases of Klinefelter's aren't diagnosed until later in life. Babies show few symptoms, although they tend to take longer to sit up and crawl than other infants. During puberty, they may have smaller testicles, less body hair, and lower energy levels than other boys their age. Men with Klinefelter's syndrome often are unable to father children, because they don't produce a normal amount of sperm. They also have an increased risk of varicose veins, osteoporosis, and abdominal fat.

To diagnose the disorder, physicians perform hormone testing and a chromosome analysis, or karyotype. Doctors often recommend testosterone treatment during puberty and, for some men, surgical removal of excess breast tissue.

ADDITIONAL FACTS

1. *Some men with Klinefelter's syndrome who wish to father children can opt for a treatment known as testicular sperm extraction, in which sperm are removed from the testicles and injected directly into the egg.*

2. *People affected by the condition have a 25 percent chance of having mental retardation.*

◆◆◆

Hepatitis

Hepatitis is an inflammation of the liver, the body's second-largest organ (after the skin), which plays an important role in metabolism and detoxification. The illness is most often caused by a viral infection, but drugs, alcohol, toxic chemicals, and physical trauma can also be to blame. Currently, there are seven known types of hepatitis viruses, labeled from A to G. Hepatitis A, E, and F are transmitted when people consume contaminated food or water, while B, C, D, and G are spread through blood or other bodily fluids.

Of these seven viruses, A, B, and C are the most common, affecting 5 to 10 percent of Americans. Hepatitis A (HVA) is found in fecal matter and is usually spread through drinking contaminated water, eating raw shellfish, or consuming food made by someone who didn't wash his or her hands after using the restroom. HVA usually lasts for 4 to 6 weeks, and usually there's no permanent damage. Hepatitis B (HVB) and hepatitis C (HVC) most often are spread through sexual contact and sharing contaminated hypodermic needles. Both of these viruses can lead to chronic hepatitis, long-term inflammation that can lead to permanent liver damage, cirrhosis, and even liver cancer. In fact, HVC is the number one cause of liver transplants in the United States. Vaccines are available for HVA and HVB. Most children and adults are administered HVB vaccines, while the HVA vaccine is recommended for people who are traveling to countries with a prevalence of hepatitis, have other forms of liver disease, or have high-risk careers, such as those in health care.

But no matter which virus is involved, the symptoms of hepatitis are the same: vomiting, abdominal pain, fever, fatigue, and loss of appetite, lasting anywhere from a few days to a few weeks. If the illness is not treated promptly, chemicals in the body that are normally secreted by the liver can lead to jaundice (a yellowing of the skin and eyes), a bitter taste in the mouth, bad breath, and dark urine. More severe cases can evolve into fulminant hepatitis, a dangerous form of the disease that develops quickly and can cause severe liver failure and impaired kidney function.

ADDITIONAL FACTS

1. *The word* hepatitis *is derived from the word* hepar *("liver") and the suffix* -itis *("inflammation").*

2. *The liver weighs about 3 pounds in adults.*

3. *Even tiny amounts of the hepatitis A virus can transmit the disease.*

✦✦✦

SAMe

Pronounced "sammy," SAMe is a chemical that is sold as a dietary supplement (and, in Europe, as a prescription medication) and has been studied extensively as a possible treatment for osteoarthritis and depression. Short for S-adenosyl methionine, SAMe is produced naturally, and small amounts are found in virtually every part of the body,

SAMe plays a role in the immune system and helps produce and break down mood-controlling brain chemicals such as serotonin, melatonin, and dopamine. It also participates in making cartilage, a tough tissue that connects to the bones, lines the joints, and helps provide structure to the body.

However, the body produces less SAMe as it ages, and scientists believe that taking a supplement of the chemical may help fight the symptoms of certain conditions and diseases. It may help alleviate pain from osteoarthritis. Preliminary research also suggests that SAMe also has potential for treating mild to moderate depression and seems to begin working more quickly and just as effectively as antidepressant medications without the side effects frequently associated with these drugs, such as headaches, sleeplessness, and sexual dysfunction. It is not clear how SAMe relieves depression, so doctors advise against taking it at the same time as antidepressants. More research about its safety and effectiveness, especially over long periods of time, is needed.

SAMe is most widely available as capsules, although injections have also been studied in clinical trials. It appears safe in doses of up to 1,600 milligrams a day, for up to 6 weeks. Side effects may include nausea, skin rashes, dry mouth, or a hot sensation or itchiness of the ear. This supplement may lower blood sugar levels, and patients with diabetes or hypoglycemia should use SAMe with caution.

ADDITIONAL FACTS

1. *Early studies suggest that SAMe may also be helpful in treating attention-deficit/hyperactivity disorder, fibromyalgia, and cholestasis—a buildup of bile in the liver.*

2. *SAMe also occurs in plants and other animals.*

3. *Although SAMe is often marketed as a "natural" cure for depression and arthritis, it is in fact a synthetic version of a chemical made in the body. Some experts believe that this makes it a drug, not a supplement, and that it should be regulated as a drug.*

◆ ◆ ◆

Amyotrophic Lateral Sclerosis

New York Yankee Lou Gehrig (1903–1941) is remembered for his major league baseball records and his consecutive game streak in the 1920s and '30s—and for his tearful retirement at age 36, when he was diagnosed with the fatal disease that now bears his name. Amyotrophic lateral sclerosis (ALS), often referred to as Lou Gehrig's disease, causes motor neurons in the brain and spinal cord to degenerate, leading to muscle weakness, coordination problems, and, eventually, total paralysis and death. Throughout the progress of the disease, mental function is not affected.

ALS attacks voluntary motor muscles, including those used for walking, talking, gesturing, and breathing. (Breathing is both involuntary and voluntary, because you *can* stop breathing—at least temporarily—on cue.) As neurons die, these muscles waste away: Limbs begin to look thinner, and people with ALS may experience weakness, twitching, cramping, slurred speech, and difficulty using their arms and legs. They may trip, drop things, or go through periods of uncontrolled laughter or crying. In more advanced stages, they may need a permanent ventilator in order to breathe.

About 15 new cases of ALS are diagnosed in the United States every day; 60 percent of these individuals are male, and 93 percent are Caucasian. Most people develop symptoms between the ages of 40 and 70 and live for 3 to 5 years after diagnosis—although for some, the disease advances less quickly or, in rare cases, may halt completely. The medication riluzole (Rilutek) can minimize the release of the chemical glutamate, an effect that appears to help slow the illness's progression in some cases. Scientists aren't sure why, but people with ALS have more glutamate in their spinal fluid than healthy people do.

Most cases of ALS are sporadic, meaning they affect people with no family history of the disease. The illness is hard to diagnose; doctors must perform blood tests, x-rays, and electrical nerve stimulation tests, and rule out all other diseases. About 5 to 10 percent of cases appear to run in the person's family, and in 1991, scientists linked this type of ALS to a gene on chromosome 21. Today, a genetic test can determine familial ALS, although diagnosis is still based mainly on symptoms.

ADDITIONAL FACTS

1. *An extremely high incidence of ALS was observed in Guam and the Trust Territories of the Pacific in the 1950s. This subset of the disease bears the name Guamanian ALS.*

2. *Gehrig played 2,130 consecutive games, earning him the nickname the Iron Horse, before his illness forced him into retirement. His farewell speech at Yankee Stadium is among the most famous moments in the history of baseball: before a packed crowd, speaking haltingly into a microphone, the first baseman declared that despite his "bad break," he considered himself "the luckiest man on the face of the earth" because of the support of his fans and the opportunity to play baseball.*

3. *The British theoretical physicist Stephen Hawking (1942–) has remarkably survived several decades with ALS. He was diagnosed at age 21, married and fathered three children after his diagnosis, and has used a computerized voice synthesizer to "speak" ever since he had a breathing device implanted in his throat.*

◆◆◆

Human Immune Deficiency Syndrome

Human immune deficiency syndrome is also known as acquired immune deficiency syndrome (AIDS) and is caused by the human immunodeficiency virus, or HIV. This virus, which affects nearly 40 million people around the globe, attacks the immune system, rendering the body less able to fight off infections, such as pneumonia, as well as certain cancers. In the early stages of HIV, infected people are often free of symptoms and their condition is known as HIV positive without AIDS.

HIV is most frequently spread through sexual intercourse, whether vaginal, anal, or oral. It can also be transmitted through blood transfusions or needle sharing, or passed from a mother to her fetus. Once inside the body, the virus lays siege against white blood cells known as CD4 lymphocytes. Like zombies in a horror film, HIV organisms inject their own DNA into the lymphocytes and destroy them. Eventually, the number of white blood cells—the immune system's first line of defense— drops so severely that the body can no longer effectively fight off viruses and bacteria. This leads to the development of AIDS, a set of life-threatening infections.

Because of the virus's complicated nature, there is no cure for it. Fortunately, however, there are a number of antiretroviral drugs that inhibit the formation of HIV. These medications can extend patients' lives—and improve the quality of their remaining years. In many cases, though, after about 20 years, the body develops a resistance to the drugs, rendering them ineffective.

ADDITIONAL FACTS

1. *HIV was first discovered in the 1980s, shortly after AIDS was identified.*

2. *Using spermicide may increase the likelihood of HIV transmission, because it may cause inflammation in the vagina that allows the virus to enter the body.*

3. *While condoms help protect against HIV, they're not foolproof.*

◆◆◆

Trace Elements

Trace elements are substances that are essential to the human diet but are needed in amounts of less than 100 milligrams per day. They include iron, iodine, copper, manganese, zinc, molybdenum, selenium, and chromium. There are probably others that have not yet been identified.

People in the United States are generally not at risk of having insufficient quantities of these elements. However, trace element deficiencies represent a major problem globally. These deficiencies impair general body function and increase the severity of common infections, such as measles and those that cause diarrhea. They also hamper intellectual growth and adult productivity.

Iron deficiency affects more than 2 billion people globally. It is one of the most common causes of anemia, and iron deficiency in children affects their mental development. We need iron for hemoglobin synthesis and function, for proper functioning of the enzymes required to produce energy, and for the production of collagen, elastin, and neurotransmitters. Iron can be found in meats, poultry, fish, and leafy green vegetables.

Iodine deficiency is another of the most prevalent micronutrient deficiencies worldwide. Fifty million infants annually are born at risk of iodine deficiency, which is the leading cause of preventable mental retardation globally. Found in seafood and iodized salt, iodine is needed for the production of thyroid hormones.

Our bodies need copper to produce hemoglobin and aid in its function; to make collagen, elastin, and neurotransmitters; and to form melanin. We get copper from fruits, nuts, organ meats, and shellfish. We also need manganese as a coenzyme to help produce energy. This mineral is found in nuts and whole grains.

Our bodies require zinc for general immunity and healing, good eyesight, and certain enzyme functions. It is found in whole grains, brewer's yeast, fish, and meats. Molybdenum helps with the detoxification of hazardous substances and is found in beans, leafy green vegetables, milk, organ meats, and whole grains.

Also needed for optimal health is selenium, which is found in broccoli, cabbage, celery, garlic, onions, organ meats, whole grains, and brewer's yeast. And chromium is required for the optimal use of sugar. We get chromium from meats, spices, whole grains, and brewer's yeast.

ADDITIONAL FACTS

1. *A balanced diet usually contains enough of all the trace elements, if it follows USDA's MyPyramid guidelines.*

2. *Iron deficiency occurs in breastfed babies unless they're given supplements, because there is insufficient iron in breast milk.*

✦✦✦

Natural Childbirth

"Natural childbirth" used to be considered the same as normal childbirth, even though in the early 1900s doctors regularly used anesthesia or sedatives to lessen pain and anxiety for mothers-to-be. Beginning at about midcentury, however, relaxation methods and childbirth education changed the way many women chose to have their babies.

The English obstetrician Grantly Dick-Read (1890–1959) first introduced the concept of natural birthing, suggesting in his 1933 book *Natural Childbirth* that fear and tension were the cause of pain during delivery. By getting rid of fear and tension—through such methods as relaxation, hypnotherapy, exercises to improve muscle tone, and better education about the process—women could make giving birth a pain free and more meaningful experience.

Fernand Lamaze (1890–1957) became perhaps the most well known proponent of natural births beginning in 1951. His methods, developed at his clinic in France, emphasized regular, controlled breathing; muscle strengthening techniques before childbirth; and a supportive role for the father. This became known as the Lamaze method, also called psychoprophylaxis. A book about this method, *Thank You, Dr. Lamaze*, helped popularize his theories in the United States. In 1960, the book's author, Marjorie Karmel (d. 1964), cofounded the not-for-profit organization ASPO/Lamaze (now Lamaze International) to spread the teachings of Lamaze and set standards for educators.

Today, Lamaze International promotes personal empowerment for women and childbirth education for both parents or other birth partners. The Lamaze approach includes allowing labor to begin on its own, using massage and aromatherapy for relaxation, applying hot and cold packs to reduce discomfort, utilizing certain positions and pushing techniques during labor and birth, and learning breastfeeding techniques.

ADDITIONAL FACTS

1. *Many of Lamaze's techniques were focused on lessening a woman's perception of pain during childbirth. This approach was partly inspired by the "conditioned reflex" theory of Russian researcher Ivan Pavlov (1849–1936), whose experiments in dogs suggested that seemingly intrinsic responses like pain, hunger, or relaxation could, in fact, be "conditioned" to occur in response to external stimuli.*

2. *In the early 1900s, natural childbirth met opposition from many physicians who felt that it denied the progress made by modern medicine and needlessly returned the birth process to a more primitive state.*

3. *Although Lamaze was originally developed to eliminate the need for medication, mothers today who practice Lamaze methods can still choose to receive an epidural (an anesthetic injection) during delivery.*

✦✦✦

Angelman Syndrome and Prader-Willi Syndrome

Human DNA is made up of 23 pairs of chromosomes: one set from the mother and one set from the father. But sometimes a genetic glitch causes a child to inherit both chromosomes from one parent, an occurrence called uniparental disomy. Angelman and Prader-Willi syndromes are examples of this malfunction on chromosome number 15.

Angelman syndrome occurs when a child's chromosome 15 pair both come from the father. Named after the British physician Harry Angelman (1915–1996), who first described it in 1965, this genetic disorder causes developmental and intellectual delays. Children with Angelman syndrome often have difficulty walking, speaking, and balancing; they also have happy, excitable personalities prone to outbursts of smiling and laughing. Other symptoms include stiff, jerky movements; seizures; and a small head size. It's estimated that this fairly rare condition affects 1 in 20,000 births. Children with Angelman syndrome may require antiseizure medication, as well as physical and behavioral therapy.

The sister syndrome to Angelman is Prader-Willi, in which a child inherits both chromosomes 15 from the mother. This condition is named after the Swiss pediatricians Andrea Prader (1919–2001) and Heinrich Willi (1900–1971), who first wrote about it in 1956. Symptoms include poor muscle tone (infants often feel like loose rag dolls when they're held), underdeveloped sex hormones, and delayed motor development. Children with the condition often have behavioral problems; they tend to be stubborn and can be prone to obsessive-compulsive disorders. Experts believe that Prader-Willi syndrome affects about 1 in 12,000 to 15,000 births.

ADDITIONAL FACTS

1. *Uniparental disomy is a completely random event.*

2. *Physicians initially diagnose Prader-Willi and Angelman syndromes based on behavior and distinctive facial features. They confirm them by ordering a karyotype, a genetic test that reveals all chromosomal sets.*

✦✦✦

Gastroenteritis

A raw oyster. A dirty fork. A sip of stream water during a hike. Each of these may contain one of the many agents that lead to gastroenteritis, an inflammation of the stomach and small intestine. Highly contagious, the "stomach flu" is the second-most-common illness in the United States after the common cold—making tens of millions of people miserable every year. Viruses, bacteria that produce toxins (such as *Staphylococcus* and *Enterococcus*), and even just the toxins in leftovers can trigger it.

So, what viruses cause gastroenteritis? There are two main groups, rotaviruses and noroviruses. They are both highly contagious and are usually spread through consuming contaminated food or drink. Some shellfish may contain a form of the virus, but the majority of the time, the microorganisms are spread when an infected person contaminates food in preparing or sharing it.

Symptoms of gastroenteritis include watery diarrhea, abdominal cramps, nausea, headache, and low-grade fever. They appear 1 to 2 days after infection and last anywhere from 3 to 10 days. Although uncomfortable, the illness is usually harmless in adults. Unfortunately, there's no cure for gastroenteritis; most people must simply wait for the irritants to leave the body. Some cases, especially those in infants and children, may lead to dehydration, in which case a visit to the doctor or hospital is necessary.

Because gastroenteritis-related diarrhea can be life threatening in infants, a rotavirus vaccine was made available in 2006. The shot, called RotaTeq, protects against at least five prevalent types of rotaviruses.

ADDITIONAL FACTS

1. *Rotaviruses and noroviruses are more active from October through April.*

2. *Noroviruses are also known as Norwalk-like viruses, named after the town of Norwalk, Ohio. That's where this type of virus was first identified after an outbreak in 1972.*

❖❖❖

Ginseng

Several types of plants are referred to as ginseng: Both American and Asian ginsengs belong to the genus *Panax,* while Siberian ginseng, or *Eleutherococcus senticosus,* is a different species in the same family. All three plants are regarded as adaptogens—substances that strengthen and normalize body functions, helping the body deal with stress.

Asian and American ginseng are both tan, gnarled roots, sometimes resembling a human body with stringy shoots that look like arms and legs—an appearance that, hundreds of years ago, led herbalists to believe that ginseng could cure human ills. In fact, the Chinese view ginseng as the most powerful of all herbs. Both types of true ginseng contain active compounds called ginsenosides. (Siberian ginseng does not, and it was originally marketed in Russia as a cheaper alternative.) Ginseng also contains peptides, B vitamins, flavonoids, and volatile oil. White ginseng (dried and peeled) and red ginseng (unpeeled and steamed before drying) are available in liquid extracts, powders, and capsules.

Ginseng may shorten the time that it takes people to recover from illness or surgery and may promote overall well-being. Preliminary research suggests that ginseng may also be helpful in speeding up metabolism and treating alcohol intoxication, slowing the progression of Alzheimer's disease, treating or preventing cancer, lowering blood sugar levels in people with diabetes, and lowering "bad" cholesterol while raising "good" cholesterol levels. Some studies have shown that ginseng can both lower and raise blood pressure, so people with hypertension or heart disease should not try ginseng without a doctor's supervision.

Ginseng is widely believed to enhance libido, and in animal studies, it increased sperm production and sexual activity. It is thought to make people feel more alert and able to concentrate or memorize things, especially when it's taken in combination with ginkgo biloba. Ginseng has even been used to increase athletic performance, although study results in this area have been inconsistent.

Ginseng may cause nervousness or sleeplessness, anxiety, diarrhea, vomiting, nosebleeds, and breast pain. To avoid low blood sugar, ginseng should be taken with food. It may act as a blood thinner and should be discontinued at least a week before surgery.

ADDITIONAL FACTS

1. *Ginseng should not be harvested for medicinal use until it reaches maturity—about 4 to 6 years.*

2. *More than 90 percent of the raw ginseng grown in the United States is harvested in Wisconsin.*

3. *Asian ginseng is almost extinct in its natural habitat but is still cultivated for medicinal use.*

✦✦✦

Personality Disorders

People are unique because of the thoughts and emotions that affect the way they react to the world. There's no such thing as a "correct" personality, whether it's good-natured or gloomy. But there are such things as personality disorders, a group of mental illnesses classified by dysfunctional ways of perceiving situations and relating to others. People with these conditions are rigid and unwavering in their strange or inappropriate behaviors, to the point where it affects their ability to relate to others and live normal lives.

Personality is formed by a combination of "nature" and "nurture" factors. Traits of temperament such as shyness or friendliness are largely inherited, but how a person grows up also has a big impact. Likewise, personality disorders seem to be caused by both genetic and environmental influences. Research suggests that some people may have predisposed vulnerabilities to developing a disorder, but a traumatic situation—such as an abusive or unstable childhood or the loss of a parent—must trigger its development.

Personality disorders affect about 10 to 13 percent of people worldwide. The American Psychiatric Association classifies them into the following three clusters:

Cluster A: Odd, eccentric thinking or behavior—including paranoid personality disorder (believing that others are trying to harm you), schizoid personality disorder (having little interest in emotional expression or social relationships), and schizotypal personality disorder (believing that you can influence people and events with your thoughts or that messages are hidden for you in public speeches or displays)

Cluster B: Dramatic, overly emotional thinking or behavior—such as antisocial personality disorder (lying, stealing, showing disregard for others, or engaging in violent behavior), borderline personality disorder (having a tendency toward volatile relationships and impulsive, risky, or suicidal behavior), histrionic personality disorder (showing a constant need for attention), and narcissistic personality disorder (believing that you're better than others and fantasizing about power and success)

Cluster C: Anxious and fearful thinking or behavior—including avoidant personality disorder (isolating oneself and being hypersensitive to criticism and rejection), dependent personality disorder (showing excessive dependence on or submissiveness toward others), and obsessive-compulsive personality disorder (having a preoccupation with orderliness, rules, and being in charge; this is not the same as obsessive-compulsive disorder)

ADDITIONAL FACTS

1. *It's not unusual to have more than one personality disorder at the same time.*

2. *A combination of psychotherapy (talk therapy and education) and medication, such as antidepressant, antianxiety, or mood-stabilizing drugs, is often used to treat personality disorders*

◆◆◆

Balanitis

Uncircumcised boys are often instructed to clean carefully around the foreskin and the area underneath it. One major reason is that bacteria trapped beneath the foreskin can lead to balanitis, a painful inflammation of the head of the penis. Men with this condition often experience pain, itching, redness, and foul smelling discharge. Experts say that balanitis is a common condition, affecting up to 11 percent of men who are treated in urology clinics.

Balanitis is often accompanied by inflammation of the foreskin (posthitis), in a double-duty infection called balanoposthitis. Although painful, these conditions aren't serious health threats if they're caught early. Most cases can be easily treated with antibiotic creams or pills, as well as steroid creams. But when the inflammation rages on for an extended period of time, it may cause permanent damage. It could scar and narrow the opening of the urethra or lead to phimosis, in which the foreskin becomes too tight to pull over the tip of the penis. Paraphimosis, in which the head of the penis swells and the foreskin can't be retracted, may also occur. When the foreskin cannot retract, erection becomes painful. In the latter two conditions, circumcision may be in order. To prevent these complications, the ultimate line of prevention is to do as your parents instructed: Wash and rinse the penis frequently, and thoroughly clean beneath the foreskin.

ADDITIONAL FACTS

1. *Some sexually transmitted infections can raise the risk of balanitis.*

2. *Balanitis may be caused by certain diseases, such as gonorrhea, lichen sclerosus et atrophicus, and uncontrolled diabetes.*

✦✦✦

Iron Supplements

Iron is essential to many proteins and enzymes your body uses to maintain good health. It is also necessary for the delivery of oxygen to your cells and the regulation of cell growth. For these reasons, iron supplements should be taken when diet alone does not restore iron to sufficient levels.

Iron supplements come in two forms: ferrous and ferric. Ferrous iron is preferred because it is better absorbed by the body. The quantity of iron absorbed by your body decreases with greater doses, so it's better to take your supplements in two or three doses spread throughout the day.

Someone who is iron deficient may develop anemia and demonstrate fatigue and decreased immunity. Supplements are particularly important if an individual is displaying symptoms of anemia. If tests indicate that a woman's level of serum ferritin—a protein that stores iron—is less than or equal to 15 micrograms per liter and she has a low red blood cell count, then she is anemic due to iron deficiency and needs iron supplements.

To treat iron deficiency anemia, it is recommended that adult women take 50 to 60 milligrams of oral elemental iron daily for 3 months. However, you should check with your doctor before taking any supplement. Iron supplements may cause side effects such as nausea, vomiting, constipation, diarrhea, dark-colored stools, and abdominal cramps.

Adult men and postmenopausal women should be careful about taking iron supplements, because iron deficiency is uncommon is these groups and they are at greater risk of iron overload, a condition in which too much iron collects in the blood and organs. This can potentially cause liver and heart problems, and even death in people with a genetic predisposition to hemochromatosis, a disease in which iron builds up in the body and causes damage to the internal organs. Additionally, people with blood disorders that necessitate frequent blood transfusions should not take iron supplements.

ADDITIONAL FACTS

1. *Iron deficiency is the most prominent nutritional disorder globally. Eighty percent of the world population may be iron deficient, and 30 percent may have iron deficiency anemia.*

2. *Pregnant women need approximately double the iron intake of women who are not pregnant. This is because of greater blood volume during pregnancy, the additional needs of the fetus, and blood loss that occurs during delivery.*

◆◆◆

Open-Heart Surgery and the Heart-Lung Machine

At Boston's Massachusetts General Hospital in 1930, a young surgeon named John Gibbon Jr. witnessed the death of a patient as a result of a massive pulmonary embolism, or a blood clot in his lung. Doctors tried for hours to save the patient with traditional surgical techniques, but failed—leaving a lifelong impression on Gibbon, who went on to develop the heart-lung machine that made possible open-heart surgery as we know it today.

Gibbon (1903–1973) left Boston soon after this incident and took a teaching position at Thomas Jefferson University in Philadelphia. There, he focused on developing a machine that could take over for the heart and lungs during surgery. He faced many challenges: how to drain the blood from the body, how to pump it back, how to keep it from clotting in the machine, and so on. Until this point in history, surgery on or around the heart was limited to what could be done while the heart was still beating, or what could be fixed in just a few minutes while the heart was stopped and the brain was deprived of oxygen.

The IBM Corporation helped Gibbon produce his first machine, which showed promise in animals but failed to pump enough blood for a human. Gibbon built a second machine in his lab and, in 1952, used it to operate on a 15-month-old girl. The patient died on the operating table, but his second operation, 3 months later, was a remarkable success and the patient made a full recovery after spending 27 minutes being kept alive by Gibbon's machine.

Gibbon's next two operations were unsuccessful, however, and he gave up performing open-heart surgery shortly thereafter. Mayo Clinic researchers, meanwhile, developed the first commercially available heart-lung machine, the Mayo-Gibbon device, modeled after Gibbon's design. This machine (along with other advancements, such as cardiac catheterization and anticlotting medication) helped doctors begin to treat heart disease, one of the most common causes of death in the United Sates, as they never could before.

ADDITIONAL FACTS

1. *After being hooked to a heart-lung machine, patients often reported cognitive decline, a condition nicknamed* pumphead. *It was thought to be a temporary symptom of surgical trauma, but recent studies have found that it may actually persist and worsen over time. Microscopic cell debris and bubbles generated by the machine are possible causes.*

2. *Before the heart-lung machine was perfected, surgeons experimented with hypothermia techniques: By cooling the patient's body before surgery, they could slightly extend the amount of time the brain could go without oxygen.*

3. *Gibbon was associated for most of his life with Jefferson Medical College in Philadelphia. He also held positions at the University of Pennsylvania, Harvard, and as an Army doctor during World War II.*

❖❖❖

Juvenile Muscular Dystrophy

Muscular dystrophy is a group of diseases in which muscles become progressively weaker with age. Some versions of this condition progress quickly and are fatal, but benign juvenile muscular dystrophy is much milder. This disease is also known as progressive tardive, or Becker, muscular dystrophy.

Both the more severe version, called Duchenne, and juvenile muscular dystrophy are genetic disorders inherited from the mother. The defective gene is recessive and resides on the X chromosome, so girls who inherit it are usually carriers—they don't show symptoms. Boys, on the other hand, with only their mother's X chromosome, do have symptoms. The condition affects about 1 in 30,000 boys.

Because of this genetic glitch, the body does not produce sufficient amounts of a protein called dystrophin. This protein helps muscle cells keep their shape and length; without it, muscles break down. Boys who have Duchenne muscular dystrophy begin experiencing symptoms at about age 2. They start to develop leg weakness, balance problems, and large calf muscles. By late childhood, they often are unable to walk; many sufferers pass away by their late teens or early twenties from pneumonia, lung weakness, or cardiac complications. Boys with benign muscular dystrophy, on the other hand, don't begin to show the effects of the disease until about age 10 or 11. Their symptoms are less severe and progress more slowly; they usually don't lose the ability to walk until late adulthood and may retain their mobility.

Unfortunately, there's no cure for muscular dystrophy. But physical therapy can help maintain the range of motion in joints, anti-inflammatory corticosteroids can help preserve muscle strength, and other prescription medications can help manage muscle spasms and stiffness.

ADDITIONAL FACTS

1. *Becker muscular dystrophy is named after the German physician Peter Emil Becker, who first reported his research on this form of the disease in 1955.*

2. *A girl who inherited an abnormal gene from a carrier mom and an abnormal gene from an affected dad would have no normal X chromosome and would be the rare case of an affected female.*

✦✦✦

Pleurisy

Before the discovery of oxygen, the lungs' function stumped physicians. Until the Renaissance, it was believed that they regulated body temperature. Since then, researchers have come a long way in learning about the lungs' anatomy and their role in oxygen transfer. For instance, they now know that each lung is encased in a thin, double-layered membrane called the pleura. When this covering becomes inflamed, that's known as pleurisy.

This ailment is brought on by a number of conditions. A viral infection, pneumonia, an autoimmune condition, or tuberculosis can cause the pleura to become inflamed. In the early stage of pleurisy, during an inhalation, the two membranes, which usually slide across each other like two sheets of satin, rub together painfully like sandpaper. Besides chest pain during breathing, symptoms include a dry cough and possibly fever and chills. In the later stages of the illness, the membranes produce an excess of fluid, which can accumulate and put pressure on the lungs. If the fluid becomes infected, the condition is known as an empyema.

To cure pleurisy, a doctor must first address the underlying issue. If a blood screening reveals that bacterial pneumonia is to blame, antibiotics will be prescribed. But if the pleurisy is caused by a virus, the most common treatment is waiting for the infection to run its course. In the meantime, over-the-counter painkillers and a prescription cough syrup with codeine can help keep the pain and symptoms under control. In rare cases, a large amount of fluid buildup requires that the fluid is drained out of the chest through a tube.

ADDITIONAL FACTS

1. *During Shakespearean times, the word* pleurisy *was often used in literature to mean a "fullness of blood."*

2. *The pressure in the pleural cavity between the two membranes is less than the atmospheric pressure, which helps keep the lungs expanded.*

✦✦✦

Macrobiotic Diet

Popular in the United States and Europe since the 1970s, the macrobiotic diet stresses simple, organic foods that proponents believe increase longevity and contribute to overall health and well-being. From the Latin words for "big life," macrobiotic diets are intended to be part of a set of lifestyle changes aimed at living harmoniously with nature.

The macrobiotic diet consists largely of whole grains, vegetables, and beans. People who follow the macrobiotic diet are also encouraged to buy local, unprocessed foods. Supporters of the macrobiotic lifestyle argue that the modern Western diet is inherently unhealthy, with its overemphasis on refined sugars and processed foods, and contributes to cancer and many other illnesses.

A macrobiotic diet is typically 50 to 60 percent whole grains—mainly brown rice— and 25 to 30 percent local vegetables. Soups, beans, and sea vegetables make up the rest of the daily diet, while fruits, nuts, seeds, and white fish are allowed two or three times a week. No meat or dairy products are allowed, and virtually all beverages aside from water and certain types of tea are frowned upon. Simple cooking methods are preferred. Where you live and the time of year also affect what you can eat in a macrobiotic diet: Foods should be grown no more than 500 miles away whenever possible. In colder seasons, macrobiotic cooks make meals with longer preparation times and more salt, while warmer weather calls for lighter cooking methods and less salt.

The effects of following a macrobiotic diet are subject to debate. It has been reported that women who follow the regime, for example, have lower circulating estrogen levels and therefore might have lower risks of breast cancer. However, there is no evidence that this diet has any effect on cancer, although it is still being investigated. What is known is that a strict macrobiotic diet can cause nutritional deficiencies, particularly among children. While some people may be able to meet their nutritional needs, it can be very difficult to get adequate protein, vitamin B_{12}, and calcium on such a regimen. Even dehydration is a risk, because tap water and any artificial drinks are to be used sparingly or not at all.

ADDITIONAL FACTS

1. *Other whole grains include barley, oats, corn, and rye. A strict macrobiotic diet forbids eating bread, however, because it contains yeast.*

2. *In a macrobiotic diet, sodium and potassium are the primary antagonistic and complementary ingredients. The amount of each that is present in a food determines its character, or "yin-yang" quality.*

3. *The macrobiotic diet discourages tropical nuts and fruits, some vegetables (such as artichokes, asparagus, beets, eggplant, and potatoes), chocolate, artificial and natural fruit sweeteners, and white sugar.*

✦✦✦

Obsessive-Compulsive Disorder

Many people have rituals they perform regularly and repetitively, such as checking several times to see whether the alarm clock is set before going to bed. But for about 2.2 million Americans, such rituals can take over their lives. These individuals suffer from obsessive-compulsive disorder (OCD): They know that their routines don't make sense, but they feel extreme anxiety if they don't follow them anyway.

To be diagnosed with OCD, a chronic anxiety disorder, a person must show certain characteristics. He or she must either suffer from repeated and persistent thoughts or feel driven to perform the same task over and over again. These obsessions and compulsions are excessive and unreasonable and significantly interfere with daily routine. Often the two are related: Someone might attempt to relieve constant worrying about germs, for example, by washing his hands until they are raw and chapped.

People with OCD may be preoccupied with shapes and patterns, lucky numbers, or counting or touching things in particular sequences. At best, these routines provide temporary relief from their obsessive thoughts, which often involve loved ones being harmed, inappropriate or unpleasant sexual acts, or thoughts that go against their religious beliefs.

Some researchers believe that OCD results from a natural change in the body's chemistry; others, that it stems from habits of behavior that a person learns over time. Studies show that an insufficient level of serotonin in the brain may contribute to symptoms.

OCD often runs in families, and scientists in recent years have found that several variations within one specific gene seem to raise the risk of the disorder. Other research suggests that it is the absence of a specific gene that causes the disorder; one group of researchers created mice with OCD tendencies by selectively breeding them without this gene. The genetic causes of OCD are being studied further.

People with OCD usually respond well to antidepressant medications that increase levels of serotonin in the brain. Cognitive behavioral therapy, in which patients are gradually exposed to items or situations that cause them anxiety (dirt, for example) until they become less sensitive to them, can also be successful.

ADDITIONAL FACTS

1. *Obsessive-compulsive behavior is commonly seen as a minor character trait, such as extreme neatness and orderliness or making daily lists of things.*

2. *The OCD mice, created by researchers at Duke University, displayed symptoms of the disorder by compulsively grooming themselves, leading to injuries. Humans with OCD may repeatedly wash their hands or scratch their skins.*

◆◆◆

Salpingo-Oophoritis
(Pelvic Inflammatory Disease)

In modern medicine, salpingo-oophoritis, or pelvic inflammatory disease (PID), has become a widespread problem. Caught early on, this infection of the fallopian tubes and adjacent pelvic organs is easily wiped out with a course of antibiotics. PID strikes an estimated 1 million women in the United States every year, leaving 100,000 women infertile and causing a large percentage of ectopic pregnancies.

PID occurs when bacteria travel up from the vagina and cervix and invade the other reproductive organs. Although a variety of bacteria can result in PID, the sexually transmitted infections (STIs) gonorrhea and chlamydia are two of the top culprits. Women under the age of 25 are most often diagnosed with PID. Men carry the bacteria and may suffer from urethritis when infected, with symptoms of urethral discharge and a burning sensation with urination. However, there may be no symptoms, or they may last only a few days and not be treated. Rarely, urethral scarring may result.

PID often goes unnoticed, both by women and by their doctors. That's because symptoms, such as odor, painful urination or intercourse, and irregular bleeding, can be mild to nonexistent. The symptoms often subside without treatment, and if a woman fails to report them, the disease remains untreated but may still progress. When left untreated, the infection attacks the reproductive organs, causing damage and leaving behind scar tissue. If this tissue harms the fallopian tubes, it can render a woman infertile. To protect against PID, doctors recommend that sexually active women get tested for STIs frequently and always use condoms.

ADDITIONAL FACTS

1. *Women who have a PID episode are at greater risk for developing the disease again.*

2. *Chronic pelvic pain is one red flag for PID.*

3. *Having multiple sex partners increases the risk of PID.*

◆◆◆

Annual Health Exam

Having annual health exams increases the likelihood of your living a long and healthy life. Annual exams are important for detecting problems before they start or when they have just begun. The earlier you identify a problem, the better your chances for treatment and a cure are.

The best place to go for your annual health exam is to your regular health care provider or doctor, usually an internist. You should undergo screenings, vaccinations, and other preventive services appropriate for your age, health, family health history, and lifestyle choices (such as diet, exercise, alcohol consumption, and smoking). Adults should be screened for cancer; bone health; and cardiovascular, reproductive, respiratory, and mental health issues.

Recommended cancer screenings for women include a Pap test at least every 3 years to check for cervical cancer and, for women ages 40 and over, a yearly mammogram to check for breast cancer. Men and women ages 50 and over should have a colonoscopy at least every 10 years to screen for colorectal cancer. For men 50 and over, an annual prostate screening is recommended.

Adults ages 60 and above should undergo a bone density test to determine whether they have osteoporosis.

Annual heart health exams include checking your blood pressure and cholesterol and monitoring your diet if you have high cholesterol or are at risk for heart disease or diabetes. Additionally, you may be prescribed low-dose aspirin to prevent a heart attack.

Sexual health screenings include testing women for chlamydia and gonorrhea. All adults at risk should be tested for HIV and syphilis.

Adults in high-risk groups should have flu shots, and men and women ages 65 and over should have pneumonia immunization and a herpes-zoster vaccination. All adults should be checked for depression.

ADDITIONAL FACTS

1. *During your annual exam, your doctor should review your health history, including previous problems you've had and whether you're taking any medications.*

2. *Children over age 2 should have an annual health examination by a pediatrician. The checkup should include monitoring growth patterns and blood pressure, performing a complete blood count, administering immunizations, and possibly checking cholesterol. Children under 2 should have regular checkups more frequently, as recommended by their pediatricians. Female children who are sexually active should have a Pap test.*

◆◆◆

Watson, Crick, and DNA

When Francis Crick announced in 1953 that he and colleague James Watson had "found the secret of life," he wasn't joking. Earlier that morning, the two scientists had decrypted the structure of life's hereditary information: deoxyribonucleic acid (DNA).

DNA is present in the nucleus of every living cell and guides the cell in making new proteins that determine biological traits. Before Watson and Crick, scientists knew that DNA carried the information that determines all of a living organism's traits and they assumed that DNA was copied from one generation to the next, but no one knew how this information was encoded or exactly how it was transmitted.

Crick (1916–2004), an English researcher, and Watson (1928–), an American postdoctoral scholar, shared a lab at Cambridge University in the 1950s. Together, they discovered that a strand of DNA looked like a twisted ladder, which they called a double helix. They also realized that each strand was made up of four building blocks, called bases. These building blocks were named adenine, thymine, guanine, and cytosine (also known as A, T, G, and C) and were bound together with hydrogen atoms to create different patterns. Working with cardboard replicas of the four bases, Crick and Watson realized that adenine and thymine always bound together, as did guanine and cytosine. These bonds form what look like rungs on DNA's twisted ladder. When a cell reproduces, this ladder "unzips," and new bases are added to each side of the helix—resulting in two new cells with identical DNA.

In 1955, the Spanish-American biochemist Severo Ochoa (1905–1993) was the first person to create, in a lab at New York University School of Medicine, a nucleic acid. He worked with ribonucleic acid (RNA), and shortly thereafter, his UCLA colleague Arthur Kornberg (1918–2007) synthesized DNA. These discoveries paved the way for genetic engineering and provided the basis for many drugs used to treat cancer and viral infections. Unraveling the genetic code depends on knowing the structure of DNA and RNA and their configuration as a double helix. Ochoa and Kornberg shared the Nobel Prize in Physiology or Medicine in 1959, while Watson and Crick were awarded the prize in 1962.

ADDITIONAL FACTS

1. *The dramatic story of James Watson and Francis Crick's discovery was chronicled in Watson's book* The Double Helix *and the movie* The Race for the Double Helix.

2. *Adenine and guanine are both made up of double-ringed nitrogen bases, while thymine and cytosine are made of single rings.*

3. *The researcher Rosalind Franklin (1920–1958), a close collaborator of Watson and Crick who showed them the first x-ray diffraction pictures of DNA and often critiqued their work, died before the Nobel Prize was awarded.*

◆◆◆

Anorexia

For centuries, certain people have purposely refused food. In medieval Europe, for instance, some women starved themselves as an act of cleansing to show their piety; some of these "martyrs" were even elevated to sainthood. In the 16th century, physicians named this phenomenon of self-starvation anorexia, after the Greek word meaning "loss of appetite." Over time, the focus of this eating disorder has shifted from showing religious devotion to attaining an imagined standard of beauty: thinness.

Today, anorexics are obsessed with their weight, their bodies, and food. They have distorted body images and starve themselves or exercise excessively to whittle themselves down to abnormally low body weights. In the majority of cases, anorexics use food and their bodies as a way to cope with emotional issues and a desire for control. That's why physicians classify this eating disorder as a mental disease.

Young women, in particular, are vulnerable. The number of 15- to 19-year-old females who suffer from anorexia has grown steadily since 1935. Today, it's estimated that as many as 10 percent of females and 1 percent of males have been affected by the disorder sometime during their lives. Experts believe that anorexia is caused by psychological, cultural, and even genetic factors. Research shows that females with a family member with the disease are more likely to develop it, as are those with low self-esteem or obsessive-compulsive personalities.

Severe weight loss causes amenorrhea (the lack of menstrual periods), infertility, thinking disorders, and even memory loss. Because the body is deprived of nutrients, people with the disorder may also suffer from anemia and malnourishment. This raises the risk of bone loss, heart problems, and even death. Treatments such as psychotherapy, nutritional counseling, and antidepressants can help correct the condition.

ADDITIONAL FACTS

1. *Besides excessive thinness, symptoms of anorexia include dry skin, downy hair covering the body, and an absence of menstruation.*

2. *Anorexia has the highest fatality rate of any mental illness.*

3. *Research shows that 81 percent of 10-year-olds are afraid of being fat.*

◆◆◆

Appendicitis

The appendix is an organ that evolution overlooked. Believed to have helped ancient species store and digest food, this 3-inch-long muscular tube has no known physiological purpose today. In fact, it's a bodily troublemaker: About 1 in 15 Americans will suffer from an inflamed appendix, or appendicitis.

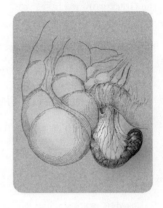

Located on the lower right side of the abdomen, the appendix extends from the beginning of the large intestine. When the appendix becomes blocked—by stool, cancer, or an infection—it becomes inflamed and fills with pus. Symptoms include pain in the lower right abdomen, nausea, abdominal swelling, cramps, and a loss of appetite. The pain increases gradually over a period of up to 12 hours, eventually becoming severe and accompanied by fever.

Because the symptoms of appendicitis overlap with those of many other conditions, physicians often conduct urine and blood tests, and possibly computed tomography scans or ultrasounds, to diagnose appendicitis. If appendicitis is suspected, doctors treat it as a medical emergency and quickly remove the organ with an appendectomy to prevent it from rupturing. During this surgical procedure, a 4-inch incision is made in the abdomen, or a minimally invasive laparoscopy is performed. A burst appendix can spill infectious materials into the body, leading to peritonitis, an inflammation of the abdominal lining. This condition may prove fatal if not treated promptly with strong antibiotics.

Although appendicitis can occur at any age, it's most common in people between the ages of 10 and 30. There is no known way to prevent the condition, but research shows that it's less common in people who eat high-fiber diets.

ADDITIONAL FACTS

1. *Scientists have found evidence of appendicitis in ancient Egyptian mummies.*

2. *The first known surgical removal of the appendix was conducted on an 11-year-old boy in 1735 by Claudius Amyand (c. 1681–1740).*

◆◆◆

Influenza Vaccination

Anyone who's ever suffered the coughs, chills, and sore muscles caused by influenza, or the flu, knows how unpleasant it can be—and to thousands of people with compromised immune systems, it can be deadly. That's why the government provides flu vaccinations each year, starting in the autumn, to help prevent the spread of influenza to the people who are most at risk.

Because the influenza virus is constantly mutating, however, scientists must tweak the vaccine every year. They use inactive (dead) viruses to produce flu vaccine, so while people won't actually catch the flu from a vaccination, they may experience flu-like symptoms. Each vaccine contains two influenza A viruses and one influenza B virus to protect against the various strains that scientists predict will be circulating during the coming months.

Because children and elderly people have weaker immune systems than healthy adults, the government recommends that everyone under age 18 or more than 50 get a flu vaccination annually. (However, babies younger than 6 months should not receive a flu vaccine.) People with chronic illnesses should be vaccinated too, as should anyone who is in close contact with these groups, such as doctors and nurses.

The flu vaccine is typically given as an injection or a nasal spray. Both types of vaccines are generally given at the beginning of flu season, in October or early November, and are available into the new year.

People who are vaccinated should not get the flu, or at worst should get a much milder version. Protection starts approximately 2 weeks after receiving the vaccine, although studies on the effectiveness of flu shots—especially among children and the elderly—have been mixed. Some research has suggested that doing physical activities, such as practicing qigong (a Chinese blend of exercise and meditation) or lifting weights, before a flu inoculation may increase the shot's effectiveness.

ADDITIONAL FACTS

1. *Mercury-free vaccines are recommended for children under 2 years old and women who expect to be past the third month of pregnancy during flu season.*

2. *Although most people recover quickly from the flu, it has historically been one of history's deadliest diseases. A flu pandemic that began in 1918 killed 25 million people across the world—more deaths than were suffered by all sides World War I, which concluded in the same year.*

3. *Anyone who has had a severe allergic reaction to chickens or egg protein should not have a flu shot.*

◆◆◆

Tourette Syndrome

A disorder characterized by involuntary utterances and motions known as tics, Tourette syndrome (TS) is named for the French doctor who first described it in 1885. About 200,000 Americans, mostly men, suffer from severe and persistent TS, and many more have milder forms of the disorder.

Symptoms of TS usually begin at age 7 to 10 and improve by early adulthood, although some cases can be lifelong. Stress or excitement can bring on or intensify tics, which are often preceded by a sensation called a premonitory urge. The individual will feel a strong and growing desire to "complete" their tic—an urge that eventually becomes unbearable.

Examples of vocal tics include throat clearing, sniffing, grunting, barking, and verbalizing words or nonsensical sounds. In about 15 percent of cases, people with TS have outbursts of obscene words—a condition called coprolalia. TS patients may also repeat the words of others or their own words. Motor tics usually appear first and include shoulder shrugging, eye blinking, and nose twitching. More complex tics appear as a series of coordinated movements, such as picking up an object to smell it, or mimicking the actions of others. Even though they seem deliberate and may be mistaken for rude behavior, the person has no control over them.

TS is linked to genetics, and a parent with the TS gene has a 50 percent chance of passing it on. However, not everyone who inherits the gene will experience severe symptoms, if any at all. Environmental factors seem to help determine the severity of TS, although their exact role is unclear.

If a person has had chronic, multiple tics for more than a year, a diagnosis of TS may be made. Most people do not need medication, but some benefit from taking neuroleptic drugs that block dopamine receptors in the brain. Medication may also be prescribed for related conditions, such as attention-deficit/hyperactivity disorder, obsessive-compulsive disorder, or depression—although treating these conditions often makes tics even worse. Talk therapy may help a patient cope with social and emotional problems, and studies show that it might help patients better control premonitory urges.

ADDITIONAL FACTS

1. *The professional baseball player Jim Eisenreich (1959–) and the basketball player Mahmoud Abdul-Rauf (1969–) both have Tourette syndrome but were able to continue playing their sports with the help of medication. Abdul-Rauf twice led the NBA in free-throw shooting percentage, a skill that some have suggested was linked to obsessive-compulsive traits brought on by TS.*

2. *The composer Wolfgang Amadeus Mozart (1756–1791) reportedly suffered from mood swings and tics and often wrote obscene letters to his cousin describing bodily functions, leading to speculation that he may have had Tourette syndrome.*

3. *In cases of twins with the TS gene, studies have shown that the twin who weighs less at birth tends to have more-severe tics later in life. This may be caused by differences in oxygen and nutrient levels in the babies' developing brains.*

◆◆◆

Dyspareunia

The act of sexual intercourse is generally thought to bring pleasure and intimacy. But, for many people, it can cause pain, a condition called dyspareunia (pronounced dis-pa-ROO-nia). Some research suggests that 15 percent of women experience this condition on a few occasions each year and that it's a regular occurrence for about 2 percent. Although dyspareunia is most frequently associated with women, it can also affect men, causing pain in the testes, seminal vesicles, penis, or lower abdomen.

Both physical and psychological factors can contribute to this condition. Common physical factors include inflammation or infection, such as yeast or urinary tract infections. Vaginal dryness, brought on by the hormonal fluctuations of menopause or a lack of foreplay, may also be a factor. For women who report a pain deep in the pelvis, endometriosis or pelvic inflammatory disease could be the underlying problem.

Typically, when a woman speaks to her doctor about dyspareunia, the physician will conduct an exam to rule out any possible physical problems. Developmental and emotional factors are far harder to pinpoint. Painful past experiences with sex or extreme guilt can block natural sexual responsiveness, reducing vaginal lubrication and increasing the chances of painful intercourse. Other emotions, such as anxiety or a lack of attraction to a partner, may have a similar effect.

ADDITIONAL FACTS

1. *The term* dyspareunia *comes from the Greek* dyspareunos, *which means "unhappily mated bedfellows."*

2. *Vaginal contraceptive creams and foams can cause painful irritation of the penis, one cause of male dyspareunia.*

◆ ◆ ◆

Pneumovax

Pneumovax is the pneumococcal polysaccharide vaccine, which protects against severe pneumonia infections caused by the bacterium *Streptococcus pneumoniae*. This bacterium often leads to pneumonia and meningitis in children, older adults, and people with chronic illnesses. The vaccine was developed by Michael Heidelberger (1888–1991) and first used on American servicemen in World War II.

For most people, the vaccine is administered by injection in a single dose, although certain people may need two doses. The vaccine is recommended for high-risk people age 2 or older, which includes people with heart disease, lung disease (excluding asthma), kidney disease, alcoholism, diabetes, cirrhosis, leaks of cerebrospinal fluid, and sickle-cell anemia. Also at risk are those age 65 or older, people who live in institutions where other people have chronic health problems, people with weakened immune systems, Alaskan natives, and some Native American populations.

The risks and side effects associated with the pneumococcal vaccine are usually minor. You might experience pain and redness at the site of the injection. And, like all medications, Pneumovax carries a small chance of an allergic reaction, a more serious reaction, or even death. If you are sick or possibly pregnant, you should let your doctor know before receiving the vaccine; he or she may opt to postpone the inoculation.

Even if you have had pneumonia or other invasive pneumococcal disease in the past, you are not immune to all types of pneumococcal infections, and you should still have the vaccine if it's recommended. However, Pneumovax does not prevent all kinds of pneumonia.

ADDITIONAL FACTS

1. *Pneumovax does not protect against pneumococcal diseases in children under age 2. Another vaccine, called the pneumococcal conjugate vaccine, is routinely given to children under 2 to protect against* Streptococcus pneumoniae.

2. *Before vaccines that protect against pneumococcal disease existed in the United States, 200 deaths in children younger than age 5 used to occur annually as a result of these illnesses.*

3. *There are more than 90 subtypes of* Streptococcus pneumoniae *bacteria. The 10 most common subtypes cause 62 percent of invasive disease worldwide.*

4. *Approximately 175,000 hospitalizations resulting from pneumococcal pneumonia occur annually in the United States, and 5 to 7 percent of those patients will die.*

✦✦✦

Lasers

Albert Einstein (1879–1955) was the first to envision the intense, powerful beams of light we know today as lasers. In 1917, he wrote that if atomic particles called photons were combined and energized in a certain way, they would emit light all in the same direction and frequency—as opposed to ordinary visible light, which is very scattered. It took several decades, however, for physicists to find out exactly how to make this technique work.

In 1954, the researchers James Gordon and Charles Townes (1915–) used microwave rays to generate the first "microwave amplification by stimulated emission of radiation," or maser, at Columbia University. Townes continued to work with Arthur Schawlow (1921–1999) at Bell Labs on a prototype device with mirrors on either side of its cavity so that photons of the desired wavelength could bounce back and forth. Four years later, calculations for a light maser, or laser, were published.

The medical community saw great potential in these lasers, although difficulty controlling the power output and delivery of early laser systems led to inconsistent and disappointing results in early human studies. One area where lasers did seem to have promise was eye surgery. In 1964, an easy-to-control, high-absorption argon ion laser was developed, and clinical systems soon became available for the treatment of retinal disease.

Also that year came the development of a carbon dioxide (CO_2) laser, which emitted an easily focused infrared beam that was well absorbed by water. Because the human body consists mainly of water, doctors found that a CO_2 laser beam could cut tissue like a scalpel—but with much less blood loss, since the beam's heat immediately cauterized the tissue.

By the early 1970s, teaching hospitals were using CO_2 lasers for sinus and gynecologic surgeries. In another 10 years, laser surgery became widespread, and smaller but more powerful devices began appearing in hospitals and even doctors' offices for everything from making laparoscopic surgical incisions to removing tattoos and birthmarks. Lasers today are also widely used for cosmetic surgery, including skin resurfacing, hair removal, and the treatment of varicose leg veins, among other procedures.

ADDITIONAL FACTS

1. *Today, dentists can use lasers to detect early-forming cavities.*

2. *Scientists at MIT are studying how a laser and a light-activated dye may be able to help heal surgical wounds and prevent scarring.*

3. *The first laser was created with a synthetic ruby crystal and produced a bright red light called a ruby laser.*

❖❖❖

Bulimia

The word *bulimia* is derived from the Greek words for "ox" and "hunger." That's because people who suffer from this eating disorder often binge, or consume large amounts of food in a short period of time. They then attempt to rid themselves of the excess calories in an unhealthy manner, such as by vomiting or abusing laxatives.

As with anorexia and other eating disorders, this mental illness is most common in adolescent and young women and is intertwined with self-image disturbances and a desire for control. People with bulimia often restrict their food intake the majority of the time and then eat to the point of discomfort—taking in thousands of calories at once—before purging. Most people suffering from the disorder have an addiction-like relationship with food. Behaviors typical of bulimics include hoarding food and going to the bathroom after meals, and typical symptoms include bloating, fatigue, weakness, dehydration, constipation, and damaged teeth.

Bulimia can also cause long-term health problems. Excessive vomiting can tear or ruptur the esophagus. It can also result in an irregular heartbeat, low blood pressure, and, in severe cases, death. What's more, bulimia is often linked to depression and feelings of shame. Because people with bulimia can have a normal body weight, the illness is not detected as easily as anorexia. That's one reason only 6 percent of sufferers receive the proper psychological treatment. To help people recover, experts recommend they undergo psychotherapy or other counseling.

ADDITIONAL FACTS

1. *In ancient Rome, wealthy men would induce vomiting at lavish banquets so they could continue eating.*

2. *People who are often on diets are 18 times more likely to develop an eating disorder.*

◆◆◆

Hemorrhoids

Hemorrhoids aren't life threatening, but they're an affliction of biblical proportions. A line in the book of Deuteronomy reads, "The Lord will strike you with the Egyptian inflammation, with hemorrhoids, boil scars and itch, from which you shall never recover." It's a fearsome threat, as the condition is embarrassing and painful.

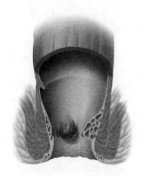

Also known as piles, hemorrhoids are a condition in which the veins around the anus and lower rectum become swollen and inflamed. Hemorrhoids can occur in either the internal or external anal membranes; although both kinds cause bloody stools, only the external kind causes severe pain and itching.

This condition is common among adults: By age 50, nearly half of people will have suffered a bout of hemorrhoids. They are usually caused by an increase in pressure in the rectum due to constipation, diarrhea, obesity, sitting for long periods of time, or pregnancy. In the majority of cases, hemorrhoids disappear on their own after a few days. To soothe the pain in the meanwhile, experts recommend using an over-the-counter hemorrhoid cream or witch hazel pads to numb the area. Applying cold compresses or sitting in a sitz bath may also provide relief.

A doctor may need to intervene if blood pools in external hemorrhoids, causing a clot. For persistent and painful cases, other treatments are also available, such as surgical removal, sclerotherapy (in which a chemical is injected to shrink the hemorrhoid), and rubber band ligation (in which a tiny rubber band is placed around a hemorrhoid to cut off its blood supply).

ADDITIONAL FACTS

1. *A high-fiber diet that promotes regular bowel movements may help fend off hemorrhoids.*

2. *The ancient Greek physician Hippocrates (c. 460–c. 377 BC) wrote of a treatment similar to the rubber band ligation procedure. He recommended tying off hemorrhoids with thick woolen thread until they dropped off.*

◆ ◆ ◆

Growth Hormone

The brain's pituitary gland produces a natural hormone that is necessary for stimulating growth. Man-made versions of this growth hormone are sometimes needed to treat children who don't grow normally or sick adults who experience dangerous weight loss and wasting of the body. Illegally, this hormone is commonly abused by athletes and older adults to increase muscle mass and reverse the effects of aging.

In normal development, human growth hormone (HGH) is secreted daily throughout childhood; production peaks during adolescence and declines afterward. The hormone helps muscles and bones, and possibly the heart. But some children—those who have Turner's syndrome, Prader-Willi syndrome, or chronic renal insufficiency—don't produce enough HGH themselves. In 1985, a synthetic, injectable version of the hormone was approved for treatment of these disorders. HGH can also be prescribed for children who have unexplained, unusually short stature and to treat weight loss and body deterioration associated with AIDS.

There are two forms of synthetic HGH: somatropin, which is identical to the natural version, and somatrem, whose chemical makeup contains one additional amino acid. Both forms are indistinguishable from naturally occurring hormones in blood and urine tests. Because HGH is so hard to detect—and because it is suspected to improve athletic performance and prevent age-related body deterioration—the hormone's illegal use among bodybuilders, athletes, and celebrities is believed to be widespread.

The use of HGH, however, is associated with negative side effects including swelling, carpal tunnel syndrome, joint and muscle pain, and numbness and tingling. HGH also increases the risk of developing diabetes and may speed the growth of preexisting cancer cells. A few patients who have taken HGH have developed leukemia, although a causal relationship has not been determined.

Synthetic growth hormones are often used illegally in combination with anabolic steroids and other performance-enhancing drugs. As part of the 1990 Anabolic Steroids Control Act, the distribution or possession of HGH for any nonprescribed use is a felony punishable with up to 5 years in jail.

ADDITIONAL FACTS

1. *Dreaming, exercise, and stress all increase the secretion of HGH.*

2. *Various sprays and pills claim to contain HGH, but the synthetic hormone molecule is actually too large for absorption when taken orally. It is effective only when given as an injection.*

3. *Illicit use of HGH in people who already have normal levels can cause enlargement of the breasts, increased growth of birthmarks, diabetes, hardening of the arteries, and high blood pressure.*

◆◆◆

Anxiety

Everyone occasionally experiences anxiety: a feeling of fear, nervousness, or dread accompanied by restlessness or tension. Its main symptoms—heart palpitations, shortness of breath, stomachaches, or headaches—are largely due to the body's involuntarily preparations to deal with a threat with a fight-or-flight response. Visible signs of anxiety may include pale skin, sweating, and trembling.

Anxiety can be useful, alerting us to danger or giving us energy to get things done. Its stressful symptoms usually fade quickly after the perceived threat is gone—when you reach the end of a dark alley or finally complete the exam you've been worried about. For many people, however, anxiety that does not fade with time can turn into one of several crippling mental illnesses known as anxiety disorders.

There are several forms of anxiety disorders. With generalized anxiety disorder, a person may worry constantly and disproportionately about something innocuous, such as the well-being of a perfectly healthy child. Shorter, repetitive, and more extreme episodes of anxiety may be classified as panic disorder—a tendency toward panic attacks that usually last about 5 to 30 minutes and may include dizziness, chest tightness, and the fear that you're going crazy or are about to die.

Other types of anxiety disorders include intense, irrational fears of specific objects or events (phobias); recurring, unwanted thoughts and repetitive behaviors (obsessive-compulsive disorder); and panic episodes stemming from troublesome events in the past (post-traumatic stress disorder). These disorders may be caused by a chemical imbalance or an unconscious memory and may be thought of as a malfunctioning alarm in the brain that is mistakenly triggered when there is no real threat. Treatment can involve medications, talk therapy, or breathing and relaxation exercises.

ADDITIONAL FACTS

1. *"Test anxiety" is a specific type of apprehension felt by students—of any age—who have a fear of failing and being evaluated negatively by teachers, superiors, and peers. Sweating, dizziness, headaches, racing heartbeat, nausea, fidgeting, and finger drumming are all common symptoms of test anxiety. In 2006, approximately 49 percent of high school students reportedly experienced this condition.*

2. *In small children, the fear of strangers is a protective developmental response toward those who are not parents or family members. Anxiety when interacting with unknown people can also be a common phase in young people. For others, it may persist into adulthood and become social anxiety or social phobia.*

3. *The "father of existentialism," Søren Kierkegaard (1813–1855), used the Danish word* angest *(meaning "anxiety" or "dread") in 1844 to describe a spiritual condition of insecurity and despair among free human beings in constant fear of failing in their responsibilities to God, to their own principles, and to others. The modern word* angst *is also commonly used to describe teenage frustration and melancholy.*

◆◆◆

Ectopic Pregnancy

By now, you're well versed in the reproductive process: The egg is fertilized in a fallopian tube and the resulting embryo attaches to the uterine wall, where it grows into a fetus. But in about 2 to 10 percent of cases, something goes awry and the egg implants outside the uterus. This is called an ectopic pregnancy. The vast majority of the time, it occurs inside one of the fallopian tubes, but the embryo can also take root in an ovary, the cervix, or the abdominal cavity.

Ectopic pregnancies are usually caused by a condition that slows or blocks the embryo's journey down the fallopian tube, giving it time to implant on the wall. Nearly half of cases are attributed to inflammation of the tubes, called salpingitis, or pelvic inflammatory disease, an inflammation of the uterus, fallopian tubes, or ovaries. Endometriosis (a condition in which uterine tissue grows outside the uterus), the sexually transmitted infections gonorrhea and chlamydia, and supplemental estrogen and progesterone (from fertility treatments, birth control pills, or the morning-after pill) are also potential causes.

For the first few weeks, a woman may believe that she has a normal pregnancy—she'll develop the same missed periods, nausea, and fatigue. But other symptoms of an ectopic pregnancy include vaginal bleeding, pain in the lower abdomen, and cramping on one side of the pelvis. Since an embryo can't grow and develop normally in a fallopian tube, about half of these pregnancies end naturally, sometimes with the rupture of the tube, which is a medical emergency. Today, most ectopic pregnancies are diagnosed early by sonograms, well before they rupture. They can be treated with the drug methotrexate or by laparoscopic surgery to destroy or remove the embryo.

ADDITIONAL FACTS

1. *In some cases, a woman can become pregnant after having her tubes tied. If the procedure fails and she becomes pregnant, chances are it will be an ectopic pregnancy.*

2. *If a woman has previously had an ectopic pregnancy, the risk that she'll have another is higher.*

3. *Ectopic pregnancies are known as tubal pregnancies, because more than 90 percent occur in the fallopian tubes.*

4. *In Greek, the word* ectopic *means "out of place."*

✦✦✦

Pap Test

A Pap test checks for changes in the cells of a woman's cervix. The cervix is the lower part of the uterus, where the uterus opens to the vagina. The test is important because it can find cancer cells or cells that may turn cancerous.

To perform a Pap test, a doctor or nurse inserts an instrument called a speculum in the vagina in order to see the cervix and take a sample of cells from inside and outside the cervix. For a satisfactory sample, it is important not to put anything, including douches or tampons, into the vagina for 2 days before the test. The cervical cells collected are smeared onto a glass slide and examined under a microscope for abnormalities.

Women should have a Pap test every 3 years at a minimum once they become sexually active or when they turn 21. However, a woman should speak with her health care professional to determine how often she should have the test based on her age, the results of previous Pap tests, her medical history, whether she has human papillomavirus (HPV), and whether she smokes. Women can stop having the tests at age 70 if the results of their Pap tests in the past 10 years have been normal, according to the US Department of Health and Human Services.

HPV infection is the main risk factor for cervical cancer and is often the cause of abnormal Pap test results. However, most women infected with HPV have normal Pap test results. Only a very small percentage of women with untreated HPV develop cervical cancer.

A woman who has an abnormal Pap test result may need further testing, such as colposcopy or biopsy. Colposcopy allows a doctor to look at the cervix through a device that is similar to a microscope. If he or she sees abnormal cells, a cervical biopsy may be needed.

ADDITIONAL FACTS

1. *The Greek-born physician George Papanicolaou (1883–1962) invented the Pap test, named for him, in 1928.*

2. *The test was first proven to be diagnostic of cervical cancer in 1943 but was not incorporated into routine gynecologic practice until the 1950s.*

3. *After the Pap test came into use, cancer of the cervix stopped being the leading cause of death from gynecologic cancer. The test's ability to detect precancerous changes and allow for early treatment has helped make the treatment of cervical cancer a model for cancer care.*

❖❖❖

Bone Marrow Transplant

Bone marrow is spongy, fatty tissue inside of bones that develops into blood cells for the rest of the body. If a person has an immune-deficiency disorder, however, or a cancer such as leukemia, bone marrow cells can become diseased or be destroyed. Such diseases are frequently fatal, which prompted researchers in the 20th century to search for ways of replacing damaged marrow.

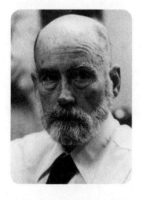

E. Donnall Thomas (1920–), a physician at Fred Hutchinson Cancer Research Center in Seattle, was the first to demonstrate a treatment for leukemia that involved removing the diseased marrow and immediately replacing it with a transfusion of healthy marrow. He performed this procedure for the first time in 1956: A leukemia patient received bone marrow cells from his identical twin brother, and the patient's body accepted those cells and used them to produce new, healthy blood cells.

Developments in immune-suppressing drugs, as well as techniques for identifying closely matched donors, allowed Thomas to perform the first transplant in 1969 on two relatives who were not twins. Although finding an unrelated donor wasn't easy, it finally proved possible: In 1973, a team at Memorial Sloan-Kettering Cancer Center in New York performed a transplant on a 5-year-old patient whose donor was found in Denmark through a Copenhagen blood bank.

Today, people with leukemia, lymphoma, sickle-cell anemia, and some other diseases may be treated with bone marrow transfusions. Finding a suitable donor remains a challenge, however, and patients are known to wait years for an appropriate match. If a person has diseased bone marrow, he or she will need a donor with a matching tissue type; this type of transfusion is called allogeneic. Another type of transfusion, called autologous, may be performed if a person's bone marrow is healthy but he or she needs to undergo a harmful procedure, such as high doses of chemotherapy or radiation for cancer. In this case, bone marrow cells are harvested beforehand and injected back into the bloodstream afterward to speed recovery.

ADDITIONAL FACTS

1. *Thomas, along with the physician Joseph Murray (1919–), who pioneered the field of kidney transplants, received the Nobel Prize in Physiology or Medicine in 1990.*

2. *The National Marrow Donor Program began connecting patients with unrelated bone marrow donors in 1987 and today has a registry of more than 7 million donors.*

3. *Baboon cells are resistant to HIV. In 1995, doctors transfused baboon bone marrow into Jeff Getty (1957–2006), a man with AIDS, in the hope that the immune cells would replace those Getty had lost. Although the transfusion did not work as well as doctors hoped, Getty lived with the disease for another 11 years.*

✦✦✦

Congenital Heart Disease

In 1 in 100 births, an infant is born with a defect or malformation of the heart, called congenital heart disease. This birth defect needs to be carefully monitored: Some cases require surgery, while others eventually heal on their own.

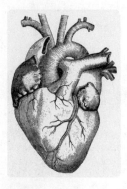

Doctors usually first pinpoint congenital heart disease by detecting a murmur, or an unusual sound, when listening to the heartbeat. Another screening, such as an echocardiogram, chest x-ray, or cardiac MRI scan, is used to make a diagnosis. But because some types of congenital heart disease don't produce any symptoms, many cases go undetected until well into adulthood.

One of the most common types of congenital heart disease is a septal defect, or a hole in the partition between the right and left atria or ventricles of the heart. Other types of disorders are heart valve problems, such as mitral, tricuspid, pulmonic, or aortic stenosis. These occur when one of the valves narrows, blocking the flow of blood into or through the heart, depriving the body or lungs of adequate bloodflow, and stressing the heart muscle. Yet another type of disorder is the transposition, or switching, of the aorta and the pulmonary artery, reducing the amount of oxygenated blood that reaches the tissues.

Experts aren't sure what, exactly, leads to congenital heart defects, but research shows that newborns with genetic abnormalities, such as Down syndrome, are at increased risk. Babies are also more likely to have a heart defect when the mother takes certain prescription medications or abuses drugs or alcohol during early pregnancy or is affected by a viral infection, such as rubella, during the first trimester. Treatments for congenital heart disease, which depend on the type and severity of the defect, include prescription medications and surgical procedures. If left untreated, congenital heart disease can lead to hypertension, heart infections, and even heart failure.

ADDITIONAL FACTS

1. *In the 1970s, nearly one in three surgeries to repair congenital heart defects ended in death. But, thanks to medical advances, deaths have dropped to only 5 percent.*

2. *Heart defects that lead to oxygen deprivation in the blood are called cyanotic, a word derived from the Greek word for "blue." When a heart defect shunts blood away from the lungs, oxygen deprivation in the blood can tint skin a blue color.*

3. *Babies with cyanotic heart disease used to be called blue babies.*

◆◆◆

Phlebitis

The meaning of *phlebitis,* an inflammation of the wall of a vein, is easy to remember if you speak Greek: It contains the word *phleb* ("vein") and the suffix *-itis* ("inflammation"). A number of factors can lead to this condition, including physical trauma, cancer, an infection of the tissues near the vein, and a lack of circulation due to bed rest or hours of prolonged sitting during a long trip.

This inflammation, over time, can lead to a blood clot—a condition called thrombophlebitis. The severity of each case depends on where the clot is located. Most often, the clots occur in superficial veins, those right under the skin's surface. This type of phlebitis, which can cause redness and tenderness, is rarely serious and usually resolves on its own. Obesity, varicose veins, and blood clotting diseases increase the risk of this condition.

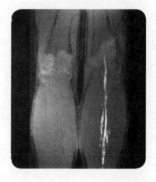

A red, swollen, painful leg can signal deep vein thrombosis. Deep vein thrombosis occurs when a larger clot clogs a vein deeper in the leg. This raises the risk of all or part of the clot breaking off and traveling to different areas of the body, causing an embolism. When an embolism blocks a vein draining to the lungs, it can result in a life-threatening pulmonary embolism.

To diagnose phlebitis, physicians usually perform an ultrasound with Doppler flow or an MRI to examine the veins. Wearing support hose to improve blood circulation and taking anticlotting drugs may be recommended. In more serious situations, a surgically inserted bypass or vein filter may be necessary.

ADDITIONAL FACTS

1. *The word* thrombo *means "clot."*

2. *Experts recommend that people with superficial phlebitis put their feet up to improve circulation.*

3. *Moving your feet, wiggling your toes, and avoiding prolonged sitting can help prevent clots from forming in your leg veins.*

◆◆◆

Osteopathy

Osteopathy is a field of medicine dedicated to treating and healing the entire patient, rather than focusing on one body part or symptom. In most parts of the world, osteopathy is considered an alternative therapy, and those who practice it are called osteopaths. In the United States, however, doctors of osteopathic medicine (DOs) are the legal and professional equivalent of medical doctors (MDs), and a majority of them use similar techniques and treatments.

Although its principles date back to Hippocrates (c. 460–c. 377 BC), osteopathic medicine officially began in the United States in 1874. Osteopathy's founder, Andrew Taylor Still (1828–1917), was a doctor who believed that many 19th-century medications and surgeries were useless. Instead, he believed that the body can largely heal itself. He studied the attributes of good health and pioneered the concepts of wellness and preventive medicine—such as eating properly and exercising—instead of just treating disease.

Still also held some beliefs that have since been disproved: He thought that all disease was caused by mechanical interference within the nerves and blood supply, that he could diagnose these diseases by feeling the body with his hands, and that these diseases could be cured by manipulation of displaced bones, nerves, and muscles. His autobiography states that he could "shake a child and stop scarlet fever, croup, diphtheria, and cure whooping cough in three days by a wring of its neck." This idea of osteopathic manipulative treatment (OMT) is still taught today, although most osteopathic physicians only use OMT in addition to conventional medical treatments.

Like an MD, a doctor of osteopathic medicine completes 4 years of basic medical education and can choose to practice in any specialty, such as surgery, emergency medicine, or pediatrics. Osteopathic physicians also receive an additional 300 to 500 hours in the study of hands-on manipulation of the body's musculoskeletal system. They are taught to evaluate patients' overall health and to act as educators about healthy lifestyle and well-being.

ADDITIONAL FACTS

1. *There are 20 accredited colleges of osteopathic medicine and about 44,000 osteopathic practitioners in the United States.*

2. *Approximately 65 percent of practicing osteopathic physicians specialize in primary care areas, such as pediatrics, family practice, obstetrics and gynecology, and internal medicine.*

3. *While osteopathy and mainstream medicine practices are similar in the United States, osteopathic organizations claim that osteopathy is a more comprehensive form of care.*

◆◆◆

Neurosis

Some people have mental disorders that affect their ability to think rationally or live a normal life. Others have slight mental imbalances that cause distress and shape their development but that don't consume them completely—call them annoying quirks or nervous habits. Though they're not as severe as psychoses (which often involve delusions and hallucinations), these quirks may still prevent people from adapting to a new environment or bettering their own lives. In the field of psychoanalysis, these tendencies are called neuroses.

In general, a neurosis is one of a group of psychological problems involving persistent negative emotions, such as anxiety, depression, anger, confusion, or low sense of self-worth. Symptoms of neurosis may include impulsive acts, lethargy, defensiveness, disturbing thoughts, habitual fantasizing, and negativity and cynicism. The personal relationships of a neurotic person are often overly dependent, aggressive, or socially or culturally inappropriate.

Scientists believe that there are hereditary conditions, including traits such as emotional instability and extremely high or low conscientiousness, that make a person more likely to develop neuroses. How well a person's upbringing and education prepares him or her for the stresses of life also plays a role. If an individual doesn't have an adequate support system, such as parents who show love and provide security, feelings of anxiety and incompleteness may begin to develop. Finally, one or more events will trigger the apprehension, anger, and defensive thinking associated with neurosis. Often the event is a situation involving personal relationships that overwhelms the person's ability to cope—an overweight teenager being repeatedly made fun of in school, for example. These situations can form lasting impressions that determine how a person views the world for the rest of his or her life.

While childhood and adolescence are the most common times to develop neuroses, people may be vulnerable into adulthood and even later in life. Anxiety about finding a partner and a successful job in order to have children and financial security or dealing with the illness and death of a loved one may trigger a neurosis at any time if a person has not been ingrained with proper coping mechanisms and support.

ADDITIONAL FACTS

1. *Neuroses seem to run in families—perhaps because of genetic predisposition and also because of similar child-raising styles passed down to new generations. But not all people with neuroses will raise neurotic children, and not all neurotic people have parents with neuroses.*

2. *The term* neurosis *was most influentially defined by Carl Jung (1875–1961) and Sigmund Freud (1856–1939), but is no longer used in psychiatric diagnosis.*

3. *Neuroses can sometimes be treated or improved with talk therapy, behavioral therapy, or antidepressant or antianxiety medications.*

Miscarriage

About one in three or four pregnancies ends with the loss of the fetus in what's called a miscarriage, or spontaneous abortion. The majority of miscarriages occur during the earliest stages—the first trimester, or 13 weeks of pregnancy. In fact, many women may not even realize they were pregnant.

Some miscarriages come from "chemical pregnancies," in which a positive test is noted but the pregnancy is lost shortly after a fertilized egg implants itself in the uterus. As a result, a woman may bleed excessively around the time of her period.

Although a number of factors increase the likelihood of having a miscarriage, experts often aren't able to pinpoint the exact cause. Miscarriages can result from chromosomal abnormalities or a health condition of the mother, such as a hormonal problem, diabetes, thyroid disease, an infection, a cervical abnormality, or an auto-immune disorder. Lifestyle factors, such as drinking alcohol, smoking cigarettes, or taking drugs, also raise the risk of pregnancy loss. Caffeine plays a role as well: A recent study found that women who took in more than 200 milligrams of caffeine daily, or more than the amount in about 2 cups of coffee, were twice as likely to have a miscarriage as those who didn't consume any.

In many miscarriages, women don't require further treatment. But if there's any remaining tissue in the uterus, a gynecologist will recommend a procedure called dilation and curettage, in which the cervix is dilated and the tissue is removed. Another option is a prescription drug called misoprostol, which helps the uterus clear itself.

ADDITIONAL FACTS

1. *About 70 percent of women who experience repeated miscarriages eventually give birth.*

2. *The risk of a couple experiencing a miscarriage increases after age 35 in women and 40 in men.*

◆◆◆

Colonoscopy

A colonoscopy is a procedure that enables a doctor to examine the lining of a person's colon, or large intestine. The screening is conducted by inserting a flexible fiber optic or video endoscope into the anus and slowly up into the rectum and colon. Sometimes patients undergo a less invasive procedure called a virtual colonoscopy, which uses MRI or computed tomography scans to produce three-dimensional images of the colon and rectum.

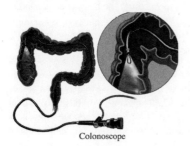
Colonoscope

Before the procedure, you will need to make sure that your colon is completely clean. Usually this requires consuming a large volume of a special cleansing solution or clear liquids and special laxatives. Some drugs interfere with the preparation or the exam, so you should make sure your doctor knows in advance if you're taking any medications.

Colonoscopies usually last 15 to 60 minutes and rarely cause any pain. It is possible that you will feel pressure, bloating, or cramping. You may be given a sedative to help you relax and tolerate any discomfort.

If your doctor thinks you need additional evaluation, during the examination he or she may obtain a biopsy to be analyzed. Sometimes polyps are found during the procedure, and the doctor is likely to remove them right then. Polyps are abnormal growths in the colon lining that are usually noncancerous. But because cancer can start in polyps, removing them is essential for preventing colorectal cancer.

ADDITIONAL FACTS

1. *After a colonoscopy, you should not drive yourself home or stay alone if you were given a sedative. You may have cramping and bloating because of the air that enters the colon during the examination. This will disappear quickly as you pass gas. You'll probably be able to eat right away, unless you had a polyp removed. In that case, your activity may be restricted as well as your diet.*

2. *Complications from colonoscopy are rare, but it is possible that a tear in the bowel wall requiring surgery could occur. Additionally, sometimes bleeding occurs at the site of a biopsy or the removal of a polyp. You should contact your doctor immediately if you have severe abdominal pain, fever and chills, or a lot of rectal bleeding.*

✦✦✦

Implantable Pacemaker

A pacemaker is a small, battery-operated device that is placed under the skin of the chest or abdomen to help control abnormal heart rhythms that may cause dizziness, shortness of breath, or fainting. The device uses electrical pulses to prompt the heart to beat at a normal, consistent rate.

The idea behind the pacemaker first surfaced in 1889, when the Scottish doctor John McWilliam suggested that electrical impulses might help regulate an irregular heartbeat. In 1928, the Australian physicians Mark Lidwell and Edgar Booth devised a plug-in device similar to a modern-day defibrillator. The American physiologist Albert Hyman first used the term *artificial pacemaker* when describing his invention of an external device powered by a hand-cranked motor.

The first pacemaker placed inside a human body—with electrodes wired directly to the heart—was implanted in 1958 at Karolinska University in Sweden. That device failed in 3 hours, and a replacement lasted 2 days. (The patient received 26 different pacemakers during his lifetime and lived to age 86.) Early pacemakers relied on mercury-zinc and rechargeable nickel-cadmium batteries, which had to be replaced often or sometimes caused death by battery failure.

In 1967 came the development of a longer-lasting lithium battery, which allowed pacemakers to last between 2 and 10 years in the body. Also that year, scientists developed a hermetically sealed metal case to hold the pacemaker—a way to prevent body fluids from leaking into it and interfering with its function.

Today, pacemakers weigh about 1 ounce and can be implanted with the use of a local anesthetic. A tiny computer generator sends electrical impulses to the leads (the wires that attach to the heart), which are inserted in a vein and fed through to the heart. These computers can even sense the changing patterns of the heartbeat and adjust automatically to the body's demands. The pacemaker's battery must be replaced periodically, but some continue working for up to 15 years. Devices such as cell phones, microwave ovens, and airport screening systems are unlikely to interfere with pacemakers, but patients should be wary of these possibilities.

ADDITIONAL FACTS

1. *The leading producer of pacemakers today released its first model—a wearable external pacemaker not much larger than a paperback book—in 1957.*

2. *Pacemaker research in the 1930s and 1940s was not well received by the public; scientists were seen to be "reviving the dead" by manipulating heart rhythms.*

3. *In 1958, researchers developed a new and improved way of attaching electrodes to the heart by using a plastic patch with two embedded, needlelike electrodes that was sutured to the heart and concentrated the electrical field where it was needed. This "Hunter-Roth electrode" required about 70 percent less current than previous pacemaker systems had.*

✦✦✦

Attention Deficit Disorder

In 1798, Alexander Crichton (1763–1856), a Scottish physician, described a mental state he had observed in people, especially children. These patients, he said, had an "unnatural degree of mental restlessness." Today, experts say this is the earliest description of attention deficit disorder (ADD), a chronic condition of poor attention and easy distractibility. It's often grouped together with impulsiveness and hyperactivity, or attention-deficit/hyperactivity disorder (ADHD).

Up to 5 percent of children have ADD or ADHD; symptoms of the condition can appear as early as infancy and usually manifest before the age of 7. They include not listening, forgetfulness, and being unable to pay attention to tasks or during play. These symptoms can interfere with social relationships and cause problems in school and activities. When the symptoms persist for 6 months or more, the diagnosis is usually ADD. ADD is easier to spot in boys; they are more prone to hyperactivity and disruptive behavior, while girls are more likely to daydream.

Although scientists aren't certain of the exact cause of ADD, they believe that genes may be a factor. It's believed that people with the disorder may have altered brain function; brain scans reveal that individuals with ADD and ADHD have less activity in the areas that control attention and concentration. Experts suggest that exposure to drugs and environmental toxins, such as polychlorinated biphenyls, during gestation or infancy may affect the development of nerve cells, raising the risk of the conditions.

Once diagnosed, ADD and ADHD are treated with counseling and prescription medications, such as methylphenidate (Ritalin) and amphetamine and dextroamphetamine (Adderall). These pills help balance out levels of brain chemicals called neurotransmitters. Many children eventually outgrow ADD and ADHD, but some 30 to 60 percent will have the condition well into adulthood.

ADDITIONAL FACTS

1. *One in four children with ADHD has at least one relative with the condition.*

2. *Research shows that children who are exposed to high levels of lead are more likely to show symptoms of ADD or ADHD.*

◆◆◆

Edema

After a long day of walking or standing, you may notice that your shoes are a little more snug than usual. That's because you're experiencing edema. Also called dropsy, this condition occurs when tiny blood vessels leak fluid. In response, the kidneys retain sodium and water, which causes more fluid to leak out. This fluid often pools in the surrounding tissue, leading to puffy, swollen body parts—most often the hands, feet, ankles, and legs.

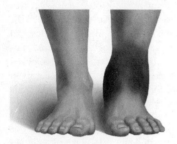

There are two main forms of this condition: The first and more common is called pitting edema. With this type, applying pressure to the swollen area for 15 seconds leaves an indentation, and the skin in the affected area is often stretched and shiny. Mild cases are caused by pregnancy, varicose veins, certain prescription medications, and sitting or standing for extended periods of time. Consuming too much sodium, which leads the body to retain water, is another factor. Other underlying causes include heart disease, kidney disease, deep vein thrombosis, varicose veins, and other medical conditions that impair circulation.

The second type is nonpitting edema, in which pressure doesn't leave a mark. Usually striking the legs or arms, it's the result of disorders of the lymphatic system, or it may stem from injury or hyperthyroidism. Both types of edema are treated by addressing the underlying medical cause of the swelling. Taking a diuretic and limiting sodium intake may also help improve symptoms. Physical therapy, massage, and wrapping or using elastic supports on the affected areas sometimes help as well.

ADDITIONAL FACTS

1. *Congenital lymphedema due to abnormal lymph vessels is known as Milroy's disease.*

2. *Sunburns is another cause of edema.*

3. *Removal of lymph nodes during cancer surgery can cause lymphedema.*

✦✦✦

Acupuncture

One of the oldest healing practices in the world, acupuncture originated in China thousands of years ago. The practice of stimulating specific points on the body, often by puncturing the skin with needles, is intended to restore health by removing blockages in the flow of chi, a person's vital energy or life force.

In the field of traditional Chinese medicine, the body is regulated by two opposing and inseparable forces: yin, which represents the cold, slow, or passive principle; and yang, which represents the hot, excited, or active principle. Good health is maintained by keeping these forces in balance, while an imbalance causes blockages in the flow of chi—the life force responsible for spiritual, emotional, mental, and physical health—and subsequently leads to illness or disease. According to traditional Chinese medicine, chi travels along pathways known as meridians and can be unblocked by stimulating points on the body connected with these meridians. There are between 14 and 20 meridians in the body, and they form a weblike matrix of at least 2,000 "acupoints."

Acupuncture became popular in America in the 1970s, incorporating traditions from China, Japan, Korea, and other countries. It is considered a form of complementary and alternative medicine and has been claimed to be helpful in treating chronic pain, osteoarthritis, infertility, and bladder control problems. A 2008 Duke University study, for example, found that acupuncture worked better than drugs such as aspirin to reduce the severity and frequency of chronic headaches. Western scientists believe that acupuncture stimulates the brain and spinal cord to release neurochemicals and hormones that can dull pain, boost immunity, and regulate body functions.

The most common form of acupuncture involves penetrating the skin with hair-thin, solid metal needles. Though the needles deter some people, acupuncture performed correctly causes little or no pain, and complications are rare.

ADDITIONAL FACTS

1. *An estimated 8.2 million US adults have received acupuncture treatment at some time in their lives.*

2. *In most acupuncture procedures, the needle is inserted less than a half inch into the body, but in some cases it may occasionally extend 3 inches or more.*

3. *Other forms of acupuncture include using physical pressure instead of needles (acupressure), needles with electrical stimulation, heat or sound waves to stimulate acupoints, and heated glass cups that stick to the skin with a vacuumlike suction (cupping). A 2008 Swiss study found that acupuncture works equally well with or without needle penetration.*

✦✦✦

Panic Disorder

A sudden, intense anxiety that leaves you feeling out of control or afraid for your life is called a panic attack. These attacks may make you short of breath or dizzy and you may feel as if you're having a heart attack or are going to be sick. If they happen often and without warning, you may have panic disorder.

People with panic disorder have frequent panic attacks without justifiable reason. Scientists aren't sure what causes them, but it seems that the body's fight-or-flight response—a defense mechanism that shortens reaction time and prepares a person to face (or flee from) a perceived threat—is activated even when there is no real danger. The attacks may result from an imbalance of chemicals in the brain, a health problem such as an overactive thyroid or depression, alcohol or drug abuse, or overuse of nicotine or caffeine.

Attacks are often triggered by agoraphobia—fear of being in a crowd or in open spaces, such as shopping malls. About one-third of people with panic disorder become homebound or cannot confront a feared situation without being accompanied by someone they trust.

Symptoms of panic attacks include feelings of intense fear or anxiety, difficulty breathing, chest pains or tightness, racing heartbeat, sweating, dizziness, nausea, and numbness that can last from 5 to 20 minutes. Attacks can occur at any time, even during sleep. When a person begins to change his or her daily activities for fear of suffering another attack—or begins to worry incessantly about when another one will occur—it's a good sign that he or she may have panic disorder. Panic attacks often begin in late adolescence or early adulthood, but not everyone who has one or two attacks will develop full-blown panic disorder.

Counseling and medication, often combined, can be effective in treating panic disorder. Early treatment can help prevent related conditions, such as depression and substance abuse, and can keep people from having future attacks and becoming further disabled by avoiding places where these attacks occur.

ADDITIONAL FACTS

1. *Symptoms of an anxiety attack typically peak at about 10 minutes, although they can last much longer.*

2. *Twice as many women as men have panic disorder. The condition affects about 1 in 75 people.*

3. *People with a depressed or bipolar parent have a higher risk of developing panic disorder.*

◆◆◆

Infertility

The act of conception is a complicated chain of events—one misstep and everything falls apart. So it's no wonder that 12 percent of women each year have trouble getting pregnant, according to the Centers for Disease Control and Prevention. When a couple doesn't succeed after a year of trying, or if the woman has repeat miscarriages, that's called infertility.

Infertility can be traced back to either the male or the female. Because of a genetic flaw, illness, or injury, a man may produce too little sperm or none at all, or produce sperm with a mobility problem. Without the normal ability to swim, sperm are unable to make their way to the egg to fertilize it. In women, infertility is often the result of an ovulation issue. A blocked fallopian tube (typically caused by pelvic inflammatory disease or endometriosis) or uterine fibroids can prevent the egg from reaching the uterus. Age is another factor for women, as the number of healthy eggs for ovulation declines slowly every year after age 35 and rapidly after age 40.

Fortunately, the field of assisted reproductive technology has grown enormously over the past decade. Doctors can now prescribe medications to regulate the hormones that govern ovulation. They are also able to perform in vitro fertilization to improve a couple's chances. These days, two out of three couples who are treated for infertility go on to have children.

ADDITIONAL FACTS

1. *Some 20 percent of women wait until after age 35 to begin families, which is one reason the number of infertile couples has risen. One in three couples in which the woman is over age 35 has problems with childbearing.*

2. *Lifestyle factors, such as diet, weight, stress, multiple sexual partners, and exposure to environmental toxins, may increase the likelihood of infertility.*

3. *Infertility is an issue of the male in about 30 percent of cases.*

✦✦✦

Mammograms

Mammograms are the best screening tool for early detection of breast cancer and other problems with a woman's breasts. The earlier breast cancer is found, the better chance a woman has of survival and the more treatment choices are available. In a mammogram, a low-dose x-ray takes pictures of both breasts. The images are recorded on x-ray film or, in the case of a digital mammogram, saved to a computer.

Mammograms are effective because they let the doctor have a detailed look within the breasts to search for lumps and breast tissue changes that may not be detectable during a breast examination. If a lump is found, your doctor will probably order other tests, such as an ultrasound or biopsy to look for cancer or indications that cancer may develop. Breast lumps and growths are not necessarily cancerous.

The two types of mammograms are screening mammograms and diagnostic mammograms. A screening mammogram is performed on women who have no symptoms of breast cancer. It is recommended that all women undergo a screening mammogram annually beginning at age 40. A diagnostic mammogram is done when a woman has breast cancer symptoms or a lump. Usually more pictures are taken during this type of mammogram.

During a mammogram, a radiologic technologist will place your breasts one at a time between two plastic plates, which will press your breasts until they're flat. Although this may be painful, it is important because the flatter your breasts are the better the picture.

Because implants can hide breast tissue, women with breast implants should make sure that the radiologic technologist administering the mammogram is trained in x-raying patients with implants. Breast tissue may need to be lifted away from the implant to get a picture.

ADDITIONAL FACTS

1. *A mammogram should be performed along with an examination by your doctor. There are some cancers that cannot be detected by a mammogram but may be detected by a physical exam.*

2. *Women should check their own breasts monthly for lumps or other changes. Breast self-exams should be performed in addition to a physical exam by a doctor and an annual screening mammogram.*

✦✦✦

Berson, Yalow, and Radioimmunoassay

Blood tests are a powerful diagnostic tool that can allow doctors to detect diseases that may be lurking in the body. One of the most important types, called a radioimmunoassay, was developed in the 1950s by two researchers who stumbled upon the idea while conducting diabetes research.

A radioimmunoassay (RIA) test uses radioactive particles to detect diseases like hepatitis in the bloodstream. When it was invented, RIA was far more sensitive than any other blood test then available to doctors. Instead of looking for the disease itself, radioimmunoassay tests work by searching for the antibodies that the body produces to fight a disease—a telltale sign of infection.

The RIA was the brainchild of American physicians Solomon Berson (1918–1972) and Rosalyn Yalow (1921–), who were co-workers at a veteran's hospital in the Bronx. The duo were seeking to solve a long-standing problem in diabetes treatment: When a patient was given animal insulin, the substance initially kept blood sugar low, but soon the patient's body developed resistance to the animal hormone, weakening its effectiveness.

Yalow and Berson theorized that animal insulin must provoke an immune reaction in the body. If so, they realized, there would be antibodies in the bloodstream. To test this hypothesis, the devised the first RIA to look for antibodies and track the effects of animal insulin in the body.

The test helped them develop a better understanding of how the body responds to animal insulin. But it soon dawned on Berson and Yalow that the same method could be used to look for antibodies directed at many other kinds of molecules associated with other hormones, drugs, diseases and infections, and many other agents. Berson and Yalow published their results in 1959, opening up a breakthrough technology to the scientific community.

The RIA test may detect a recent or chronic infection because it can take weeks or months for antibodies to appear, and antibodies may still be present after an infection has passed. Radioimmunoassay remains helpful in many medical settings and in medical research, although numerous new technologies are being used as well.

ADDITIONAL FACTS

1. *Along with Andrew Schally (1926–) and Roger Guillemin (1924–), Rosalyn Yalow received the Nobel Prize in Physiology or Medicine in 1977 for pioneering work in the field of diabetes. Berson did not live to share the prize with her; he died of a heart attack in 1972.*

2. *Berson and Yalow could have worked with any number of hormones in their early work, but they chose insulin because it was readily available and easy to work with—and possibly because Yalow's husband had diabetes, which gave her a special interest in the research.*

3. *Berson and Yalow never patented their invention. "Patents are about keeping things away from people for the purpose of making money," Yalow explained. "We wanted others to be able to use [radioimmunoassay]."*

✦✦✦

Black-and-Blue Mark

Maybe your child took a spill during a bike ride or bumped into a table while running around the living room. For whatever reason, there's an ugly black-and-blue mark on her leg. These common injuries occur when the connective tissue and muscle are damaged. Blood from small vessels called capillaries leaks out and pools beneath the skin, forming a bruise. It's probably the most common childhood injury, but we seldom stop to ask why it goes through all those changes.

As the body reabsorbs the blood, the bruise changes colors accordingly. At first, it appears reddish as the blood gathers, but as the iron-containing blood substance hemoglobin breaks down, the mark becomes blue or purplish black. As the blood continues to disintegrate, a green pigment called biliverdin forms after about a week, making the skin appear green or yellow. Eventually, the bruise completely fades away, usually in about 2 weeks.

How easily you bruise depends on a variety of factors. Some people have more delicate tissue than others, leaving them more vulnerable. Children have thinner skin than adults and are more likely to bruise because they are more active. Certain medications, such as blood thinners and aspirin, also lead to bruising, and older people are at an increased risk because capillary walls weaken with age and break more easily. Low blood platelet levels and certain diseases, such as Cushing's syndrome, may predispose a person toward bruising.

To slow bloodflow to the area and speed healing, apply an ice or cold pack to the injured area as soon as a bruise begins to form. You can also elevate the bruised area in order to slow the influx of blood. But if your child suddenly experiences large or painful bruises for no known reason, or black-and-blue marks are accompanied by abnormal bleeding elsewhere, such as from the nose or gums, consult a physician. These symptoms may signal a more serious issue, such as a blood-related disease or blood clotting problem.

ADDITIONAL FACTS

1. *Black-and-blue marks are also known as contusions or ecchymoses. The term* ecchymosis *comes from the Greek words* ekchymousthai *("to pour out") and* chymos *("juice").*

2. *There are three types of bruises: The most common, subcutaneous, occur directly beneath the skin. Intramuscular bruises happen in the underlying muscle, while periosteal ones occur on the bones.*

◆◆◆

Hypertension

Hypertension, or high blood pressure, is often called a silent killer, because the condition usually has no symptoms. If left untreated, high blood pressure can lead to heart disease and stroke. That's worrisome, considering that one in three Americans currently has the condition—but nearly a third of them don't know it.

Blood pressure is a measure of the force in the arteries when the heart muscle contracts (called systolic pressure) and when the heart relaxes (called diastolic pressure). Hypertension occurs when blood vessels narrow or become less flexible, a condition called arteriosclerosis, which increases resistance and requires the heart to work harder to pump blood throughout the body. This raises the risk of heart disease.

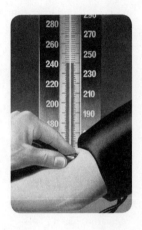

Measured in millimeters of mercury, or mmHg, hypertension is divided into different stages. Normal blood pressure in adults is 100 to 119 mmHg systolic over 70 to 79 mmHg diastolic (expressed as 100/70 to 119/79), while prehypertension (a precursor to the condition) ranges from 120/80 to 139/89. Stage 1 hypertension is 140/90 to 159/99, and stage 2 is 160/100 and above.

Several factors contribute to the development of high blood pressure, including kidney and adrenal disease, smoking, being overweight, genetics, and stress. Regularly consuming too much sodium is another major factor. Because blood pressure screenings are part of a general physical exam, doctors are able to detect the condition early on. If hypertension is found, a number of medications can help control it. Diuretics, beta-blockers, angiotensin converting enzyme inhibitors, and calcium channel blockers all work in different ways to relax blood vessels or reduce blood volume.

ADDITIONAL FACTS

1. *Although the Reverend Stephen Hales (1677–1761) was a botanist who primarily studied plants, he was the first person to effectively measure blood pressure, in 1733.*

2. *Following a diet that's rich in vegetables, whole grains, low-fat dairy, and lean protein and low in saturated fat and sodium can help tame blood pressure. This diet is known as the DASH diet (Dietary Approaches to Stop Hypertension); find out more at www.dashdiet.org.*

◆◆◆

Reflexology

In 1913, an ear, nose, and throat specialist named William Fitzgerald (1872–1942) introduced to the United States a practice he called zone therapy. He used vertical lines to divide the body into 10 zones, each of which was represented by specific areas on the hands and feet. The belief that massaging or pressing these areas can stimulate the flow of energy and nutrients, thereby healing ailments in the corresponding zone, is today known as reflexology.

The purpose of reflexology is not to treat or diagnose any specific medical disorder, but to promote better health and well-being in the same way that an exercise program or diet does. Reflexologists believe that pressure on the hands and feet (and sometimes the ears and face) triggers a release of stress and tension in the corresponding area or body zone, unblocking nerve impulses and improving blood supply to the entire body. The heart, for example, can be stimulated by putting pressure on the ball of the left foot, according to reflexologists.

Some reflexology proponents also believe that the practice can cleanse the body of toxins, improve circulation, assist in weight loss, improve organ health, and treat chronic health conditions, although there is no evidence to support these ideas and the field has many critics. Studies on asthma and premenstrual syndrome, for instance, have found no benefit from reflexology.

Since it is not legally recognized as a field of medicine, no formal training is required to practice reflexology—although some nurses and massage therapists offer reflexology as part of their licensed practices. Some schools, such as the International Institute of Reflexology in St. Petersburg, Florida, grant "certified member" status. And in 1995, the Reflexology Association of America was formed to help standardize the ethics and practices of reflexology across the country.

ADDITIONAL FACTS

1. *The most popular type of reflexology practiced in America is the Ingham method, named after Eunice Ingham (1889–1974), who coined the term* reflexology *in 1938.*

2. *Sandals, shoe inserts, and foot massage devices have been marketed based on reflexology theory. Manufacturers of these products are not allowed to make medical claims, however, and the products' benefits have not been studied.*

3. *Reflexology theory associates the big toe with the brain, the heel with the lower back, and the foot's arch with the kidneys.*

✦✦✦

Psychosis

Psychosis occurs when a person has trouble telling the difference between what is real and what's not. A person with psychosis may have delusions and hallucinations that cause strange behavior and changes in personality. The condition may be caused by alcohol or drug abuse, a brain tumor, dementia, stroke, depression, or other serious illness.

Symptoms of psychosis include confusion, disorganized thoughts and speech, mania, depression, and paranoia. Psychosis may be a temporary symptom of an illness, infection, or injury or it may be the primary indicator of a chronic psychotic disorder, such as schizophrenia. Scientists hypothesize that these disorders develop because the brain overreacts to certain neurotransmitter chemicals and sends the wrong signals. Doctors identify causes of psychosis by reviewing drug records and family history, testing for syphilis (one potential cause of mental illness), and performing brain scans and blood tests. Medications such as opioids, benzodiazepines, and digoxin may also be to blame, and some psychotic disorders tend to run in families. Even extreme stress or sleep deprivation can cause temporary psychosis.

A person with schizophrenia may develop psychotic symptoms as a young adult or during middle age. Many people with psychotic disorders, however, first develop symptoms during old age. As many as 1 out of every 50 elderly people has a psychotic disorder. Though many people function quite well in spite of having a psychotic disorder, others may become withdrawn, hostile, or depressed. They may believe that friends and family are plotting against them or lose the ability to take care of their personal hygiene.

People with psychosis often respond well to treatment with antipsychotic drugs, which can reduce auditory hallucinations (voices in a person's head) and delusions and help control thinking and behavior. Group or individual therapy may also be helpful. When psychosis develops as part of another problem, such as depression or sleep deprivation, appropriately treating that condition may lessen or stop the psychosis.

ADDITIONAL FACTS

1. *Temporary psychosis can be triggered by excessive alcohol use. If heavy drinking continues over the long term, psychosis can become chronic.*

2. *People with psychosis living in long-term care facilities such as nursing homes have better control of their symptoms when the staff remind them of who everyone around them is and reassure them of their safety.*

3. *Antipsychotic medications can have many side effects, including sedation, muscle stiffness, tremors, weight gain, restlessness, and increased risk of stroke. They may also cause tardive dyskinesia, a disorder in which a person exhibits one or more types of involuntary movements, such as puckering of the lips or writhing of the arms and legs.*

◆◆◆

Sperm Donor

For infertile couples or for women wishing to have children without a male partner, sperm banks are often the answer. These facilities supply sperm for use in in vitro fertilization or artificial insemination. The men who donate the semen specimens, which are later frozen, are called sperm donors.

To become a sperm donor typically requires a series of screening tests. In fact, it's estimated that 90 to 95 percent of applicants are rejected. The ideal candidate is a man between the ages of 18 and 35 who doesn't drink or smoke and is free of sexually transmitted infections. Sperm banks perform a full physical examination and ask to see a man's medical history to make sure he doesn't have any serious hereditary diseases swimming in his gene pool. Further testing for transmissible diseases, including HIV, is done, and repeated annually if the donor continues to provide his semen. After a semen sample is collected through masturbation, the sperm donor is usually compensated with a cash payment.

These men can choose between anonymous and non-anonymous sperm donation. When a man chooses to remain anonymous, his identity is fully withheld; the couple receiving the sperm may receive a limited amount of information, such as the donor's height, hair color, weight, and other physical attributes. In a non-anonymous donation, the donor allows his information to be revealed. Once the child turns 18, he or she may learn the identity of a non-anonymous genetic donor.

ADDITIONAL FACTS

1. *In the United States, sperm banks are regulated by the Food and Drug Administration.*

2. *Each state has its own law stipulating how many children can be born from one donor's sperm.*

✦✦✦

CA-125

CA-125 is a protein that is found in higher amounts in ovarian cancer cells than in other kinds of cells. This protein enters the bloodstream and can be measured with a CA-125 test, which consists of taking a blood sample from a vein and then measuring the level of CA-125 in the sample.

The test is usually used to evaluate ovarian cancer treatment for a woman who has already been diagnosed or to check on a woman whose cancer is in remission. Normal CA-125 values vary depending on the lab running the test. In general, levels below 35 units per milliliter are considered normal. In a woman who has been diagnosed with ovarian cancer, a decrease in CA-125 usually means the disease is responding to treatment. An increase in CA-125 typically indicates that the disease has gotten worse or has come back.

The CA-125 test is not an effective method of screening healthy women for ovarian cancer because the test has a high false positive rate—in other words, an elevated CA-125 level usually does not indicate ovarian cancer. But it can point to many problems, such as other types of cancer and many other conditions, including uterine fibroids, endometriosis, benign ovarian cysts, pelvic inflammatory disease, cirrhosis of the liver, and a first-trimester pregnancy.

If a healthy woman has an abnormal CA-125 test result, she will need further tests to confirm it and make a specific diagnosis. These tests could include surgical procedures that involve additional risks. Studies are being conducted to determine whether the CA-125 test can be effective for early diagnosis of ovarian cancer in healthy women if used in combination with other blood tests and sonograms. When the cancer is detected at its earliest stage and has not spread from the ovaries, more than 90 percent of women will live at least 5 years.

ADDITIONAL FACTS

1. *Only 1 in 3,000 women has ovarian cancer. However, 21,000 new cases of ovarian cancer are diagnosed in the United States annually.*

2. *Only 20 percent of ovarian cancer cases are detected early. When ovarian cancer is first detected at a later stage, after it has spread, only about 30 percent of women with this cancer will survive 5 years.*

3. *In the United States, 15,000 women die of the disease each year.*

♦♦♦

Stem Cells

Stem cells can be described as shape-shifters: They are young, undeveloped cells that have not yet been assigned an adult role. They are a biological blank slate that can be turned into almost any kind of tissue. For this reason, stem cells hold enormous medical potential—to create insulin-producing cells for people with diabetes or new brain cells for those with Parkinson's disease, for example. But because harvesting stem cells often involves the destruction of human embryos, research involving them has met with controversy.

In the early 1960s, the Canadian scientists James Till (1931–) and Ernest McCulloch (1926–) began experimenting with bone marrow cells injected into mice that had been weakened by radiation, much as humans would be after treatment for a cancer such as leukemia. They observed that tiny lumps grew on the spleens of the mice, and Till and McCulloch speculated that these "spleen colonies" arose from marrow cells they called colony-forming, or multipotent, cells. In 1961 and again in 1963, the pair published its results.

There are two main types of stem cells: Embryonic stem cells are not yet "differentiated" and are generally able to develop into more types of cells. Adult stem cells, which are found in the bone marrow, the brain, and other areas of the body, are less flexible and therefore not as highly valued by researchers. Stem cells can also come from the umbilical cord of a baby or the amniotic fluid of a pregnant woman.

The first stem cells grown in a lab were those of mice. In 1998, researchers at Johns Hopkins University in Baltimore and the University of Wisconsin in Madison successfully extracted and cultured the first human stem cells. One experiment used donated eggs and sperm to create blastocysts (3- to 5-day-old embryos consisting of about 100 cells); the other used cells from aborted fetuses.

Embryonic stem cell research has been opposed by people who believe that blastocysts are human life and are against abortion. This has created controversy and has led to a search for other sources of stem cells, including attempts to induce mature cells to revert to stem cells in the laboratory.

ADDITIONAL FACTS

1. *Congress restricted the study of stem cells in 1996, rules that were reinforced by President George W. Bush (1946–) in 2001 and limited federally funded researchers to using only existing stem cell lines. Some of those restrictions were lifted by President Barack Obama (1961–) in 2009.*

2. *In 2008, researchers at the University of California, San Francisco, created the first human embryonic stem cells developed without the destruction of a human embryo.*

3. *In 2009, University of Wisconsin–Madison researchers announced that they had changed skin cells back into stem cells, which they then turned into heart muscle cells.*

◆◆◆

Fracture

The human skeleton is quite an impressive feat of architecture: Our bones, though lightweight, are as strong as the reinforced concrete in a man-made bridge. But if too much force is applied—in a fall or car accident, for instance— those bones can split or break, resulting in a fracture.

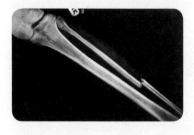

A broken bone leads to swelling, pain, bruising, and a misshapen or out-of-place limb or joint. The person can't apply pressure to the injured area and often can't move it without feeling extreme pain. A physician can diagnose the break by taking an x-ray or an other imaging test. There are three common types of fractures. In a closed, or simple, fracture, the skin around the bone isn't broken. An open, or compound, fracture occurs when the bone is part of an open wound, which raises the risk of infection. Lastly, stress fractures are small cracks in the bone caused by repetitive movements that put pressure on the bone, such as running.

Treatment for a fracture depends on the severity of the break, as well the patient's age. Stress fractures, which can heal on their own, may require only rest, ice packs, and painkillers. Closed and open fractures, however, may call for a sling or cast to reset the bone. In severe cases, devices such as screws, rods, or plates may be needed to replace lost bone or hold the bone in place as it heals. This act of bone setting can be traced throughout history: As far back as 10,000 BC, ancient Egyptians formed splints from tree bark wrapped in linen. Blacksmiths in medieval Europe made casts out of egg whites, flour, and animal fat. Thankfully, today's casts are fabricated from plaster or fiberglass.

ADDITIONAL FACTS

1. *A full break is called a complete fracture, while a partial one is called an incomplete fracture or greenstick.*

2. *Certain conditions, such as osteoporosis and other bone diseases, can increase the likelihood of fractures.*

✦✦✦

Hardening of the Arteries

Arteries are the freeways of the body, transporting food and oxygen in the bloodstream to the tissues. When healthy, these blood vessels are flexible, strong, and elastic. But hypertension, or high blood pressure, along with high cholesterol can cause them to become thick, stiff, and hard—a condition called arteriosclerosis.

The most common form of arteriosclerosis is atherosclerosis, although the terms are often used interchangeably. Derived from the Greek words *athero* ("gruel" or "paste") and *sclerosis* ("hardness"), it's a condition in which fatty substances, cholesterol, calcium, and other materials collect on the arteries' inner walls. This buildup, called plaque, hardens and may grow large enough to block bloodflow in an artery. If a plaque ruptures, a blood clot can form at the site, and if this clot blocks a small blood vessel that feeds the heart or brain, it can trigger a heart attack, embolism, or stroke by closing off the feeding vessel and so depriving the tissue of oxygen.

Hardening of the arteries is slowly progressive and takes years to develop, but it begins in late childhood. Although the exact cause of atherosclerosis is unknown, experts believe that it results from damage to the endothelium, the lining on the arteries' inner walls. This causes the blood to deposit platelets to repair the artery. Inflammation occurs, and a blood clot followed by organization into plaque can form. This damage is most frequently caused by high cholesterol, high blood pressure, smoking, and certain diseases, such as diabetes.

Atherosclerosis itself has few symptoms until its later stages. That's why physicians routinely screen for high cholesterol and blood pressure, two common signs of the condition. Doctors prescribe lifestyle changes, such as eating a healthful diet and exercising, to improve bloodflow and help control the arteries' deterioration. But there are also a variety of medications available, such as blood-thinning and anti-platelet drugs, as well as those for high cholesterol and high blood pressure.

ADDITIONAL FACTS

1. *More than 16 million Americans have atherosclerotic heart disease.*

2. *Chronic stress can raise blood pressure and, in turn, set the stage for atherosclerosis.*

3. *The German physician Felix Marchand (1846–1928) first introduced the term* atherosclerosis *in 1904.*

✦✦✦

St. John's Wort

An ancient remedy for depression, anxiety, and other mental disorders, *Hypericum perforatum,* a plant commonly known as St. John's wort, is still sometimes used as a supplement today. It should be taken cautiously, however, as it can interact with many medications.

Medicinal applications for St. John's wort were first recorded in ancient Greece, when its yellow flowers were used to prepare teas and tablets containing concentrated extracts. It has been used to treat wounds, burns, insect bites, and malaria, among other ailments.

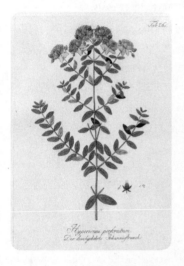

There is conflicting evidence about the herb's effectiveness against depression. Two large studies found that it was ineffective, while other evidence suggests it has a modest effect on mild cases.

Generally, St. John's wort is well tolerated in recommended doses for up to 3 months. However, because it affects the way the liver's cytochrome P450 enzyme system processes many drugs, the herb can speed up or slow down the breakdown of certain medications, including antidepressants, birth control pills, blood thinners, and drugs used to treat cancer or HIV infection. This can keep medications from working properly or may increase the severity of side effects such as high blood pressure, suicidal thoughts, or serotonin syndrome—a potentially fatal condition associated with the antidepressant MAO inhibitors, selective serotonin reuptake inhibitors, and serotonin-norepinephrine reuptake inhibitors. St. John's wort can also cause anxiety, dry mouth, gastrointestinal symptoms, fatigue, headache, decreased sexual function, and increased sensitivity to sunlight.

Early studies of *Hypericum* cream in the topical treatment of mild to moderate dermatitis (dry, irritated skin) have shown positive results. St. John's wort may also help calm nerve pain, premenstrual syndrome, and seasonal affective disorder, although more research is needed.

ADDITIONAL FACTS

1. *The flower of St. John's wort blooms in late June, close to the feast day of St. John the Baptist on June 24—hence the first part of the plant's name.* Wort *is an archaic term for medicinal plants.*

2. *St. John's wort is also known as amber touch-and-heal, balm-of-warrior's-wound, balsana, devil's scourge, and witcher's herb.*

3. *The flowers and stems of St John's wort have been used to produce red and yellow dyes.*

✦✦✦

Depression

Experiencing sadness or grief when an unhappy event occurs is normal. Being unable to bounce back from the situation, even after several weeks, is not. Depression is a mental illness that causes a person to feel sad and hopeless much of the time, to the point where it interferes with normal activities. It's more than just a bad mood: Studies have shown that physical changes in the brain contribute to depression, and many patients can't just "snap out of it."

Depression often runs in families, but it can happen to anyone at any time. A depressive episode may begin during an illness or a stressful event—such as childbirth or a death in the family—or may be linked to medication, alcohol, or illegal drug use. These triggers can interfere with the production of brain chemicals that regulate mood, causing people to become irritable, forgetful, or uninterested in things they used to enjoy. They may gain or lose weight, sleep too much or too little, or complain about pains that don't have a physical cause. Severe depression can lead to thoughts about or attempts at suicide. If a person experiences these symptoms consistently for more than 2 weeks, he or she may be diagnosed with depression.

Treatment for depression typically involves psychotherapy or cognitive behavioral therapy, in which patients talk to mental health professionals about potential causes of and solutions for their problems. More severe depression may require antidepressant medications that normalize chemicals in the brain, but it can take several tries to find a drug that's effective for a certain individual, and it usually takes a few weeks for the drug to start working. Some people need to take medication for the rest of their lives, because it's likely that they will relapse even after they've recovered. For extreme cases of depression that don't respond to other treatments, electroconvulsive therapy (ECT) may be used. The safety and effectiveness of ECT—electrical currents sent through the brain that trigger brief seizures—has improved, so this treatment can now provide hope where previously there was very little.

ADDITIONAL FACTS

1. *Women are twice as likely to suffer from depression as men are, but men are more likely to commit suicide because of it.*

2. *Specific diagnoses include psychotic depression (characterized by hallucinations or delusions), postpartum depression (occurring within a month after giving birth), and seasonal affective disorder (triggered by dark, cold winters). Having mild symptoms of depression for 2 years or longer is known as dysthymic disorder.*

3. *St. John's wort, an ancient herbal remedy for depression, is widely used as a supplement to fight depression; however, studies have shown that is ineffective against major depression.*

❖ ❖ ❖

Egg Donor

There are a variety of reasons why a woman might choose to become an egg donor: She might want to help an infertile couple bear children. Or, she might wish to further the advancement of science, or simply score the monetary compensation (about $3,000 to $5,000 per cycle). Whatever the motivation, her eggs are used for in vitro fertilization—they are fertilized by sperm to form an embryo, which is then implanted in another woman's uterus.

Becoming an egg donor is a long and complicated process, requiring several visits to the fertility clinic. Physicians screen for sexually transmitted and other infections and run blood tests to check for any genetic or psychiatric disorders. Most egg donors are healthy women between the ages of 21 and 35 who don't smoke or drink. After a woman is chosen, she must undergo fertility treatments to prepare her body for the harvesting of eggs. Women release only one egg per cycle, so doctors give egg donors hormones that stimulate the growth of multiple eggs for about 3 weeks. As a result, donors produce anywhere from 5 to 20 eggs in one cycle. These oocytes are removed from the ovary with a hollow needle in a process called follicular aspiration.

Like sperm donors, egg donors have the choice of remaining anonymous or having their identities made available to couples and their children. Sometimes couples ask a friend or relative to donate her eggs; such donors are called known donors.

ADDITIONAL FACTS

1. *More than half of the time, the donated eggs do not result in a successful pregnancy.*

2. *After being fertilized by the sperm, two or three of the healthiest-looking embryos are placed in the woman's uterus.*

3. *Twins and triplets are more common in such cases than in a normal pregnancy because multiple embryos are transferred.*

✦✦✦

PSA Testing

A PSA (prostate-specific antigen) test is a blood test commonly used to screen men for prostate cancer. PSA is a protein is made by the prostate gland. The test measures how much PSA is in a man's blood.

The prostate gland is found in men only and is about the size of a walnut. It produces and stores the fluid that carries sperm. The prostate is positioned just below the bladder, near the rectum (the last part of the bowel before the anus), and surrounds the urethra, which is the tube that drains urine from the bladder.

When there is a higher-than-normal level of PSA in a man's blood or his PSA level has increased over time, it is an indication that he may have prostate cancer or a noncancerous enlargement of the prostate. If a PSA test is abnormal, a doctor may order other tests, including a prostate gland biopsy to check for cancerous cells. This is because the PSA test is not specific for cancer.

PSA testing can help find cancer at an early stage, when it is relatively small and before it causes symptoms. The PSA test is also used to monitor existing prostate cancer to determine whether it has spread. A serial PSA blood test is usually given every 3 months to 1 year as part of the Gleason score, a cancer grading system, to evaluate the severity of prostate cancer.

Another kind of common prostate cancer screening is a digital rectal exam. This is performed by a doctor or nurse, who uses a finger to feel the prostate gland through the rectum in order to check the gland's shape and to search for hard spots.

ADDITIONAL FACTS

1. *Nine out of 10 men diagnosed with prostate cancer have localized cancer that has not spread outside the prostate gland. Most men with localized prostate cancer survive the disease, no matter what the treatment.*

2. *There are four common treatments for prostate cancer. These are (1) watchful waiting, which means carefully monitoring the cancer with regular checkups; (2) surgical removal of the prostate called radical prostatectomy; (3) radiation, administered in the form of either external beam or brachytherapy (seeding); and (4) hormone treatment.*

3. *Doctors are debating whether PSA screening is necessary for men over age 70, because most prostate cancers grow very slowly and spread only after many years.*

✦✦✦

Artificial Heart Valves

The heart contains four valves that open and close to maintain the flow of blood in one direction. If one or two of those valves become diseased, narrowed, or unable to close all the way, bloodflow can become limited and pressure can build up in the lungs. Sometimes a valve can be repaired, but often it needs to be replaced to keep the heart pumping smoothly.

In the early 1950s, scientists began replacing diseased heart valves with acrylic ones. Surgeons performed the procedure on several patients, but the valves failed to regulate bloodflow properly and clotting and swelling often occurred. Over the next few years, scientists attempted other artificial implants to replace the mitral and aortic valves—the two harder-working valves on the left side of the heart, which pumps blood through the body. Design criteria were important: The materials had to be compatible with human tissue, and the valves had to open and close rapidly and be able to function for many years.

The advantages of using human tissue to create heart valves became evident in 1962, when the English surgeon Donald Ross implanted the first heart valve harvested from a dead body: The immune system proved less likely to reject human tissue, and clotting was less likely to occur. The limited supply of cadavers, however, necessitated a search for other tissue substitutes, and in 1965, scientists first reported on five successful surgeries in which they'd implanted heart valves made from pig organs.

Today, patients have a choice between mechanical and biological valves. Mechanical valves are made from synthetic materials such as carbon, polyester, and titanium. They are durable and reliable and they last a long time, although patients need to take blood-thinning drugs to prevent clots from forming. Biological valves, made from cow or pig tissue (called a xenograft) or a donated human heart (called an allograft or homograft), must be replaced every 10 to 15 years. They are generally recommended for elderly patients or patients who cannot take blood-thinning medication. Sometimes a patient's own tissue can be used for valve replacement (called an autograft or a Ross procedure).

ADDITIONAL FACTS

1. *The noise made by the acrylic heart valve replacements of the early 1950s was disconcerting to patients—reminiscent, some said, of a ticking time bomb.*

2. *The average heart beats 60 to 90 times per minute, or more than 31 million times a year.*

3. *Before the heart-lung machine was developed (see page 280), surgery on heart valves could attempt repair but not replacement. The surgery had to be done very rapidly on a still-beating heart*

✦✦✦

Congenital Hip Dysplasia

Each time we walk, sit down, or dance, we have the ball-and-socket hip joint to thank. But about 1 in 1,000 infants is born with a defective joint. In some cases, the socket may be too shallow, allowing the ball to fall out of the joint. This condition is called congenital hip dysplasia or developmental dysplasia of the hip (DDH) and occurs in newborns.

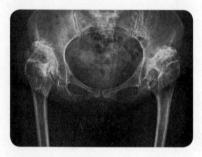

Most parents and physicians can spot congenital hip dysplasia; one leg may be shorter than the other, or the leg from the dislocated hip may splay outward. The space between the legs may seem wider than usual, giving the child a bow legged appearance, or the folds of fat on the thighs may appear uneven. To diagnose the condition, physicians perform an x-ray, ultrasound, or MRI scan.

Congenital hip dysplasia is caused by both genetic and environmental factors. The condition tends to run in families, and a breech birth may also increase risk. To correct the hip joint, physicians put the ball back into its socket to allow the hip to develop normally. The first method is usually a Pavlik harness, which has two slings to hold the hip in place. The cast is worn around the clock for 6 weeks and then 12 hours a day for another 6 weeks.

If this treatment isn't successful, a cast, traction, or surgery may be necessary. With traction, a series of pulleys and weights helps stretch the soft tissues around the hip and keep the bones aligned properly. A baby typically remains in traction for 2 weeks, either at home or in the hospital. As a last resort, surgeons can correct the hip and a cast can hold it in place.

ADDITIONAL FACTS

1. *Because the uterus tends to be smallest in a woman's first pregnancy, firstborn children are more likely to have congenital hip dysplasia.*

2. *Girls have a greater chance of developing congenital hip dysplasia than boys do.*

❖❖❖

Heart Disease

The heart beats some 35 million times a year, making it one of the hardest-working parts of the human body. So, when this organ falters, serious problems can arise. In fact, heart disease is the leading cause of death, killing 700,000 Americans every year.

Heart disease, which is also known as cardiovascular disease, is actually an umbrella term for several specific heart conditions. Coronary artery disease (a hardening of the arteries that supply blood to the heart, caused by atherosclerosis), high blood pressure, heart attack, heart failure, and angina are the most common forms of the condition. Heart disease tends to run in families and strike older people; more than 80 percent of people who die of cardiovascular disease are 65 years of age or older.

Still, the good news about heart disease is that much of it is preventable: Research shows that 82 percent of heart disease can be averted with lifestyle changes. Smokers, for instance, are up to four times more likely to develop the condition, since chemicals in the smoke can damage blood vessels and lead to fatty buildup within them. Since high blood pressure and elevated cholesterol levels are two main players in heart disease, keeping these two factors in check is crucial. A diet high in vegetables, fiber, low-fat dairy, omega-3 fatty acids, and lean protein, as well as low in sodium and saturated fat, is thought to safeguard the ticker. A regimen of exercising regularly and maintaining a healthy weight has also been proven to be beneficial. And because chronic exposure to stress can damage the heart, learning to cope, avoid stress when possible, and relax promotes well-being and reduces the risk of a heart attack.

ADDITIONAL FACTS

1. *Heart disease is responsible for 40 percent of deaths in the United States, more than are caused by all forms of cancer combined.*

2. *Anger and fear raise the heart rate by 30 to 40 beats per minute.*

❖❖❖

Echinacea

There are nine known species of echinacea, also known as purple coneflower, all native to the United States and Canada. This herb has been used to treat or prevent colds and flu for hundreds of years and is a common ingredient, along with vitamin C, goldenseal, astragalus, and other herbs and nutrients, in immune-boosting remedies.

Echinacea teas and extracts are made of all parts of the plant, from the flower and stems to the roots. The most commonly used species, *Echinacea purpurea,* is believed to be the most potent, although *Echinacea pallida* and *Echinacea angustifolia* are also used frequently. While plenty of research has found echinacea to be ineffective in treating colds, a review of more than 700 studies conducted in 2007 reported that the herb reduced the risk of catching a cold by 58 percent and significantly shortened a cold's duration. A few small trials have found echinacea to decrease the duration and severity of upper respiratory infections. Echinacea has also been used to treat wounds and skin problems, such as acne or boils, and vaginal yeast infections.

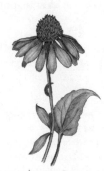

purple coneflower
Echinacea purpurea

Side effects of echinacea are rare but tend to be more common in people who are allergic to related plants in the aster family, such as chrysanthemums, daisies, marigolds, and ragweed. Ill effects can include rashes and gastrointestinal symptoms or, rarely, anaphylaxis and shock. Also, people with asthma may experience increased symptoms when taking echinacea. Use by children is not recommended because of reports of rash and apparent lack of benefit, according to several studies.

ADDITIONAL FACTS

1. *Echinacea's genus name comes from the Greek word* echino, *meaning "spiny" and referring to the flower's spiny central disk.*

2. *According to the National Institutes of Health, about 10 percent of all dietary supplements sold in the United States are echinacea.*

3. *Some herbal medicine experts discourage the use of echinacea because long-term use of this herb may cause low white blood cell counts (leukopenia).*

❖❖❖

Mania

In the 2002 book *Electroboy: A Memoir of Mania,* author Andy Behrman describes "the most perfect prescription glasses with which to see the world . . . life appears in front of you like an oversized movie screen." Behrman suffers from bipolar disorder, a condition in which people cycle between extreme highs called mania and extreme depressive lows. He adds, "When I'm manic, I'm so awake and alert that my eyelashes fluttering on the pillow sound like thunder."

The word *mania* comes from the Greek *mainomai,* meaning "to rage" or "to be furious." Mania is most commonly associated with bipolar disorder and can vary in intensity from periods of mild happiness (known as hypomania) to extreme euphoria. This may not sound like such a bad thing, but the other symptoms that accompany a manic episode, such as hypersensitivity, loss of concentration, and extreme risk taking, can make mania a scary and unpleasant experience.

People experiencing mania may speak rapidly, have racing thoughts, and have an elevated sex drive. Severe episodes of mania can also be accompanied by symptoms of psychosis, including hallucinations and delusions of grandeur. When an elevated mood is accompanied by three of these symptoms for most of the day, every day, for a week or more, it is considered a manic episode.

During manic episodes, people may feel full of energy and ideas. They may perform creative tasks such as writing, drawing, or painting for hours on end and feel that they're "in the zone." But they also might be irritable, aggressive, and easily distracted. They may become argumentative or take impulsive actions such as going on spending sprees, giving away money, driving too fast, or abusing drugs or alcohol.

People with bipolar disorder who are incorrectly diagnosed with depression and given antidepressant medications are at risk for manic states. Instead, mood-stabilizing medications such as lithium and valproate should be used to keep patients stable.

ADDITIONAL FACTS

1. *Mania and hypomania have been associated with creative talent, and it is hypothesized that Vincent van Gogh (1853–1890), Rudyard Kipling (1865–1936), Ludwig van Beethoven (1770–1827), and other famous artists, writers, and composers had mental disorders and did much of their work during manic episodes.*

2. *The TV journalist Jane Pauley (1950–) was diagnosed with bipolar disorder at age 50; she has said that during her first manic episode, she "enjoyed a few weeks of high-octane creativity and confidence, but after that, it was just an idling engine on overdrive."*

3. *A deficiency of the vitamin B_{12} may also cause symptoms of mania.*

✦✦✦

Insemination

Artificial insemination is the act of placing semen into a woman's reproductive tract without sexual intercourse. This fertility treatment is used by people who have trouble conceiving because of a problem such as low sperm count, impotence, or vaginismus (painful spasmodic contractions of the vagina). For most physicians, artificial insemination is a first-line option for an assisted reproductive technology because it's minimally invasive and less expensive than other procedures. What's more, success rates are respectable: With each cycle, there's a 15 percent chance a couple will become pregnant, compared with 20 percent for natural conception.

The procedure is relatively fast and painless for both males and females. First, a physician tracks a woman's ovulation by measuring her basal body temperature and performing sonograms, as well as examining cervical mucus and using other tests. If she has an irregular menstrual cycle, ovulation-inducing drugs are administered to guarantee the release of an egg. Next, at the expected time of ovulation, a fresh semen sample from the man is procured through masturbation and then injected with a syringe and catheter into the cervix. In cases in which sperm will be injected into the uterus, it is prepared with a procedure called washing, in which the seminal fluid is removed and replaced with a small volume of a nutrient solution. This creates a concentrated sample of active sperm, increasing the chance of fertilization and eliminating the uterine cramps the seminal fluid would cause if introduced into the uterus.

The woman is then instructed to remain supine for about 5 to 10 minutes to allow the sperm to swim up into the fallopian tubes in hopes that it will reach and fertilize the egg. If the man is sterile or if a woman wishes to become pregnant without a male partner, donor sperm are used. These sperm are donated by men and then frozen and stored in licensed sperm banks around the country.

ADDITIONAL FACTS

1. *Artificial insemination was developed in the early 1900s in Russia for the breeding of livestock. With one bull's sperm, thousands of calves can be produced every year.*

2. *A donor insemination from a normal male is more likely to be successful than one from a man with sperm abnormalities.*

3. *The procedure still remains the subject of religious and ethical controversy, despite more than half a century of clinical use.*

◆◆◆

Perspiration

Perspiration, or sweat, is a clear, salty liquid produced by glands in your body to cool itself. When sweat evaporates from your skin, it cools your body down.

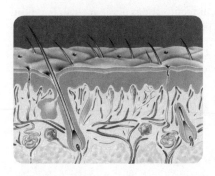

You perspire mainly under your arms, on the palms of your hands, and on the soles of your feet. When sweat mixes with bacteria found on your skin, it may cause an unpleasant odor. Bathing regularly and using an antiperspirant or deodorant can reduce or prevent this odor.

It is normal and healthy to sweat more heavily when it's hot, when you're exercising, when you're anxious, or when you have a fever. Menopausal women may perspire a lot, as well. However, some people sweat too much, in a condition called hyperhidrosis. This may stem from low blood sugar or a disorder of the thyroid or nervous system. Other people sweat too little, which is called anhidrosis. This can be life threatening, because your body may overheat. Anhidrosis is caused by dehydration, burns, or a disorder of the skin or nerves.

Your skin has two kinds of sweat glands: eccrine glands and apocrine glands. You have between 2 million and 5 million eccrine glands, which can be found all over your body and open directly to the surface of your skin. When you get hot, your autonomic nervous system stimulates these glands to secrete sweat onto the surface of your skin.

Apocrine glands secrete a fatty sweat into the tubule of the gland. When you're emotionally stressed, the sweat is pushed to the surface of your skin. Usually, it is apocrine sweat that produces the worst odor when it comes in contact with the bacteria on your skin.

ADDITIONAL FACTS

1. *It is normal to lose several quarts of fluid through perspiration when it's hot or you are working out.*

2. *A bead of sweat the size of a pea can cool approximately 1 quart of blood by 1°F.*

3. *The way your sweat smells can be influenced by your mood, diet, medications, medical conditions, and hormone levels.*

◆◆◆

RhoGAM

For centuries, women with a certain rare blood type suffered mysterious miscarriages or delivered stillborn babies due to an unexplained condition known as hemolytic disease of the newborn (HDN). The development of Rh immune globulin (brand name RhoGAM) in 1968 is estimated to have prevented the deaths of 10,000 babies each year in the United States alone.

Between 1 and 15 percent of US females have Rh-negative blood—meaning they lack a certain protein, D antigen, on the surface of their red blood cells. If an Rh-negative woman carries a baby who is Rh-positive, the mother's immune system will recognize the baby's blood cells as foreign and produce antibodies to destroy those cells. Usually a first baby is not affected, because the antibodies need time to multiply and strengthen. During subsequent pregnancies, however, the antibodies can lower babies' red blood cell counts and cause jaundice, anemia, mental retardation, heart failure, and death.

In 1939, doctors first discovered that HDN stemmed from an incompatibility between a mother's and baby's blood; they were tipped off when a woman had a stillborn birth and then, later, a bad reaction to a transfusion of her husband's blood. At that time, HDN affected about 10 percent of all pregnancies, and the infant's only chance of survival was a massive transfusion involving total replacement of the baby's blood immediately after birth. In the 1960s, scientists proposed giving Rh-negative pregnant women an injection of antibodies instead.

The medicine Rh immune globulin was developed in 1968 by doctors at Columbia University in New York City and a Johnson and Johnson laboratory in Raritan, New Jersey. RhoGAM blocks the mother's immune system from identifying the foreign fetal blood cells so she will not become "sensitized" and make antibodies. Millions of doses have been administered since, and the incidence of Rh-negative pregnant women becoming sensitized today has dropped to approximately 0.1 percent.

ADDITIONAL FACTS

1. *The American College of Obstetrics and Gynecology has hailed the development of RhoGAM as one of the top achievements in 50 years of women's health.*

2. *One famous historical personage who may have been Rh-negative was Catherine of Aragon (1485–1536), the first wife of King Henry VIII (1491–1547). Five of her six children were either born stillborn or died in infancy, telltale signs of the disease. Whatever the reason, Catherine's inability to bear a male heir had a momentous impact on history: when the pope refused to allow Henry to divorce Catherine to seek a more fertile queen, he responded by repudiating Roman Catholicism and founding the Church of England, a major event in the Protestant Reformation of the 16th century.*

3. *Rh factor is short for rhesus factor, because the antigen was first identified in rhesus monkeys.*

◆◆◆

Osgood-Schlatter Disease

Although it sounds frightening, Osgood-Schlatter (pronounced "oz-good SLOT-er") disease is a harmless and passing condition of knee pain in growing children. It occurs mainly between the ages of 11 and 12 for girls and 13 and 14 for boys, when they're growing and their bones are developing rapidly. As a result, kids who frequently run or jump can develop this overuse condition. About one in five adolescent athletes is affected.

The problem is named after the American orthopedist Robert Osgood (1873–1956) and the Swiss surgeon Carl Schlatter (1864–1934), who described it in 1903. They found that a lot of activity pulls at the tendons attached to the shinbone and kneecap, causing the shinbone's growth plate to swell. This leads to a tender bone bump about 2 inches below the knee. Kneeling, jumping, or running—or performing any activity in which the leg is fully extended—leads to pain.

A physician will diagnose the condition with an examination and, in some cases, an x-ray. Fortunately, Osgood-Schlatter usually goes away on its own without harmful side effects or complications. Children with the condition are advised to cut back on the athletic activities that aggravate the problem. In the meantime, icing the affected areas and taking over-the-counter pain relievers can help reduce the pain. Warming up properly before engaging in exercise may also lower the risk of inflammation.

ADDITIONAL FACTS

1. *Osgood-Schlatter disease is also known as tibial tuberosity apophysitis.*

2. *Usually, only one knee is affected.*

✦✦✦

Diabetes

Call it the epidemic of the 21st century: One in three Americans has either diabetes or its precursor, prediabetes. The full-blown disease, also known as diabetes mellitus, occurs when the body has either a deficiency or a malfunction in the action of insulin. This hormone, which is produced by the pancreas, helps cells convert sugar into energy. As a result, people with diabetes struggle with maintaining healthy blood sugar levels.

There are two major forms of diabetes: type 1 and type 2. Type 1 diabetes, previously called juvenile diabetes, makes up about 5 to 10 percent of cases. It's usually diagnosed in children or young adults, although it can occur at any age. In type 1, the body stops synthesizing insulin or makes only a small amount due to autoimmune destruction of the cells that produce it. Because the body requires insulin to survive, people with this disease need to monitor their blood sugar levels constantly and must give themselves daily injections of insulin. Without this insulin supplement, the body breaks down fat for energy. As a result, ketones—acidic by-products of fat breakdown—flood the bloodstream, resulting in a dangerous condition called ketoacidosis. This blood imbalance causes nausea and rapid breathing; if it's not treated promptly, a coma or even death can occur.

In type 2 diabetes, the body doesn't produce enough insulin or is unable to utilize the insulin properly. (The latter condition is called insulin resistance.) As a result, the sugar from foods builds up in the bloodstream instead of fueling the cells. Studies show that uncontrolled diabetes raises the risk of Alzheimer's disease, heart disease, nerve and kidney damage, and eye problems.

For those with type 2 diabetes, losing weight, exercising regularly, and eating a diet high in fiber and protein can lower blood sugar levels. Physicians also prescribe medication that helps reduce blood sugar levels by stimulating insulin release and improving insulin action. Patients with type 2 very rarely develop ketoacidosis.

ADDITIONAL FACTS

1. *Insulin was first discovered in 1921.*

2. *About 5 percent of women who don't have diabetes develop the disease during pregnancy, in which case it's called gestational diabetes. Although the condition usually goes away after childbirth, these new moms are at greater risk for developing type 2 diabetes later in life.*

◆◆◆

Red Clover

Trifolium pratense, commonly known as red clover, is an herb that grows in Europe, Asia, and North America and belongs to the legume family, a group that also includes peas, alfalfa, peanuts, and beans. Red clover contains isoflavones—compounds with properties similar to those of the female hormone estrogen—and is used to treat menopausal symptoms, breast pain associated with menstrual cycles, high cholesterol, and osteoporosis

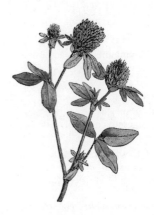

Historically, the flowering tops of the red clover plant have been used to treat cancer and respiratory problems such as asthma, bronchitis, and whooping cough. It has also been used as a folk remedy for skin problems. Today, researchers believe red clover's estrogen-like properties may be helpful in treating hormonal conditions such as menstrual pain and menopause. However, there is also concern about the safety of isoflavones, as they appear to contribute to the growth of certain types of female cancer in the same way that estrogen does.

Red clover also provides many nutrients, including vitamin C, niacin, and calcium. Because of its high isoflavone content, it's suggested that red clover may also reduce hot flashes in menopausal women, although the largest study showed no effect. Preliminary evidence has shown that an extract of the plant may slow bone loss and may even boost bone mineral density to protect against osteoporosis.

ADDITIONAL FACTS

1. *Red clover is native to Europe and Asia and has been naturalized to grow in the United States. It is frequently used for grazing cattle and other animals.*

2. *Traditionally, red clover was thought to improve circulation, cleanse the liver, and purify the blood by ridding the body of excess fluid and helping clear the lungs of mucus.*

3. *Side effects of red clover are usually mild and include headache, nausea, and rash. However, infertility has been noted in grazing animals that consume large amounts of the plant.*

◆◆◆

Manic-Depressive Disorder

Everyone goes through ups and downs in terms of mood and energy levels. But when these shifts in behavior and emotion become so extreme that they affect a person's ability to function normally, the condition may be considered bipolar disorder, also known as manic-depressive illness—a serious disorder requiring lifelong care.

Bipolar disorder generally develops in late adolescence or early adulthood, but symptoms are sometimes experienced as early as childhood. The disorder affects about 5.7 million American adults, or about 2.6 percent of the population ages 18 and older. The condition is often overlooked or misdiagnosed as regular depression, and people can go for years without proper treatment.

Dramatic mood swings are the hallmark symptoms of bipolar disorder: People experience "high" periods—known as manic episodes—that last for a week or longer in which they feel extremely energetic, creative, and invincible. During these episodes, they may go for days without sleeping, make risky sexual decisions, abuse drugs, and spend money wildly.

These phases are countered by periods of extreme depression, irritability, anxiety, and hopelessness. Depressive episodes last for 5 days or longer and can include chronic pain, unintended weight loss or gain, and thoughts of death or suicide.

For most people with bipolar disorder, there are breaks between the episodes. But a small percentage of people with the condition experience unremitting symptoms all the time in what's known as rapid-cycling bipolar disorder.

Without treatment, bipolar disorder tends to worsen over time. In most cases, mood-stabilizing medication and talk therapy can help control symptoms and allow patients to lead normal, productive lives.

ADDITIONAL FACTS

1. *Children with bipolar disorder (an increasingly common diagnosis) often experience very fast mood swings between mania and depression, several times within a day. Children whose parents have bipolar disorder are more likely to develop the disease.*

2. *The exact cause of bipolar disorder is unknown, but it is believed to be linked to genetics. But genetics alone are not thought to cause the disorder, and an identical twin may develop bipolar disorder while his or her sibling does not.*

3. *People with bipolar disorder often suffer from related conditions as well, such as abnormal thyroid function, ongoing anxiety, or post-traumatic stress disorder.*

◆◆◆

In Vitro Fertilization

In 1974, Landrum Shettles (1909–2003), a New York City–based gynecologist, fertilized a woman's egg by mixing it with her husband's sperm in a test tube. He believed that he could implant the embryo in the mother's womb. But before he could attempt the procedure, the head of his department heard about the experiment and instructed him to stop, fearing the creation of a genetically deformed child and concerned about the religious and ethical implications. Nonetheless, 4 years later the first baby created using this laboratory process, called in vitro fertilization (IVF), was born, in Norfolk, England. That baby, Louise Brown (1978–), went on to become an administrative worker and mother.

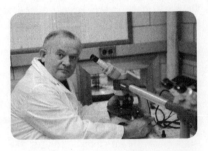

To conduct IVF, a sperm specimen is taken from the man and eggs are harvested from the woman. They're placed in a laboratory dish, where fertilization occurs. Over the next few days, the embryo divides repeatedly until it becomes a ball of cells, called a blastocyst. Meanwhile, the woman receives the hormone progesterone to prepare her uterine lining for an embryo. At this point, the blastocyst is placed in the uterus, where it floats free for up to 3 days until it attaches to the wall of the uterus. IVF is successful when the embryo implants in the uterine lining and begins to grow into a fetus.

Since it became available to the public, IVF has often been a topic of religious and ethical arguments. In 1987, the Roman Catholic Church released a statement opposing the procedure, because IVF removes procreation from the marital context. What's more, embryos not used for implantation are sometimes destroyed, which the Church considers abortion.

ADDITIONAL FACTS

1. *The experts who carried out the first successful IVF birth were Patrick Steptoe (1913–1988) and Robert G. Edwards (1925–).*

2. *The term* in vitro *means "in glass"; natural conception is called* in vivo, *or "in the living."*

◆◆◆

Yawning

Yawning is opening your mouth involuntarily while taking a long, deep breath. It is usually a response to drowsiness, fatigue, or boredom. Excessive yawning occurs when yawning happens more often than is typical.

Everyone yawns at all ages. It is normal to yawn when someone else yawns.

Most mammals and some birds and reptiles yawn. The action is not very well understood, probably because it is rarely a health problem. It is known that the hypothalamus, in the brain, plays an important role in yawning. Research has revealed that several neurotransmitters increase yawning when they are injected into an animal's hypothalamus.

One theory regarding yawning is that we yawn to get rid of extra carbon dioxide and to take in more oxygen. When people are bored or tired, they breathe more slowly, and less oxygen makes it into the lungs. Theoretically, as carbon dioxide builds up in the blood, the person yawns to take a deep breath and let in more oxygen. However, some research has shown that there is no relationship between breathing and yawning.

It has also been proposed that yawning and stretching are related. They both increase blood pressure and heart rate and flex muscles and joints. You may have observed that the stretching of jaw and face muscles is needed for a "good" yawn.

Sometimes, excessive yawning happens as a result of vasovagal reaction, which is the action of the vagus nerve on your blood vessels. This can be a sign of a heart problem. You should contact a medical professional if you experience unexplained, excessive yawning or you yawn frequently and are extremely sleepy during the day.

ADDITIONAL FACTS

1. *The average yawn lasts about 6 seconds. Yawns in males may last longer than those in females.*

2. *The earliest occurrence of a yawn happens at about 11 weeks after conception, before the baby is born.*

3. *Human beings start yawning in response to other people's yawns between the ages of 1 and 2.*

✦✦✦

LASIK Surgery

When a young boy in 1970s Russia cut his eye on a shard of his broken glasses, an incredible thing happened: His eyesight improved in the injured eye. This stroke of luck paved the way for the revolutionary vision-correction surgeries we know today.

In a LASIK surgery, doctors improve a patient's eyesight by permanently altering the shape of the cornea. (The term stands for *laser-assisted in situ keratomileusis*.) A tiny blade or laser (called a microkeratome or laser keratome) is used to cut a flap in the cornea, leaving a hinge at one end so it can be folded back. The doctor then wields a laser to vaporize a portion of the cornea's middle section, called the stroma, shaping it to correct vision problems such as nearsightedness, farsightedness, and astigmatism.

Corrective lenses work by changing the angle at which light enters the eye. For much of the 20th century, doctors wondered how they could produce a similar result by changing the curvature of the cornea instead. Japanese scientists in the 1930s attempted corneal incisions, but it wasn't until the accidental injury of the young patient's eye in Moscow (the glass merely shaved off a piece of the cornea) that the ophthalmologist Svyatoslav Fyodorov (1927–2000) began to regularly and success-fully perform a procedure called radial keratotomy using tiny knives. The American ophthalmologist Leo Bores studied with Fyodorov in Russia and brought the tech-nique back to the United States in 1978.

The first laser-assisted eye surgery—known as photorefractive keratectomy (PRK)—took place in Germany in 1988. A device called an excimer laser produces a cool beam of ultraviolet light that breaks down the carbon bonds in corneal tissue mol-ecules with a degree of safety and precision that was unattainable with traditional tools. LASIK surgery, first approved in the United States in 1998, also uses an excimer laser but does not scrape away outer layers of the cornea as PRK does, so recovery is usually quicker and side effects are less severe. Since its approval, hun-dreds of thousands of people in the United States have undergone LASIK surgery.

ADDITIONAL FACTS

1. *Some patients experience side effects from LASIK such as double vision, dry eyes, or seeing halos around bright objects.*

2. *Between 5 and 10 percent of patients need follow-up procedures to fix over- or undercorrection. Results can also diminish over time for some patients.*

3. *Fyodorov apparently became determined to find a way to avoid wearing glasses when he saw the 1973 Woody Allen (1935–) comedy* Sleeper. *Allen's character wakes up in the 22nd century surrounded by doctors, one of whom is wearing glasses; apparently even after all that time, no cure for poor eyesight had been developed.*

◆◆◆

Hirsutism

At 19th-century circus sideshows, bearded ladies were often labeled freaks. But these women simply suffered from extreme cases of hirsutism, an excessive growth of coarse, colored hair in areas where such hair is typically associated with males, such as the upper lip and chin. Up to 10 percent of women have this condition to some degree.

Named for the Latin word *hirsutus,* or "hairy," the condition is often caused by high levels of androgens. Androgens are the main male sex hormones, but all women naturally have small amounts of them. Certain medications, such as steroids and some progestins, can lead to a spike in androgens. Some prescription drugs that treat endometriosis, schizophrenia, and migraine headaches may do the same.

In some cases, the excess androgens stem from an abnormality of the ovaries, adrenal glands, or pituitary glands. The most common culprit is polycystic ovarian syndrome (PCOS), a hormonal disorder that affects some 10 percent of girls and women of childbearing age. The next most common is congenital adrenal hyperplasia, in which the adrenal glands pump out excessive amounts of male hormones. Cushing's syndrome, involving excess cortisol and androgens, is another culprit. And in a significant number of instances, there's no discernible cause of the hair growth; these cases are called idiopathic hirsutism.

Although the excessive hair doesn't have any side effects, the condition that causes it—such as PCOS—may have complications if left untreated. Hirsutism itself may be treated with oral contraceptives, which inhibit androgen production in adolescent girls; antiandrogen medications; and topical creams. Laser therapy and electrolysis can also permanently remove unwanted hair. Cortisol treats girls and boys with congenital adrenal hyperplasia, but boys seldom require treatment for the excess hair.

ADDITIONAL FACTS

1. *Women of Mediterranean, Middle Eastern, and South Asian descent are more likely to develop idiopathic hirsutism.*

2. *Excessive hair growth that doesn't occur in specifically male hair-growth areas is called hypertrichosis. This disorder may be caused by anorexia or thyroid problems.*

✦✦✦

Lyme Disease

Old Lyme is a small, charming town on the coast of Connecticut. It's from this otherwise unassuming city of 8,000 that Lyme disease takes its name. That's because in 1975, American researchers first studied and wrote a full description of the tickborne condition there—in spite of the fact that European scientists had documented the disease nearly a century earlier.

Lyme disease is caused by a bacterium called *Borrelia burgdorferi,* which is carried by deer ticks (found in the northeastern and north-central United States) and black-legged ticks (found on the West Coast). The infection can spread from animals to humans through tick bites; each year, more than 200,000 people are affected. Within a month of the bite, a rash generally appears. It starts as a red spot and then, as it spreads, the center fades, leaving behind a bull's-eye ring.

Other symptoms of early-stage Lyme disease include fever, chills, fatigue, headaches, a stiff neck, and muscle and joint pain. In rare cases, the infection may spread to the heart, resulting in an irregular or slow heartbeat. If it attacks the nervous system, numbness or facial droop can occur. A doctor can prescribe a course of antibiotics to kill the infection.

But if Lyme disease is not detected soon enough, it can lead to painful, swollen joints and wreak havoc on the nervous system, causing memory loss, concentration problems, and mood changes. In a small number of cases, the disease or its complications can prove fatal.

The best protection against the disease is to avoid exposure to ticks and their bites. Experts recommend wearing long pants and long-sleeved shirts and using a DEET-based insect repellent when out in grassy, wooded areas. If a tick bites you, it's best to grasp the insect near its head with a pair of fine-tipped tweezers and pull it out carefully and slowly. Slathering a tick with Vaseline or nail polish, or applying a match to it, will only cause the tick to burrow in further, increasing your risk of contracting the disease.

ADDITIONAL FACTS

1. *The longer a tick is attached to you, the greater your risk of getting Lyme disease.*

2. *To diagnose the disease, physicians administer a series of tests that detect antibodies to* B. burgdorferi.

◆◆◆

Nurse-Practitioner

Many patients are introduced to their first nurse-practitioner because their regular doctors aren't available for an urgent appointment. These people generally learn that nurse-practitioners provide services similar to those of physicians. In fact, some people prefer seeing a nurse-practitioner, because he or she can often spend more time with patients and provide a more personal experience.

Although common today, the profession of nurse-practitioner was unknown until 1965, when a national physician shortage inspired the University of Colorado to offer the training. Programs soon spread across the country. More than 120,000 nurse-practitioners serve patients today, and hundreds of universities offer degree programs.

Most nurse-practitioners earn master's degrees or doctorates and go to work in clinics, hospitals, emergency rooms, urgent care sites, nursing homes, schools, and private practices. Nurse-practitioners perform many of the same tasks as doctors, and in many states they can prescribe medications. They also practice in specialties such as allergies and immunology, cardiovascular health, dermatology, and emergency medicine. For example, pediatric nurse-practitioners educate children and their families about growth and development issues such as toilet training, temper tantrums, and biting.

According to the American Nurses Association, it is estimated that nurse-practitioners can perform approximately 60 to 80 percent of primary and preventive care. They learn a unique approach that stresses both care and cure, and their practice focuses on health promotion, disease prevention, and education.

ADDITIONAL FACTS

1. *Some of the first nurse-practitioner training programs were inspired by the military's effort in World War II to rush doctors through medical school to ensure that there would be enough medics on the front lines.*

2. *Nurse-practitioners may also be referred to as advanced practice nurses, or APNs.*

3. *Some states require a doctor to cosign prescriptions written by a nurse-practitioner.*

❖❖❖

Schizophrenia

People who suffers from schizophrenia may hear voices in their heads, suffer from hallucinations, or develop paranoid fears. They may have delusions of grandeur, engage in bizarre social behavior, and use illogical or odd speech.

What these symptoms have in common is the fundamental marker of schizophrenia—an inability to distinguish what is real from what is not. The crippling disorder is one of the most prevalent mental illnesses in the United States, with an estimated 3 million cases.

For many schizophrenics, the disease makes it difficult to lead a normal life, and schizophrenia is the leading cause of institutionalization in mental hospitals. However, the disease can be successfully controlled in many people with a combination of psychotherapy and antipsychotic drugs.

Schizophrenia is typically diagnosed in men in their late teens and women in their twenties and thirties. It is though to be caused by a chemical imbalance in the brain that results from a combination of genetic factors and environmental stresses such as illness or malnutrition.

Schizophrenics are grouped into several subcategories according to the type and severity of their symptoms. Paranoid schizophrenics develop delusions that they are being persecuted by grand conspiracies. Catatonic schizophrenics lose their ability to move and sometimes to talk, assuming a zombielike mein. Hebephrenic schizophrenics report hallucinations, delusions, and unusual or inappropriate behavior.

Although this condition has a reputation for being dangerous, most people with schizophrenia are not prone to violence. They are, however, more likely to attempt suicide and abuse alcohol and drugs than the normal population. If people with this illness do become violent, their anger is most often directed at family members in their own home. The "split personality" popular in movies is based on a rare form of schizophrenia.

ADDITIONAL FACTS

1. *People with schizophrenia are addicted to nicotine at three times the rate of the general population, and research shows that quitting smoking can be especially difficult for someone with this disorder.*

2. *A 2009 study found that schizophrenia is linked to a higher risk of dying from cancer, in part because schizophrenics are less likely to follow treatment programs.*

3. *Famous schizophrenics include author Jack Kerouac (1922–1969), Green Bay Packers defensive end Lionel Aldridge (1941–1998), and Nobel Prize-winning mathematician John F. Nash Jr. (1928–), the subject of the 2001 biopic* A Beautiful Mind.

◆◆◆

Embryo Storage

When a woman chooses fertility treatment by in vitro fertilization, the physician creates a number of extra embryos as a safety net. These embryos are usually destroyed, but a technology called embryo storage, or embryo cryopreservation, allows couples to freeze and store the leftover embryos for future attempts at pregnancy. As a result, some families have siblings born years apart that were conceived from the same batch of embryos.

Although research shows that fresh embryos tend to have a higher success rate, the benefit of embryo storage is that the couple doesn't have to repeat the fertility treatments and processes required to harvest the egg and sperm. In a best-case scenario, up to 70 percent of embryos survive the freezing and thawing procedure. As with egg storage, water molecules may turn into ice when the embryo is placed in the cooling machine. These ice crystals can expand, stretching the embryo, or may act as knives and slice through cell membranes.

To protect the embryo, water is removed and a special freeze-proof cryoprotectant chemical—sort of like a cellular antifreeze—replaces it. When it's time to thaw, this cryoprotectant is replaced with water. Embryos may be stored frozen for an indeterminate amount of time. Some reports have detailed cases in which embryos frozen for up to 10 years have resulted in healthy pregnancies. Among the serious concerns about this technique are who "owns" these extra embryos and what is to become of them when they are unwanted.

ADDITIONAL FACTS

1. *The first reported case of a frozen embryo generating a healthy pregnancy was in 1983.*

2. *The optimal embryo to freeze is one that is 3 days old.*

3. *In some states, these extra embryos can be adopted by prospective parents.*

◆◆◆

Botox

You have probably heard of Botox as a drug that is injected into parts of the face to temporarily remove facial wrinkles. It works by paralyzing the muscles that cause wrinkles, and its effects usually last for 3 to 4 months.

Botox is made from a toxin produced by the bacterium *Clostridium botulinum*. This is the same toxin that causes botulism, a life-threatening kind of food poisoning that leads to paralysis. Botox is a purified form of this toxin that triggers paralysis in a limited area of the body without causing the disease.

Botox is most useful for lines that form between the eyebrows, across the forehead, and around the eyes (crow's-feet). It is less effective for smile lines around the mouth. This is partially because paralyzing those muscles may interfere with a person's ability to eat and talk.

The process of having a Botox treatment is quick and easy. Usually a dermatologist injects the affected areas during an office visit. Sometimes Botox is used in combination with other cosmetic skin procedures, such as chemical peels, laser resurfacing, and dermal fillers. These combination therapies can prevent the formation of new wrinkles.

Doctors also use Botox to remedy severe underarm sweating, uncontrollable blinking, misaligned eyes, and cervical dystonia, a neurological problem that causes severe neck and shoulder muscle contractions. Possible side effects include pain at the site of the injection, flulike symptoms, headache, and upset stomach. Injections in the face may temporarily cause drooping eyelids. Women who are pregnant or breastfeeding should not use Botox.

ADDITIONAL FACTS

1. *In the United States, no form of botulinum toxin can be used on humans unless it has been approved by the Food and Drug Administration (FDA). At this time, the only kind of botulinum toxin approved by the FDA to temporarily reduce frown lines between the eyebrows is Botox Cosmetic, made by Allergan.*

2. *As of July 2008, the FDA's Office of Criminal Investigations has arrested 68 and convicted 29 people of purposely injecting unapproved botulinum toxin into almost 1,000 patients.*

◆◆◆

CT Scan

Since its invention in the 1970s, computed tomography technology—commonly known as CT or CAT (computed axial tomography) scanning—has revolutionized the way doctors find and diagnose problems inside the body.

Today's CT scanners enable doctors to view the internal structures of patients' bodies by taking very thin (fractions of a millimeter thick) x-ray slices across the head or body. The cross-sectional images provide a greater contrast and better view of internal organs and soft tissues such as the heart, lungs, arteries, and brain, so abnormalities can be more easily detected and diagnosed.

X-rays were discovered in 1895, and for the next several decades, scientists worked to develop ways to produce clearer images. In 1914, the Polish doctor Carol Mayer was able to capture a reasonable image of the heart by blurring out the shadows of the ribs and leaving one remaining plane, or slice, of the heart. This technique soon became known as tomography—*tomo* being Greek for "section" or "cut"—and primitive tomography machines were developed over the next few decades. The Tufts University professor Allan Cormack (1924–1998) was the first to combine computers and x-ray tomography, which he used to construct three-dimensional images of mannequins in 1963. Like his predecessors, however, he was unable to drum up funding or support from the medical community.

It wasn't until 1971 that a successful CT scanner was put into use, by London-based Electrical and Musical Industries (EMI) Limited. The EMI scientist Godfrey Hounsfield (1919–2004) performed the first head-only scan—a 15-hour process—on a woman suspected of having a brain tumor. The scanner recorded more than 28,000 readings on magnetic tape, which was sent to a computer across town to be processed. The computer produced a cross-sectional image of the brain, revealing a tumor in the patient's left frontal lobe.

After the EMI scanner went into production, improvements came rapidly. Newer machines were developed to scan the entire body, and slices got thinner and more accurate while scans got quicker. Spiral CTs, widely used today, rotate the patient at the same time as the x-ray beams, reducing radiation exposure and speeding up the process.

ADDITIONAL FACTS

1. *It's been suggested that the invention of computed tomography was made possible by the success of the British rock band the Beatles. EMI was the Beatles' record label, and the company made so much money from their album sales that it was able to donate laboratory space and funding to CT research.*

2. *Cormack and Hounsfield won a Nobel Prize in 1979 for their work in developing CT scans.*

3. *The number of CT scans performed in the United States tripled between 1995 and 2007, and some researchers fear they are ordered too frequently. In 2009, the American Heart Association urged limits on the use of cardiac CT scans because of cancer risk.*

✦✦✦

Nearsightedness

Some accounts claim that the Roman emperor Nero (AD 37–68) would gaze through an emerald in order to see gladiator fights more clearly. Nero's jewel is believed to be one of the earliest remedies for nearsightedness, a common vision condition in which one can see nearby objects clearly but things that are farther away appear blurry.

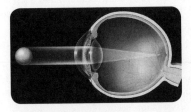

Some one in three Americans suffers from nearsightedness, which is also known as myopia. The changes that cause the problem usually begin in childhood and progress until about age 20. Most often, the cornea, which is the clear cover on the front of the eye, becomes too curved. As a result, the light that enters the eye doesn't focus properly, which makes objects in the distance appear blurred. Genetics usually dictates whether someone develops myopia, although research suggests that the stress of too much close work, such as reading small type or staring at a computer screen on a regular basis, can exacerbate the condition.

Nearsightedness can range from mild cases, in which people can see objects several feet away, to more severe instances, in which people can clearly see only objects that are a few inches away. Refractive lenses in glasses and hard or soft contact lenses are easy and inexpensive ways to correct this vision problem. Surgery can also reshape the cornea to improve vision. Some of the most common eye procedures include laser-assisted in situ keratomileusis, photorefractive keratectomy, and anterior intraocular lens implants.

ADDITIONAL FACTS

1. *Contrary to popular belief, sitting too close to the television or reading in dim lighting does not increase the risk of nearsightedness.*

2. *If you don't wear glasses or contacts and have no eye trouble, experts recommend having an eye exam once between the ages of 20 and 39, every 2 to 4 years from age 40 to 64, and every 1 to 2 years beginning at age 65.*

◆◆◆

Glaucoma

During your last visit to the eye doctor, he or she probably measured the internal pressure of your eyes and then administered a few drops to dilate your pupils. Both of these tests screen for glaucoma, a disease that strikes as many as 4 million Americans. Unfortunately, since the condition doesn't cause any symptoms in its early stages, nearly half of those people don't realize that they have it.

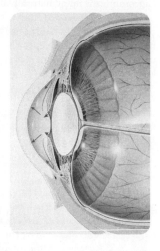

Although generally thought of as one disease, glaucoma is actually a group of conditions that harm the optic nerves. Most of the time, this damage is the result of fluid buildup in the eye. Normally, the eye's fluid, or aqueous humor, exits from the front of the eye. A meshlike drain sits at an angle where the iris and cornea meet. But when this area becomes clogged, pressure builds and wears away at the optic nerve—causing open-angle (chronic) glaucoma. The other form of the disease, called angle-closure (acute) glaucoma, occurs when the iris bulges forward and blocks the angle. Because the optic nerve's job is to transmit images from the retina to the brain, damage can lead to vision loss. As a result, glaucoma is the second-leading cause of blindness. (Cataracts are the most frequent cause.)

Glaucoma typically develops slowly, with a gradual loss of peripheral vision that leads to tunnel vision. The condition can appear suddenly, however, and can bring on blurred vision, eye reddening, halos of light, and eye pain. Experts recommend that, beginning at age 18, everyone receive a glaucoma test every 2 years; people at greater risk, such as African Americans and those with a family history of the condition, may need to be tested more frequently. Because diabetes, heart disease, eye injuries, and the frequent use of corticosteroid eyedrops can also leave you vulnerable to the disease, people with these factors should also keep close watch on their vision. If glaucoma is diagnosed, pressure-lowering eyedrops or oral medications can protect the eyes. In more serious cases, surgery to drain the fluid may be necessary.

ADDITIONAL FACTS

1. *British researchers found that men who wear tight neckties have higher intraocular pressure, putting them at greater risk for glaucoma.*

2. *About 120,000 Americans are blind as a result of glaucoma.*

3. *One in four Americans says he or she does not have an eye exam every 2 years.*

◆◆◆

Glucosamine and Chondroitn

Two nutritional supplements that some believe may help treat the degenerative disease osteoarthritis, glucosamine and chondroitin are widely used by elderly people who suffer from the pain and stiffness associated with the disease. While studies have had contradictory results, some doctors and patients believe strongly in the supplements' healing potential.

Glucosamine is found naturally in the body, but production decreases with aging. Supplements are derived from the shells of shrimp, crabs, and other shellfish. Glucosamine has also been suspected (though not proven) to help treat diabetes, inflammatory bowel disease, psoriasis, leg pain after injury, and chronic venous insufficiency (a syndrome that includes leg swelling, varicose veins, pain, itching, and skin ulcers).

Chondroitin typically comes from cow or shark cartilage and is often marketed under the name chondroitin sulfate. A carbohydrate, chondroitin appears to improve water retention, fight inflammation, and counter the breakdown of cartilage in the human body.

Study results on the effectiveness of glucosamine and chondroitin have not always been favorable: The largest and best-designed clinical trial on this topic—the ongoing Glucosamine/Chondroitin Arthritis Intervention Trial (GAIT), funded by the National Institutes of Health—has found no benefit compared with a placebo in reducing pain or loss of cartilage (as measured by x-rays) in osteoarthritis patients. However, smaller studies have shown significant improvement in patients taking the supplements, especially for osteoarthritis of the knee. Whether glucosamine and chondroitin offer any advantages over pain relief medications such as acetaminophen, traditional nonsteroidal anti-inflammatory drugs, or COX-2 inhibitors has not been determined.

Glucosamine and chondroitin tend to be well tolerated, although side effects can include upset stomach, drowsiness or insomnia, headache, sun sensitivity, and nail toughening. Based on some research, glucosamine may increase the risk of bleeding when taken with blood-thinning medications, and it may increase the risk of cataracts. Taking glucosamine and chondroitin with bromelain, manganese, or vitamin C may enhance the supplements' beneficial effects on osteoarthritis, but this remains unproven.

ADDITIONAL FACTS

1. *Animal research has raised the possibility that glucosamine may worsen insulin resistance, a major cause of diabetes. No human studies have substantiated the risk so far, but to be safe, people with diabetes should monitor their blood sugar levels while using the supplement.*

2. *There have been no reports of allergies to glucosamine, but because it is made from shellfish shells, people with seafood allergies should use it cautiously and watch for reactions.*

3. *In 2008, a Scottish newspaper reported that a few people had died of liver failure within weeks of taking glucosamine. Though physicians weren't sure why this happened, they issued a warning about glucosamine.*

✦✦✦

Post-Traumatic Stress Disorder

Often a problem for war veterans, post-traumatic stress disorder (PTSD) is a delayed and long-term psychological reaction to a disturbing event. While very common in soldiers who have experienced combat, PTSD can happen to anyone of any age who has experienced a bad accident, natural disaster, or violent crime in which they endured or were threatened by physical harm.

PTSD affects about 7.7 million American adults. People can develop post-traumatic stress after being harmed themselves or witnessing a harmful event happening to someone else. They may seem fine or emotionally detached from the event at first, but usually within 3 months they begin to exhibit symptoms. The disorder is more common in women than in men.

People who suffer from PTSD display a variety of symptoms, including skittishness, emotional numbness toward loved ones, and loss of interest in hobbies and other activities they once enjoyed. Some who have PTSD become aggressive and violent. They avoid places and situations that remind them of the original incident. They may experience vivid flashbacks, sometimes triggered by unrelated noises that remind them of the original incident, such as a car backfiring that sounds like gun-fire, which then cause them lose touch with reality. PTSD patients may also relive their past experiences in nightmares while sleeping.

Symptoms must last for more than a month to be considered PTSD. Occasionally, the symptoms don't emerge until several years after the original incident. Some people recover within 6 months, while others never fully escape the effects. People with PTSD are also at risk for depression, substance abuse, other anxiety disorders, and sometimes suicide.

Treatment includes antidepressants or antianxiety medications, talk therapy sessions, or both. Another type of therapy, called eye movement desensitization and reprocessing (EMDR), encourages patients to talk about their memories while focusing on distractions, such as eye movements, hand taps, and sounds; studies have shown that this technique may help people change the way they react to their traumatic memories so they experience fewer PTSD symptoms.

ADDITIONAL FACTS

1. *Symptoms of post-traumatic stress disorder tend to be worse if the traumatic event that triggered them was deliberately initiated, as in a rape, mugging, or kidnapping.*

2. *Children with PTSD may temporarily be unable to talk or may revert to behavior from when they were younger, complain of stomach problems or headaches, or refuse to play with friends.*

3. *Nearly one in five military service members who have returned from Iraq and Afghanistan has reported symptoms of PTSD or major depression, according to a 2008 study, yet only slightly more than half of those have sought treatment.*

❖❖❖

Ova Storage

A woman's fertility begins to decline in her thirties, so that by her forties, there's a one-in-six chance that she'll conceive. Given that more and more women are waiting to start families until later in life, many have hoped for a procedure that would allow them to push the pause button on the march of time. Enter ova storage, also called the freezing of eggs or, in medical terms, oocyte cryopreservation. In this procedure, a woman's egg is removed from her body and frozen until a later point, when it is thawed. After undergoing in vitro fertilization, the new embryo can be implanted in the woman's uterus to make her pregnant.

This technology was first applied in the mid-1990s for young women with cancer who had to undergo chemotherapy or radiation that destroyed their egg supplies. Before the cancer treatment, fertility treatments are needed to stimulate egg production. Then a needle is inserted through the vagina to retrieve the eggs. They are placed in thin tubes, which are then placed in a machine that freezes them. After freezing, the eggs are transferred to a storage bank cooled with liquid nitrogen to a temperature of $-321°F$.

The trouble with ova storage is that eggs are more fragile than sperm: Water in the cell can turn into ice, putting pressure on the cell and damaging or even rupturing it. One study found a pregnancy rate of about 17 percent with the use of frozen ova.

ADDITIONAL FACTS

1. *It costs about $10,000 to $15,000 to harvest and freeze a batch of eggs.*

2. *Storage costs about $500 a year.*

3. *There are two methods of freezing the egg: dropping the temperature rapidly or slowly lowering the temperature while protecting the egg with solutions called cryoprotectants, a process called vitrification.*

✦✦✦

Contact Lenses

Contact lenses are thin pieces of clear plastic that float on the surface of the eyes. They are usually used to correct a person's vision, but may be worn for purely cosmetic reasons. Contact lenses provide a safe alternative to glasses as long as the wearer's eyes are healthy and the person has the ability to care for the lenses properly.

The two major types of contact lenses are soft lenses and rigid gas permeable (RGP) lenses. Soft contact lenses are made of soft, pliable plastics that permit oxygen to pass through to the cornea. These lenses are usually easier to adjust to and more comfortable than RGP lenses. Most soft contact lenses are designed to be replaced daily, weekly, or monthly.

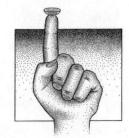

RGP contact lenses are longer lasting and more resistant to deposit buildup and tearing. They usually provide clearer vision correction. They're also likely to be less expensive in the long run, because they don't need to be replaced as frequently as soft contact lenses do.

There are risks associated with wearing all types of contact lenses, including conjunctivitis (pinkeye), corneal ulcers, corneal abrasions, vision impairment, and even blindness. This is why it is both important and required by law that you have a valid prescription for contact lenses, even cosmetic ones. Your eye care professional should be experienced with contact lenses. He or she will need to fit your lenses and diagnose and treat any problem that might interfere with your wearing them.

ADDITIONAL FACTS

1. *Some of the specific vision conditions that contact lenses can correct are myopia (nearsightedness), hyperopia (farsightedness), astigmatism (blurred vision caused by the shape of the cornea), and presbyopia (inability to see close up).*

2. *More than 24 million people in the United States wear contact lenses.*

3. *Cosmetic lenses are designed to change the appearance of the eye. For example, they can make a brown-eyed person's eyes look blue or any other color.*

◆◆◆

MRI Machine

Today's magnetic resonance imaging, or MRI, machines create body scan images almost instantly and can be used to diagnose disorders such as multiple sclerosis and cancer or injuries such as strained or torn muscles. The technology certainly has come a long way from the first MRI machine, which took almost 5 hours to produce one grainy image.

Raymond Damadian (1936–), then a physician at the State University of New York Downstate Medical Center, began experimenting with nuclear magnetic resonance in the 1960s. He proposed the first magnetic resonance scanner, which could presumably use magnetic waves to produce images of the body based on the radio frequencies emitted by atomic nuclei in the body. Experimenting on rats, Damadian had discovered dramatic differences in the signals emitted by cancerous as opposed to healthy human tissue, leading him to suspect that this could help diagnose disease.

The first MRI performed on a human, in 1977, provided a grainy (by today's standards, at least) image of the heart, lungs, and chest wall, and the patient suffered no side effects. Since then, countless advances have been made to render MRIs faster, less claustrophobic, and more able to show minute details and chemical compositions of human tissue. The first commercial version was unveiled 3 years later. Recent developments include the FONAR 360, a full-size room with two magnetic poles projecting from the ceiling and the floor, and Stand-Up MRI, the only machine that allows patients to be scanned while standing.

Most MRI machines are about 7 feet by 7 feet by 10 feet, although models are becoming smaller, lighter, and less uncomfortable for the patient. They consist of a giant magnet with a horizontal tube (called the bore) running through the center. Patients lie on their backs and are slid into the bore so that they are in the center of the magnetic field. Alternating magnetic fields are then sent out to explore the body, building a two-dimensional or three-dimensional map of its structures and tissues by computer processing of changes in the fields caused by the shifting responses of the body's atoms.

ADDITIONAL FACTS

1. *Damadian named his first MRI prototype Indomitable, in reference to the obstacles and skepticism he'd had to overcome. It is now on display at the Smithsonian Institution.*

2. *Metal objects such as paper clips, pens, and keys can become dangerous projectiles when an MRI magnet is turned on, and they are strictly forbidden in hospital scanning rooms.*

3. *Patients with implantable pacemakers, steel aneurysm clips in the brain, or certain dental or orthopedic implants may not be able to undergo MRIs because the magnet may cause the objects to shift out of place or malfunction.*

✦✦✦

Strabismus

When most people gaze at an object, both of their eyes focus on it to create a single image. But for roughly 4 percent of Americans, their eyes point in different directions some or all of the time. This condition is known as strabismus.

In many cases, children are born with unaligned eyes, called congenital strabismus. Although experts aren't sure of the exact physiological reason, they believe that a genetic factor may lead to a problem in the nervous system. Severe farsightedness could also play a role; children may cross their eyes in order to focus. As a result, the muscles that control the eyes don't function properly, leading to eyestrain, headaches, poor peripheral vision, and inadequate depth perception. If strabismus is not treated promptly, the brain may learn to suppress the image from the weaker eye, leading to amblyopia, or the permanent loss of vision in one eye.

Adults can also develop strabismus, most often as a result of an underlying cause, such as a stroke, a thyroid problem, or other illness. Adults with strabismus usually suffer from double vision because they aren't able to adapt.

There are a few different treatments for strabismus. Some children may wear a patch over the dominant eye in order to strengthen the weaker one, while glasses to correct vision problems are also prescribed. But for most significant cases, surgery is recommended. First performed in 1839 by a German physician, the surgery either "strengthens" or "weakens" the muscles that control vision. During the procedure, an incision is made into the eye, and an eye muscle is either shortened with a suture or lengthened with an incision to align the eyes. Strabismus surgery is typically safe and effective.

ADDITIONAL FACTS

1. *The word* strabismus *is derived from the Greek* strabismos, *which means "to squint."*

2. *There are different types of strabismus: Esotropia, or crossed eyes, is the turning in of one or both eyes; exotropia, or walleye, is the turning outward of one or both eyes; hypertropia occurs when one eye aims higher than the other; and in hypotropia, one eye points lower than the other.*

◆◆◆

Cataract

As far back as the 5th century BC, healers performed rudimentary eye surgery to correct cataracts. By 1743, the English physician Samuel Sharp (1700–1778) was able to remove them by making an incision in the eye and then applying pressure with his thumb. More than a century later, cocaine-based eyedrops were developed as anesthesia. Thanks to modern science, this procedure has become much less painful—and much more successful.

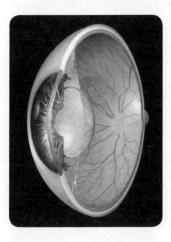

A cataract is a painless, cloudy area in an eye's lens. Because it blocks the passage of light to the retina, a cataract can cause fuzzy vision, much like staring through a foggy car window. Cataracts can also lead to glare from lamps or sun, as well as double vision.

So, what exactly causes cataracts? Aging is a major factor. That's because age causes the eyes' lenses, which are made of water and protein fibers, to become less flexible and transparent. The protein fibers break down and clump together, causing the clouding. Other risk factors include prolonged exposure to sunlight, a family history of the condition, diabetes, and smoking. In the United States, cataracts affect 22 million people.

Cataracts can form in any part of the lens, including the center (in which case the cataract is described as nuclear); the outside of the lens, on the cortex (cortical); and at the back, or under the capsule of the lens (subcapsular). The only remedy for cataracts is a safe outpatient surgical procedure. A doctor makes a small incision in the eye and uses an ultrasound probe to break up the protein fibers. If the cataract is too big, the surgeon must make a larger incision and remove it. More than 90 percent of people who undergo this type of surgery experience an improvement in their vision.

ADDITIONAL FACTS

1. *August is National Cataract Awareness Month.*

2. *Because of a growing baby boom population, it's estimated that 30 million Americans will have cataracts by the year 2020.*

◆◆◆

Hypnosis

In movies, hypnosis is often used to manipulate people into doing illegal or foolish things they wouldn't normally do. You may have also seen hypnosis used as an entertaining trick at a party or comedy show. But in a medical context, hypnosis can be a useful, helpful way to overcome obstacles to good health.

The use of hypnosis for medical reasons is referred to as hypnotherapy. The goal of hypnotherapy is to bring about deep relaxation and an altered state of consciousness known as a trance. When in this deeply focused state, people are usually responsive to an idea or image, and they can learn to affect their bodily functions and psychosocial responses.

Hypnotherapy was endorsed by the American Medical Association in 1958, and today it is commonly used to help treat chronic pain, anxiety, and addiction and to assist in weight loss. It has even been shown to lower blood pressure and heart rate. Hypnosis can also be performed before an operation or before childbirth or to reduce the need for medication during certain types of recovery. Studies on children in emergency treatment centers show that hypnotherapy reduces fear, stress, and discomfort and improves cooperation with medical personnel.

To put a patient under hypnosis, she is led through a series of steps to make her feel relaxed. The patient should feel physically at ease but mentally very awake. At this point, patients are very responsive to the hypnotherapist's suggestions—that they don't like the taste of cigarettes, for example, or that they can turn down the "volume" of their pain the way they can a radio. The brain stores these physical and emotional feelings as long-term memories, and when a cigarette is presented at a later time, that memory comes flooding back into the person's consciousness. It may take as many as 10 sessions before people begin to respond to hypnosis. Self-hypnosis, often with the help of an audiotape or compact disc, can help patients re-create at home the feelings they experience during a hypnotherapy session.

ADDITIONAL FACTS

1. Hypnos *means "sleep" in Greek. The term* hypnosis *was coined in the 19th century.*

2. *In the 1700s, a German physician named Franz Anton Mesmer (1734–1815) claimed that hypnosis through magnets and other techniques could cure blindness, joint pain, and paralysis. Though Mesmer was dismissed as a fraud by the medical community, the word* mesmerize *lives on.*

3. *Very rarely, hypnotherapy leads to the development of false memories fabricated by the unconscious mind, called confabulations.*

✦✦✦

Multiple Sclerosis

Multiple sclerosis (MS) is a chronic autoimmune disease in which the body attacks proteins in the myelin sheath, a fatty substance that insulates nerve fibers in the brain and spinal cord. Damage to the sheaths—and then to the fibers that they surround—causes scarring and blocks nerve signals that control muscle coordination, sensation, and vision.

An estimated 300,000 people in the United States have MS, and two-thirds of those are women. Most people experience their first symptoms—which include numbness, tingling, or weakness in limbs; pain during eye movement; or electric shock sensations that occur during head movements—in early adulthood. Genetic factors play a small role in the development of MS, but researchers believe that most cases are brought on by viruses or prolonged periods of sickness.

The disease occurs in four main patterns: people with **relapsing remitting MS** may experience long periods without symptoms punctuated by abrupt relapses. Many people with this variety will eventually develop **secondary progressive MS**, in which those symptoms become permanent. Less common is **primary progressive MS,** which usually appears in people older than 40. People with this version of the disease do not experience intermittent symptoms, but instead a gradual deterioration. When these symptoms are coupled with periods when symptoms intensify, it is known as **progressive relapsing MS.**

There are no specific tests for MS, although MRI scans may reveal lesions in the brain or spinal cord caused by myelin loss. An injected dye can highlight lesions that have formed within the past 2 months, which may help a doctor decide whether the MS is in an active phase.

Medications for early stage MS include beta interferons—genetically engineered proteins that help regulate the immune system—and corticosteroids to fight inflammation. Regular exercise and physical therapy can help patients strengthen their muscles and continue to live independently, often with the use of a cane, wheelchair, or mobility scooter. The worst cases of MS can progress so far that a person can no longer write, speak, or walk, but the majority of cases can be controlled with medications and lifestyle modifications.

ADDITIONAL FACTS

1. *One complementary treatment for MS is plasma exchange, in which blood is removed from the patient, blood cells are separated and mixed with a replacement solution, and the mixture is returned to the body. Plasma exchange may dilute the concentration of destructive antibodies, although it has no proven benefit if performed more than 3 months after symptoms first appear.*

2. *Many people with MS experience muscle weakening on extremely hot days or in hot showers or baths. Cooling down for a few hours in an air-conditioned room or a tepid bath may provide relief.*

3. *Many viruses and bacteria—including the Epstein-Barr virus, which also causes mononucleosis—have been suspected of causing MS, but none has been shown to be causative so far.*

✦✦✦

Surrogate Pregnancy

The medical term *surrogate pregnancy* has existed since the 1970s, but the concept of one woman having another's baby is as old as time: In the Bible's book of Genesis, the infertile Sarah gives her servant, Hagar, to her husband, Abraham, to bear a child for Sarah and Abraham to raise as their own. Today, however, the procedure is far more technical: A surrogate mother is usually hired by a couple that are unable to have a child and artificially impregnated with the couple's embryo or with the husband's sperm (typically the case when the woman of the couple is infertile). After giving birth, the surrogate normally gives up all parental rights to the child.

The first legal case involving surrogate pregnancy was brought by the Michigan lawyer Noel Keane (1939–1997) in 1976. An infertile couple named Tom and Jane hired a woman, Carol, to bear their baby. A decade later, Keane again stepped into the spotlight in the infamous "Baby M" trial, in which a New Jersey woman, Mary Beth Whitehead (1957–), signed a contract accepting $10,000 to carry the baby of another couple using her egg and the father's sperm. During the pregnancy, Whitehead changed her mind and sued the couple; the court deemed the surrogacy contract illegal and granted her visiting rights.

Although the practice has grown in popularity—with an estimated 300 to 400 or more instances per year—surrogacy is still a controversial topic. Some people consider it tampering with nature; some states, such as Michigan and Arizona, penalize surrogate pregnancy or ban it altogether.

ADDITIONAL FACTS

1. *Surrogate mothers are generally paid $20,000 to $25,000 for their services; the entire process, including medical and legal bills, can cost parents more than $100,000.*

2. *Some celebrities, such as Marissa Jaret Winokur (1973–) of* Hairspray, *a cervical cancer survivor, have used surrogate mothers.*

✦✦✦

Tanning

Tanning occurs when your skin darkens from exposure to ultraviolet A (UVA) radiation, either from the sun or from a commercial tanning machine or lamp. UVA radiation goes through your skin to the lower layers, where it triggers cells called melanocytes to produce melanin, the brown pigment that causes your skin to tan.

You get a sunburn when you're exposed to ultraviolet B (UVB) radiation, which burns the upper layers of your skin. Melanin helps prevent your skin from burning.

However, even if your skin tans without a burn, you are still being exposed to both UVA and UVB radiation. You are not protected from skin cancer, wrinkles, sun spots, eye problems, or damage to your immune system. UVA radiation can also lead to melanoma, which is the most deadly form of skin cancer. Melanoma can spread from your skin to your body's other organs and to lymph nodes near the site of the cancer.

Melanoma can occur anywhere on the body but is most common in the areas frequently exposed to sunlight. Skin cancers are usually treated by excision, which means cutting the tumors out.

UVA damage is also the main factor in premature aging. The majority of wrinkles are caused by exposure to the sun. UVA rays also contribute to cataracts of the eye.

To protect yourself from sun damage from either tanning or burning, stay out of the sun between 10:00 a.m. and 4:00 p.m., use sunscreen with an SPF of at least 15, wear protective clothing, wear wraparound sunglasses that provide 100 percent UV protection, and avoid sunlamps and tanning beds. You should also check your skin for changes in the size, shape, color, or feel of birthmarks, moles, and spots. Such changes can be an indication of skin cancer, which can be cured when detected early.

ADDITIONAL FACTS

1. *More than 1 million new cases of skin cancer are diagnosed annually in the United States.*

2. *Darker-complexioned people tan more easily than lighter-skinned people because the melanocytes in people with darker skin produce more melanin.*

3. *You can get a suntan or sunburn at any temperature.*

4. *Up to 80 percent of Americans under age 25 think they look better tanned.*

✦✦✦

Robotic Surgery

In most aspects of medicine, nothing can take the place of an expert doctor with the compassion of the human touch. In some others, however, the efficiency of computer-driven treatment is quite useful. Today, when it comes to surgery, for example, robotic technology can reduce healing time and improve patient recovery. Minimally invasive laparoscopic surgery is supplemented by robotic instruments directed by the surgeon.

Although robotic surgery may not literally be "hands on" for doctors, they are still very much involved in the process by programming information about the surgery and the patient into a computer ahead of time and by operating the robotic tools themselves during the surgical procedure. These robotic tools can reduce human error and allow finer movement of instruments. Robots also make possible the concept of telesurgery—a surgeon in Canada operating on a patient in Mexico, for example, although current technology hasn't yet been able to eliminate a significant time lapse within such systems.

In 2000, the Food and Drug Administration approved for sale the first robot for use in American hospitals, the da Vinci Surgical System. The device can be used for minimally invasive laparoscopic surgery. The da Vinci system consists of a viewing and control console and three or four stainless steel "arms" that can hold tiny cameras or surgical instruments. Instead of cutting a patient's chest completely open to perform heart surgery, for example, a surgeon makes just three or four tiny incisions in the patient's chest. Using handheld remote controls, the surgeon steers the thin arms below the skin to perform the surgery. The system magnifies the operative field to increase what can be seen, as well.

These devices are very expensive, but they potentially may reduce costs by shortening hospital stays, minimizing complications, and permitting a more rapid return to work with less time to full recovery.

ADDITIONAL FACTS

1. *To date, the da Vinci Surgical System has been used to treat conditions including prostate cancer, endometrial cancer, morbid obesity, and heart disease.*

2. *Several universities are developing microscopic robots, including cameras and surgical devices, that can travel through the bloodstream.*

3. *Laparoscopic surgery may also be known as Band-Aid, keyhole, or pinhole surgery because incisions are $\frac{1}{2}$ to 1 centimeter (about a $\frac{1}{5}$ to $\frac{1}{3}$ of an inch) long.*

◆◆◆

Bullying

Teasing is a normal and inevitable part of childhood. But when taunting becomes hurtful, intentional, and constant, it crosses the line into bullying. It can take the form of name-calling, threats, shoving, hitting, and extortion. Unfortunately, bullying is commonplace: Researchers estimate that some 25 percent of children are bullied at school, and 60 percent of them witness occurrences of bullying every day.

Unlike typical arguments, bullying has less to do with a conflict and more about a person or group's struggle for power. Bullies often target people they believe don't fit in, either because of their physical appearance or behaviors, for a variety of reasons. Some children act out because they are insecure or have been targets themselves. Others simply enjoy mistreating others. In fact, some research reveals that certain individuals may be wired for it: Brain scans of bullies suggest that their empathetic response seems to be overruled by the areas of the mind associated with pleasure, making them more likely to enjoy others' pain or discomfort.

Both girls and boys participate in bullying, although they seem to take different approaches: Girls tend to engage in group teasing and psychological attacks, while boys are more apt to use physical violence. But no matter the sex, bullying takes a psychological—and sometimes, physical—toll on both aggressors and victims. Bullying has been linked with anxiety, depression, and even suicide.

Many children hide from adults the fact that they're being tormented because they're ashamed, afraid of being a "tattletale," or worried that a parent's intervention may make the situation worse. Symptoms of being bullied include a sudden drop in interest in school or grades, frequent nightmares, a change in appetite, and unexplained bruises or injuries. If a child says he or she is being bullied, experts recommend praising him or her for being honest and considering approaching the bully's parents or school administrators. In some cases, legal action may be required; at least 16 states have passed laws to address bullying and harassment.

ADDITIONAL FACTS

1. *Today, children are becoming involved in cyber-bullying, or bullying via the Internet. This form can involve cruel texts, instant messages, or Web page posts.*

2. *According to the World Health Organization, the rates of bullying tend to be consistent across the globe.*

3. *Animals also bully each other; sheep and chickens, for example, intimidate each other to establish a social hierarchy.*

◆◆◆

Index

A

Acetaminophen, 185
Acetylcholine, 129
Acne, 204
Acquired immune
    deficiency syndrome
    (AIDS), 271
Acupuncture, 311
ADD, 78, 309
Addiction, 167
Adenoids, 232
Adrenogenital syndrome,
    187
Aesculapius, 28
AIDS, 271
Alcohol, 195
Allergy, 72, 122
Alzheimer's disease, 242,
    249
Ambulance, first, 84
Amino acids, 6, 171
Amygdala, 32
Amyotrophic lateral
    sclerosis, 270
Anatomy, 49, 105
Anemia, 51, 272, 279
Aneurysm, cerebral, 186
Angelman syndrome, 274
Annual health exam, 286
Anorexia, 288
Anosmia, 214
Antibiotics
    cephalosporins, 10
    penicillin, 10, 59, 224, 259
    quinolones, 31
    sulfa drugs, 52, 259
    tetracycline, 66
Antibodies, 30
Anticholinergics, 129
Antidepressants, 101, 115,
    178, 325, 326
Antihistamines, 87
Antioxidants, 223
Antisepsis, 140
Anxiety, 298
Apgar, Virginia, 1
Apgar score, 1
Appendicitis, 289
Arteries, hardening of, 324
Arteriovenous
    malformations, 200

Artificial heart valves, 329
Artificial insemination, 334
Artificial joints, 217
Artificial sweeteners, 48
Asklepios, 28
Asperger's syndrome, 221
Aspirin, 17
Asthma, 79
Atherosclerosis, 324
Attention deficit disorder
    (ADD), 78, 309
Autism, 50, 221
Autoimmune disease, 86
Autonomic nervous system,
    25
Ayurvedic therapy, 199

B

Balanitis, 278
Banting, Frederick, 210
Barker, David, 64
Barker hypothesis, 64
Bellevue Hospital, 84
Benzodiazepines, 108
Berson, Solomon, 315
Best, Charles, 210
Bipolar disorder, 333, 340
Birth control, 264
Birthmarks, 57
Black-and-blue mark, 316
Black cohosh, 220
Black Death, 35
Blindness, 179
Blood circulation, 70
Blood clotting, 44
Blood pressure drugs, 73
Blood transfusion, 77
Blood typing, 175
Body mass index (BMI),
    146, 153
Bone, broken, 323
Bone age, 239
Bone marrow transplant,
    301
Booth, Edgar, 308
Bores, Leo, 343
Botox, 349
Bozzini, Philip, 238
Brain atrophy, 228
Brain surgery, ancient
    Incan, 21

Brain tumor, 193
Breast cancer, 156, 283, 314
Bronchitis, 100
Brown, Louise, 341
Bubonic plaque, 35
Bulimia, 295
Bullying, 365

C

Calcium, 251
Calor, dolor, rubor, and
    tumor, 7
Cancer
    breast, 156, 283, 314
    cervical, 257
    colon, 142
    Hodgkin's disease, 135
    leukemia, 9, 128, 301
    lung, 184
    macrobiotic diet and, 283
    ovarian, 321
    pancreatic, 191
    prostate, 163
    skin, 198
CA-125, 321
Carbohydrates, 20, 27
Cardiac catheterization, 231
Cardiovascular training, 90
Carotid artery, 18
Cataract, 359
Cavities, tooth, 181
Celiac disease, 212
Celsus, Aulus Cornelius, 7
Cephalosporins, 10
Cerebellum, 46
Cerebral aneurysm, 186
Cerebral angiogram, 109
Cerebral cortex, 39
Cerebrospinal fluid (CSF),
    11, 116
Cervical cancer, 257
Cervix, 33, 40
Charnley, John, 217
Chickenpox, 99, 121
Childbed fever, 119
Children and adolescents
    acne, 204
    adenoids, 232
    Angelman syndrome, 274
    anorexia, 288
    Apgar score, 1

❖❖❖

Children and adolescents (*cont.*)
attention deficit disorder, 309
autism, 50
Barker hypothesis, 64
birthmarks, 57
black-and-blue mark, 316
bone age, 239
bulimia, 295
bullying, 365
chickenpox, 99
chills, 134
congenital heart disease, 302
congenital hip dysplasia, 330
cryptorchidism, 246
dehydration, 148
developmental delay, 71
Down syndrome, 253
febrile seizure, 43
fever, 141
fifth disease, 127
fracture, 323
German measles, 106
growth hormone, 218
growth plate, 183
growth spurt, 211
hirsutism, 344
hives, 176
juvenile muscular dystrophy, 281
Klinefelter's syndrome, 267
measles, 113
menarche, 197
mononucleosis, 169
mumps, 120
nearsightedness, 351
necrotizing enterocolitis, 22
oppositional defiant disorder, 78
Osgood-Schlatter disease, 337
Prader-Willi syndrome, 274
prematurity, 8
puberty, 190
rash, 92
respirator therapy, 29
respiratory distress syndrome, 15
SIDS, 36
strabismus, 358
strep throat, 162

thyroid, 225
tonsillitis, 155
Turner syndrome, 260
vaccination, 85
Chills, 134
Chiropractic, 24
Chlamydia, 229
Chloroform, 112
Cholesterol, 62, 76, 125, 164
Chondroitin, 353
Chromosomes, 12, 89, 96, 103, 110, 253, 260, 267, 274
Circle of Willis, 4
Colds, 58
Colitis, 261
Colon cancer, 142
Colonoscopy, 307
Common cold, 58
Computed tomography, 350
Congenital heart disease, 302
Congenital hip dysplasia, 330
Contact dermatitis, 92
Contact lenses, 356
Contraception, 264
Cormack, Allan, 350
Cortisone, 94
Cournand, André-Frédéric, 231
Crichton, Alexander, 309
Crick, Francis, 287
Crohn's disease, 261
Cryptorchidism, 246
CT scan, 350
Curie, Marie, 161, 168
Cyst, 149
Cystitis, 233

D

Damadian, Raymond, 357
Deafness, 144
Decker, Albert, 189
Deep vein thrombosis, 303
Dehydration, 148
Dementia, 249
Depression, 326
Desormeaux, Antoine Jean, 238
Developmental delay, 71
DHA (docosahexaenoic acid), 69, 255
Diabetes, 210, 338
Diazepam, 108
Dick-Read, Grantly, 273

Diets
heart healthy, 125
macrobiotic, 283
Mediterranean, 132
Pritikin, 262
Digitalis, 38
Dihydrotestosterone deficiency, 180
Dilantin, 80
Diseases and ailments
allergy, 72
anemia, 51
antibodies, 30
appendicitis, 289
asthma, 79
autoimmune disease, 86
blood clotting, 44
breast cancer, 156
bronchitis, 100
cataract, 359
celiac disease, 212
colitis, 261
colon cancer, 142
common cold, 58
cyst, 149
cystitis, 233
diabetes, 338
diverticulitis, 226
edema, 310
embolism, 177
emphysema, 170
gastroenteritis, 275
germs, 16
glaucoma, 352
hardening of the arteries, 324
heartburn (GERD), 240
heart disease, 331
hemorrhoids, 296
hepatitis, 268
Hodgkin's disease, 135
hypertension, 317
immunity, 2
kidney stones, 247
lactose intolerance, 205
leukemia, 128
lung cancer, 184
Lyme disease, 345
meningitis, 107
osteoporosis, 219
pancreatic cancer, 191
phlebitis, 303
pleurisy, 282
pneumonia, 93
prostate cancer, 163
red blood cells, 37
shingles, 121

✦✦✦

sinusitis, 65
skin cancer, 198
tuberculosis, 114
ulcer disease, 254
virus, 23
white blood cells, 9
Diuretics, 45, 73
Diverticulitis, 226
DNA, 96, 287
Down, John Langdon, 253
Down syndrome, 253
Dreaming, 102
Drinker, Philip, 29
Drugs and alternative
treatments
acupuncture, 311
anticholinergics and
acetylcholine, 129
antihistamines, 87
aspirin, 17
Ayurvedic therapy, 199
black cohosh, 220
blood pressure drugs, 73
cephalosporins, 10
chiropractic, 24
cortisone, 94
DHA/omega-3 fatty acids,
255
digitalis, 38
Dilantin, 80
diuretics, 45
echinacea, 332
Effexor, 115
endorphins, 143
epinephrine, 122
ginseng, 276
glucosamine/chondroitin,
353
green tea, 213
growth hormone, 297
homeopathy, 150
hypnosis, 360
indomethacin, 192
influenza vaccination,
290
macrobiotic diet, 283
MAO inhibitors, 178
midwife, 227
morphine, 3
Nexium, 136
nurse-practitioner, 346
osteopathy, 304
penicillin, 59
physical therapy, 241
Pritikin Program, 262
Prozac, 101
quinolones, 31

red clover, 339
reflexology, 318
Rolfing, 234
SAMe, 269
St. John's wort, 325
statins, 164
steroids, 206
sulfa drugs, 52
tetracycline, 66
tryptophan, 171
Tylenol, 185
Valium, 108
vegetarianism, 248
Viagra, 157
Dyspareunia, 292

E
Echinacea, 332
Ectopic pregnancy, 299
Eczema, 92
Edema, 310
Edinburgh Medical School,
grave robbers and,
105
Effexor, 115
Egg donor, 327
Einstein, Albert, 294
Embolism, 177, 303
Embryo storage, 348
Emphysema, 170
Endorphins, 143
Endoscopy, flexible, 238
Enriched foods, 41
EPA (eicosapentaenoic
acid), 69
Epilepsy, 137
Epinephrine, 122
Epstein-Barr virus, 169
Erectile dysfunction, 157
Exercise
cardiovascular training,
90
fitness, 83
Pilates, 104
stretching, 111
weight-bearing, 97
yoga, 118

F
Fallopian tube, 26, 33, 68,
197, 299
Falloppio, Gabriele, 26
Fats, 55, 125
Febrile seizure, 43
Fertilization, 75
Fever, 141
Fiber, 139

Fifth disease, 127
Fitness, 83
Fitzgerald, William, 318
Fleming, Alexander, 59, 224
Flemming, Walther, 82
Flexible endoscopy, 238
Flu
influenza epidemic of
1918, 203
influenza vaccination,
290
Folic acid, 34
Food poisoning, 202
Forssmann, Werner, 231
Fracture, 323
Fragile X syndrome, 110
Freud, Sigmund, 124
Fyodorov, Svyatoslav, 343

G
Galen, 7, 49
Gardasil, 250
Gastroenteritis, 275
Gehrig, Lou, 270
Gender identity, 159
Genetics, 133
GERD, 100, 136, 240
German measles, 106
Germs, 16
Gibbon, John, Jr., 280
Gingivitis, 188
Ginseng, 276
Glaucoma, 352
Glucosamine/chondroitin,
353
Goldberger, Joseph, 196
Gonorrhea, 236
Gordon, James, 294
Grave robbers, 105
Green tea, 213
Growth hormone, 218, 297
Growth plate, 183
Growth spurt, 211
Grubbe, Emil, 161
Gum disease, 188

H
H. pylori, 254
Haboush, Edward, 217
Hahnemann, Samuel, 150
Halsted, William, 154
Hand washing, childbed
fever and, 119
Hardening of the arteries,
324
Harvey, William, 70, 77
Headaches, 158

Health exam, annual, 286
Hearing loss, 144
Heartburn, 136, 240
Heart disease, 62, 331
    congenital, 302
Heart healthy diet, 125
Heart-lung machine, open-
    heart surgery and, 280
Heart valves, artificial, 329
Hemorrhoids, 296
Hepatitis, 268
Hermaphroditism, 208
Herpes, 243
High blood pressure, 317
Hip dysplasia, congenital,
    330
Hippocampus, 32
Hippocrates, 14, 17, 233,
    304
Hirsutism, 344
HIV, 271
Hives, 92, 176
Hodgkin, Thomas, 135
Hodgkin's disease, 135
Hoffman, Felix, 17
Homeopathy, 150
Homosexuality, 166
Hounsfield, Godfrey, 350
HPV, 250
Human immune deficiency
    syndrome (HIV), 271
Human papillomavirus
    (HPV), 250
Huntington, George, 256
Huntington's disease, 256
Hydrocephalus, 130
Hyman, Albert, 308
Hypertension, 317
Hyperthyroidism, 225
Hypnosis, 360
Hypothalamus, 32
Hypothyroidism, 225

I
Immunity, 2, 9
Imperato-McGinley,
    Julianne, 180
Implantable pacemaker, 308
Indomethacin, 192
Infertility, 313, 320, 327,
    334, 341, 348
Inflammation, cardinal
    signs of, 7
Influenza epidemic of 1918,
    203
Influenza vaccination, 290
Insall, John, 217

Insemination, 334
Insomnia, 95
Insulin, 210
Intelligence, 88
In vitro fertilization, 341,
    348, 355
IQ test, 88
Iron supplements, 279
Ivanovsky, Dmitry I., 23

J
Jacobaeus, Hans Christian,
    189
Jenner, Edward, 85, 98
Johnson, Virginia, 152
Juvenile muscular
    dystrophy, 281

K
Kallmann syndrome, 214
Kidney stones, 247
Kinsey, Alfred, 145, 166
Klinefelter's syndrome, 267
Koch, Robert, 114
Krafft-Ebing, Richard
    Baron von, 117
Kussmaul, Adolf, 238

L
Lactose intolerance, 205
Lamaze, 273
Landsteiner, Karl, 175
Langerhans, Paul, 210
Laparoscopy, 189
Lasers, 294
LASIK surgery, 343
Learning, 81
Lejeune, Jérôme-Jean-
    Louis-Marie, 253
Lesbianism, 173
Leukemia, 9, 128, 301
Leukocytes. See White
    blood cells
Libido, 124
Lidwell, Mark, 308
Lifestyle and preventive
    medicine
    addiction, 167
    alcohol, 195
    amino acids, 6
    annual health exam, 286
    antioxidants, 223
    artificial sweeteners, 48
    body mass index, 146
    Botox, 349
    calcium, 251
    CA-125, 321

carbohydrates, 20
cardiovascular training, 90
cholesterol, 62
colonoscopy, 307
contact lenses, 356
DHA and EPA, 69
enriched foods, 41
fats, 55
fiber, 139
fitness, 83
folic acid, 34
food poisoning, 202
heart healthy diet, 125
iron supplements, 279
mammograms, 314
Mediterranean diet, 132
mercury contamination,
    209
obesity, 153
Pap test, 300
periodontal disease,
    188
perspiration, 335
Pilates, 104
Pneumovax, 293
protein, 13
PSA testing, 328
smoking, 174
stretching, 111
sugar, 27
tanning, 363
tooth cavities, 181
trace elements, 272
trans fats, 76
vitamin A, 265
vitamin B_{12}, 258
vitamin C, 230
vitamin D, 244
vitamin E, 237
vitamins, 216
weight-bearing exercise,
    97
weight loss drugs, 160
yawning, 342
yoga, 118
Limbic system, 32
Lind, James, 91
Lister, Joseph, 140
Lou Gehrig's disease, 270
Lung cancer, 184
Lyme disease, 345
Lymphoma, 135, 301

M
Macrobiotic diet, 283
Magnetic resonance
    imaging, 357

♦ ♦ ♦

Mammograms, 314
Mania, 333
Manic-depressive disorder, 333, 340
MAO inhibitors, 178
Marshall, Barry J., 254
Masters, William, 152
Mayer, Carol, 350
McCulloch, Ernest, 322
McWilliam, John, 308
Measles, 113
  German, 106
Medical milestones
  Aesculapius, 28
  antisepsis, 140
  artificial heart valves, 329
  artificial joints, 217
  Banting, Frederick, 210
  Berson, Solomon, 315
  Best, Charles, 210
  Black Death, 35
  blood circulation, 70
  blood transfusion, 77
  blood typing, 175
  bone marrow transplant, 301
  cardiac catheterization, 231
  Celsus and signs of inflammation, 7
  childbed fever, 119
  chloroform, 112
  Crick, Francis, 287
  CT scan, 350
  Curie, Marie, 168
  Dick-Read, Grantly, 273
  DNA, 287
  Edinburgh Medical School and grave robbers, 105
  first ambulance, 84
  Fleming, Alexander, 224
  flexible endoscopy, 238
  genetics, 133
  Goldberger, Joseph, 196
  Halsted, William, 154
  Harvey, William, 70
  Hippocrates, 14
  implantable pacemaker, 308
  influenza epidemic of 1918, 203
  insulin, 210
  Jenner, Edward, 98
  Lamaze, 273
  Landsteiner, Karl, 175
  laparoscopy, 189

lasers, 294
LASIK surgery, 343
Lister, Joseph, 140
Mendel, Gregor, 133
microscope, 63
modern surgery, 154
MRI machine, 357
open-heart surgery and heart-lung machine, 280
organ transplants, 266
Paracelsus, 42
Paré, Ambroise, 56
Pasteur, Louis, 126
pasteurization, 126
pellagra, 196
penicillin, 224
polio vaccine, 245
radioimmunoassay, 315
radiotherapy, 161
radium, 168
rehabilitative medicine, 252
RhoGAM, 336
robotic surgery, 364
Rusk, Howard, 252
Sabin, Albert, 245
Salk, Jonas, 245
Semmelweis, Ignaz, 119
smallpox, 98
stem cells, 322
sulfa drugs and World War II, 259
surgical ligature, 56
trepanation (ancient Incan brain surgery), 21
ultrasound, 147
Van Leeuwenhoek, Antoni, 63
Vesalius and anatomy, 49
vitamin C and scurvy, 91
Watson, James, 287
Wiener, Alexander, 175
Yalow, Rosalyn, 315
yellow fever, 182
Mediterranean diet, 132
Medulla oblongata, 53
Meiosis, 89
Melanoma, 198
Memory, 74
Menarche, 197
Mendel, Gregor, 133
Meningioma, 207
Meningitis, 107, 116
Menstrual cycle, 68, 197
Mental retardation, 110

Mercury contamination, 209
Microscope, 63
Midwife, 227
Mind
  Alzheimer's disease, 242
  amyotrophic lateral sclerosis, 270
  anosmia (Kallmann syndrome), 214
  anxiety, 298
  arteriovenous malformations, 200
  Asperger's syndrome, 221
  autonomic nervous system, 25
  blindness, 179
  brain atrophy, 228
  brain tumor, 193
  carotid artery, 18
  cerebellum, 46
  cerebral aneurysm, 186
  cerebral angiogram, 109
  cerebral cortex, 39
  circle of Willis, 4
  deafness, 144
  dementia, 249
  depression, 326
  dreaming, 102
  epilepsy, 137
  headaches, 158
  Huntington's disease, 256
  hydrocephalus, 130
  intelligence, 88
  learning, 81
  limbic system, 32
  mania, 333
  manic-depressive disorder, 340
  medulla oblongata, 53
  memory, 74
  meningioma, 207
  multiple sclerosis, 361
  muscular dystrophy, 263
  neurosis, 305
  obsessive-compulsive disorder, 284
  panic disorder, 312
  paralysis, 151
  Parkinson's disease, 235
  peripheral neuropathy, 172
  personality disorders, 277
  post-traumatic stress disorder, 354
  psychiatrists and psychologists, 123

✦ ✦ ✦

Mind (*cont.*)
  psychosis, 319
  reflexes, 60
  schizophrenia, 347
  sleep, 95
  spinal tap, 116
  stroke, 165
  taste, 67
  Tourette syndrome, 291
  ventricles, 11
Miscarriage, 306
Mitosis, 82, 89
Modern surgery, 154
Money, John, 215
Mononucleosis, 169
Monounsaturated fats, 55, 125
Morphine, 3
MRI machine, 357
Multiple sclerosis (MS), 361
Mumps, 120
Murray, Joseph, 266
Muscular dystrophy, 263
  juvenile, 281

N
Natural childbirth, 273
Nearsightedness, 351
Necrotizing enterocolitis, 22
Neuropathy, peripheral, 172
Neurosis, 305
Nexium, 136
Nurse-midwives, 227
Nurse-practitioner, 346

O
Obesity, 153
Obsessive-compulsive disorder (OCD), 284
Omega-3 fatty acids, 69, 255
Open-heart sugery, heart-lung machine and, 280
Oppositional defiant disorder, 78
Organ transplants, 266
Orgasm, 131
Osgood, Robert, 337
Osgood-Schlatter disease, 337
Osteopathy, 304
Osteoporosis, 219, 251
Ovarian cancer, 321
Ovary(ies), 5, 19, 26, 33, 68, 197

Ova storage, 355
Ovulation, 5
Ovum, 5, 68, 75, 89, 197

P
Pacemaker, implantable, 308
Palmer, Daniel David, 24
Palmer, Raoul, 189
Pancreatic cancer, 191
Panic disorder, 298, 312
Papanicolaou, George, 257
Pap test, 257, 300
Paracelsus, 42
Paralysis, 151
Paré, Ambroise, 56
Parkinson's disease, 235
Parvovirus B19, 127
Pasteur, Louis, 119, 126, 140
Pasteurization, 126
Pellagra, 196
Pelvic inflammatory disease (PID), 285
Penicillin, 10, 59, 224, 259
Periodontal disease, 188
Peripheral neuropathy, 172
Personality disorders, 277
Perspiration, 335
Phenytoin, 80
Phlebitis, 303
Physical therapy, 241
PID, 285
Pilates, 104
Pleurisy, 282
Pneumonia, 93
Pneumovax, 293
Polio vaccine, 245
Polyunsaturated fats, 55, 125
Post-traumatic stress disorder, 354
Prader-Willi syndrome, 274
Pregnancy. *See also* Sexuality and reproduction
  surrogate, 362
Prematurity, 8
Priapism, 138
Prilosec, 136
Pritikin, Nathan, 262
Pritikin Program, 262
Prostate cancer, 163
Prostate gland, 61
Protein, 6, 13
Prozac, 101

PSA testing, 163, 328
Psychiatrists, 123
Psychologists, 123
Psychosis, 319
Puberty, 190

Q
Quinolones, 31

R
Radioimmunoassay, 315
Radiotherapy, 161
Radium, 161, 168
Rash, 92
Red blood cells, 37
Red clover, 339
Reflexes, 60
Reflexology, 318
Rehabilitative medicine, 252
REM sleep, 102
Respirator therapy, 29
Respiratory distress syndrome, 15
RhoGAM, 336
Richards, Dickinson, 231
Robotic surgery, 364
Rokitansky, Baron Karl von, 201
Rokitansky syndrome, 201
Rolf, Ida P., 234
Rolfing, 234
Röntgen, Wilhelm Conrad, 161
Ross, Donald, 329
Rubella, 106
Rusk, Howard, 252

S
Sabin, Albert, 245
Salk, Jonas, 245
Salpingo-oophoritis, 285
SAMe, 269
Sappho, 173
Saturated fats, 55, 125
Schawlow, Arthur, 294
Schizophrenia, 347
Schlatter, Carl, 337
Scurvy, 91, 230
Seizure(s), 80
  epileptic, 137
  febrile, 43
Semen, 61
Seminal vesicle, 54
Semm, Kurt, 189
Semmelweis, Ignaz, 119

❖ ❖ ❖

Sertürner, Friedrich
  Wilhelm Adam, 3
Sex change surgery, 215
Sex-linked disease, 103
Sexual desire, 124
Sexuality and reproduction
  adrenogenital syndrome,
    187
  balanitis, 278
  birth control, 264
  cervical cancer, 257
  cervix, 40
  chlamydia, 229
  chromosome, 96
  dihydrotestosterone
    deficiency, 180
  dyspareunia, 292
  ectopic pregnancy, 299
  egg donor, 327
  embryo storage, 348
  fallopian tube, 26
  fertilization, 75
  fragile X syndrome, 110
  gender identity, 159
  gonorrhea, 236
  hermaphroditism, 208
  herpes, 243
  homosexuality, 166
  HPV, 250
  human immune
    deficiency syndrome,
    271
  infertility, 313
  insemination, 334
  in vitro fertilization,
    341
  Kinsey, Alfred, 145
  Krafft-Ebing, Richard
    Baron von, 117
  lesbianism, 173
  libido, 124
  Masters and Johnson,
    152
  meiosis, 89
  menstrual cycle, 68
  miscarriage, 306
  mitosis, 82
  Money, John, 215
  orgasm, 131
  ovary, 19
  ova storage, 355
  ovum, 5
  priapism, 138
  prostate gland, 61
  Rokitansky syndrome,
    201

salpingo-oophoritis
  (pelvic inflammatory
  disease), 285
seminal vesicle, 54
sex change surgery, 215
sex-linked disease, 103
sperm, 12
sperm donor, 320
surrogate pregnancy, 362
syphilis, 222
testicular feminization,
  194
testis, 47
uterus, 33
Shettles, Landrum, 341
Shingles, 121
SIDS, 36
Sinusitis, 65
Skin cancer, 198
Sleep, 95, 102
Smallpox, 85, 98
Smith-Petersen, Marius,
  217
Smoking, 174, 184
Sperm, 5, 12, 47, 54, 75, 89
Sperm donor, 320
Spinal tap, 116
St. John's wort, 325
Statins, 164
Stem cells, 322
Steroids, 206
Still, Andrew Taylor, 304
Strabismus, 358
Strep throat, 162
Stretching, 111
Stroke, 165
Sudden infant death
  syndrome (SIDS), 36
Sugar, 27
Sugar substitutes, 48
Sulfa drugs, 52
  World War II and, 259
Surgery
  ancient Incan brain, 21
  LASIK, 343
  modern, 154
  open-heart, 280
  robotic, 364
  sex change, 215
Surgical ligature, 56
Surrogate pregnancy, 362
Syphilis, 222

T
Tanning, 363
Taste, 67

Tea, green, 213
Testicular feminization,
  194
Testis, 12, 47, 246
Tetracycline, 66
Thomas, E. Donnall, 301
Thyroid, 225
Till, James, 322
Tonsillitis, 155
Tooth cavities, 181
Tourette syndrome, 291
Townes, Charles, 294
Trace elements, 272
Trans fat, 55, 76, 125
Trepanation (ancient Incan
  brain surgery), 21
Tryptophan, 171
Tuberculosis, 114
Turner syndrome, 260
Tylenol, 185

U
Ulcerative colitis, 261
Ulcer disease, 254
Ultrasound, 147
Uterus, 26, 33

V
Vaccination, 85
Vaccines
  autism and, 50
  chickenpox, 99
  Gardasil, 250
  immunity from, 2
  influenza, 290
  MMR, 106
  Pneumovax, 293
  polio, 245
Valium, 108
Van Leeuwenhoek, Antoni,
  63
Vegetarianism, 248
Ventilators, 29
Ventricles, 11
Vesalius, Andreas, 49
Viagra, 157
Virchow, Rudolf Ludwig, 7,
  177
Viruses, 2, 23
  cold, 58
  Epstein-Barr, 169
  hepatitis, 268
  herpes, 243
  HIV, 271
  HPV, 250
  measles, 113

❖❖❖

Viruses (*cont.*)
  parvovirus B19, 127
  rubella, 106
Vitamin A, 265
Vitamin B_{12}, 258
Vitamin C, 91, 230
Vitamin D, 244
Vitamin E, 237
Vitamins, 216

W
Water pills, 45, 73
Watson, James, 287
Weight-bearing exercise, 97
Weight loss drugs, 160
White blood cells, 2, 7, 9, 30
Whitehead, Mary Beth, 362
Wiener, Alexander, 175
Willis, Thomas, 4

Y
Yalow, Rosalyn, 315
Yawning, 342
Yellow fever, 182
Yoga, 118
Young, Bruce, 189

✦✦✦

Image Credits

❖❖❖